Central Sensitization
and Sensitivity Syndromes

McFarland Health Topics Series

Central Sensitization and Sensitivity Syndromes

A Handbook for Coping

AMY TITANI

Foreword by Ric Arseneau, M.D.

MCFARLAND HEALTH TOPICS

McFarland & Company, Inc., Publishers
Jefferson, North Carolina

To the reader:
While I hope something I say can help you manage your
illness and improve your life, I am not a doctor, a licensed vocal
therapist, or a counselor. Far from it. I have no medical training,
and though I have years of professional singing experience, I have
only minor vocal training, and that happened decades ago.
I do not give medical advice in any way.
This book shares my research findings, my own experience, and
strategies and treatments that have worked for me. That doesn't mean
these things are good for *you* or guaranteed to help you.
Always check with a medical professional before making any changes
in physical activity, diet, prescriptions or other
health-related aspects of your life.
If you require medical attention, please contact medical
professionals, and if you are in danger
of hurting yourself or others, call 911.

Library of Congress Cataloguing-in-Publication Data

Names: Titani, Amy, 1969– author.
Title: Central sensitization and sensitivity syndromes : a handbook
for coping / Amy Titani ; foreword by Ric Arseneau, M.D.
Description: Jefferson, North Carolina : McFarland & Company, Inc.,
Publishers, 2017. | Series: McFarland health topics |
Includes bibliographical references and index.
Identifiers: LCCN 2017022286 | ISBN 9781476668635
(softcover : acid free paper) ∞
Subjects: LCSH: Central nervous system—Diseases—Treatment.
Classification: LCC RC361 .T58 2017 | DDC 616.8/3—dc23
LC record available at https://lccn.loc.gov/2017022286

British Library cataloguing data are available

ISBN (print) 978-1-4766-6863-5
ISBN (ebook) 978-1-4766-2780-9

Front cover image © 2016 SIphotography/iStock

Printed in the United States of America

*McFarland & Company, Inc., Publishers
Box 611, Jefferson, North Carolina 28640
www.mcfarlandpub.com*

Acknowledgments

This book wouldn't be here if a lot of people hadn't done some extraordinary things. I am ever so grateful. To my good friends Clélie and Peter, thank you for feeding and housing me and providing laughter aplenty in the best and worst of times. Thanks to Jody, Sheila, Suz, and Sam, who read an early draft and provided essential feedback. *Ma chére amie* Sarah, for reading and editing essay drafts and for sending me to healing places, *merci mille fois*. Barb, you tucked your support into my pocket one day and refused to take it back—thank you. Thanks to Jen C., for your healing compassion, and to Suzanne S. and BJ, for fielding countless questions. Jim, thank you for showing up for me time and again (and again). Thanks to all at the CCDP, and Doctors Shoja, Hamm, Morrison, Yang, and Rammage, for all your care. Thanks also to all at McFarland.

Much gratitude to Daniel Ladinsky, for permitting me to include your wonderful work in this project. Ric, thank you for being a brilliant doctor and lovely human. Your wisdom plucked me from the CFS maelstrom, your generosity springs eternal, and your foreword rocks!

Many more have supported me in writing this book and in my related efforts towards education, compensation, and healing. I can't possibly name you all, but I remember you. You are my shining stars, and you all have my abundant gratitude.

Table of Contents

Foreword
by Ric Arseneau, M.D.

I am grateful for the opportunity to write the foreword to Amy's book. While reviewing the manuscript, I was astounded by Amy's transformation as she struggled with the challenges of dealing with chronic illness. More impressive is that she managed to thrive and find meaning in her new circumstance.

Accepting and adapting to a new life with chronic illness is difficult enough. Having an "invisible" illness makes the predicament even more trying. When that illness is not well understood and science is lacking, the tribulations magnify exponentially. Many patients feel judged, dismissed, and misunderstood. Outright ridicule is not uncommon. Frustration with physicians and the health care system is the norm. Dealing with others who think you are malingering or have misperceptions about your illness only adds to the stress. Sometimes it can seem that even friends and family need constant reminding of your limitations. Suddenly everyone you know has a Google M.D. degree. Subjected to unsolicited advice from well-meaning people, you are left feeling frustrated, isolated and unsupported.

The family of conditions under the rubric "Central Sensitivity Syndromes" (CSS) fall into the unfortunate category of chronic illnesses that are both invisible and poorly understood. Having cared for patients with such conditions for over 20 years I am optimistic that things are starting to change. For instance, Fibromyalgia (FM) now has several evidence-based treatment options. Also, a 2015 report by the Institute of Medicine on Myalgic Encephalomyelitis/Chronic Fatigue Syndrome (ME/CFS) has done much to legitimize the disease and raise awareness on the need for better care and increase funding for research. Unfortunately, not all CSS have fared so well. Multiple Chemical Sensitivities remains an "orphan" condition that is often relegated to the psychologic realm and for which little support is available.

Amy provides a thorough overview of CSS, including ME/CFS, FM, and MCS. She makes the topic accessible to those without a science background without compromising the integrity of the science itself. She takes you on a journey from what is well established scientifically, to interesting hypotheses awaiting more rigorous research, to her own personal theories. Unlike many books, she qualifies her assertions accordingly rather than presenting everything as "truth." She acknowledges that everyone is different and that each situation presents its own unique challenges, rather than prescribing a one-size-fits-all solution. It is an excellent primer for those newly diagnosed with a CSS, and an invaluable resource for those already well-versed in their condition. More importantly, if fills a need for those with MCS; I have yet to come across a better patient guidebook.

Acceptance is an important aspect of living with chronic illness. For many, acceptance is a dirty word—it means giving up. Nothing could be further from the truth. Acceptance is finding the resolve to do the best you can with what you have. Amy guides you through this process with her keen insight. We are reminded that acceptance is a process, not a decision.

Patients with chronic conditions often have an unarticulated agreement with themselves: my life is on hold until I get better. But what if this is it? Chronic illness and happiness don't have to be mutually exclusive. Amy addresses the complicated relationship between illness and happiness; she underscores the fact that happiness does not have to be contingent on getting better.

Acceptance, actually the lack thereof, is a common source of suffering for many patients. Paradoxically, "fighting" rather than accepting your illness can be a barrier to feeling better. Buddhists make a distinction between primary and secondary suffering. Pain, for instance, is an example of primary suffering. Secondary suffering arises from the meaning, emotions, and distress caused by the pain. Science has finally caught up with Buddhist thinking: functional MRI studies show that these two types of suffering reside in distinct parts of the brain. Interestingly, these two areas communicate with each other; secondary suffering can feed back and amplify pain. What does this have to do with acceptance? Although you may not have control over your pain itself, you can take steps to deal with and reduce secondary suffering. Acceptance helps you understand and take control of your situation. It allows you to focus your limited energy where it will have the most impact. Nothing captures this concept better than the Serenity Prayer, well known to those who have participated in 12-step programs:

> Grant me the serenity to accept the things I cannot change
> The courage to change the things that I can, and
> The wisdom to know the difference.

Amy demonstrates a creative approach to the process of acceptance. She avoids "all or none thinking." She has learned to embrace the shades of gray. She embodies the *wisdom* required to distinguish between accepting and giving up. She is a model for adapting to change while cultivating an attitude of gratitude.

Redefining your identity is one of the many tasks inherent in the process of acceptance. One of my patients, let's call him John, uses humor to deal with this process of *de-identification*: the process by which someone with chronic illness lets go of their old identity and accepts a new reality for themselves. John, a man with comedic tendencies, now refers to himself as "John-lite." Now, when a friend calls him to go out for a beer, he quips, "John would love that. But John-lite would prefer if you came over and brought some Starbuck's so we could chat for a half-hour." Although Amy doesn't use the term de-identification, her story outlines how she managed to re-create her life and identity without falling into the common trap of playing the sick role or victim role.

Among the many tools provided in this book, cognitive behavior therapy (CBT) is likely the most powerful. Some of you will chafe at the idea of CBT—especially if your condition was once blamed on psychological or psychiatric problems. Others will discount CBT given the discredited and now infamous PACE trial, where CBT and Graded Exercise Therapy were used as *treatments* for ME/CFS. It is important to point out that neither Amy nor I are suggesting that CBT will treat your CSS. CBT is a tool and a skill that helps you cope with life whether or not you are ill. Living with a chronic disease is stressful. Furthermore, patients with CSS are especially sensitive to stress—this can lead to a vicious cycle. Also, many patients with chronic illness develop depression and anxiety. These are the result of living with chronic illness—not the cause. CBT can help patients deal with stress and suffering, and may even have an impact on the illness itself. For instance, in patients with coronary heart disease, CBT reduces the rate of fatal and non-fatal cardiovascular events (e.g., heart attacks) by over 40 percent—yet no one would blame heart attacks on psychological issues. Finally, a significant percentage of patients with CSS have a history of abuse or trauma. These can predispose to illness in general, but are more specifically related to chronic pain and CSS. The trauma need not be one (or more) major traumatic event. So-called *developmental* trauma can arise from repeated intense situations that lead to the fight, flight, or freeze responses. Persistent activation of the autonomic sympathetic nervous system (i.e., adrenaline system) physically changes the brain. It "sensitizes" the brain and predisposes it to future illnesses including CSS. Many patients with CSS also have *autonomic dysfunction*—a dysfunctional adrenal system. This can lead to, or exacerbate, many symptoms related to CSS. Amy does a great job explaining how CBT and mindfulness can help you calm this response.

Using CBT to tame negative *automatic thoughts* is a useful skill. Otherwise, these thoughts often lead to self-defeating and paralyzing behaviors that get in the way of self-care. For instance, difficulty with pacing rarely stems from a lack the knowledge; instead, negative thoughts and emotions raise barriers to pacing, and self-care including: acceptance, overwhelm, perfectionism, and difficulties with boundaries. Amy helps you navigate and challenge your beliefs and automatic ways of thinking, thereby helping you avoid self-defeating and paralyzing behaviors.

Of the CSS, MCS is arguably the most isolating; many patients are literally quarantined. We are social animals; we all long to belong and feel connected. In prison, the worst punishment for inmates is solitary confinement. Too often, patients turn to mood regulating substances (e.g., alcohol or food) and behaviors (e.g., gambling or spending money they don't have) that only further complicate a difficult situation. Amy steers us through the difficult process of letting go, maintaining important friendships, and even forming new relationships.

Throughout this book, Amy provides you with useful ideas and tools. The primacy of self-management should be your guiding principle—you need to be in charge. Living with a complex and chronic illness can leave you feeling overwhelmed and helpless. Amy has been there. Learn from her story. I urge you to not only read this book, but to *do it*—use it as a workbook. The old saying that knowledge is power is incorrect: Knowledge acted upon is power.

Ultimately this book is about many things. But most of all, it's about living your best life now. An aphorism I often use captures the essence of the idea I presented in the beginning of this introduction—the unarticulated pact of patients with chronic illness: my life is on hold until I get better.

> *Life isn't about waiting for the storm to pass…*
> *it's about learning to dance in the rain.*

It's time to get wet! I hope you enjoy this book as much as I did.

Ric Arseneau, M.D., is an academic internist and clinical associate professor at the University of British Columbia. He is also the director of program planning at the Complex Chronic Diseases Program at BC Women's Hospital, an innovative new program with a focus on ME/CFS, FM, MCS and related CSS. He has more than 20 years of experience working with patients with CSS.

Preface

In 2012, I was exposed to unsafe levels of Volatile Organic Compounds and a mélange of particulates, fumes, dust and unidentified stuff (let's say the air quality was super substandard) while working at an internationally known green architecture corporation. (Yep, I said *green* architecture. I know, the irony.) I'll call that corporation "Green and Sustainable," or "GAS," for short. The workplace incident left me with Asthma, Central Sensitization, and three Central Sensitivity Syndromes: Multiple Chemical Sensitivities, Irritable Larynx Syndrome, and Chronic Fatigue Syndrome.

GAS did not take responsibility. It misinformed the provincial workers compensation corporation and my short- and long-term disability insurers, misrepresented the indoor air quality, and laid me off. Thrust into a battle for compensation (four years and counting), I lost my home, hundreds of thousands of dollars, and an active life rich with athletic pursuits, stories, songs, and people. Due to Central Sensitization (CS) and the Central Sensitivity Syndromes (CSS) it helps manifest, I also lost my ability to breathe in many public places. This took a toll on my sense of safety for quite some time.

It has taken years, in fact, for me to adjust to life with CS and CSS, and I'm not done yet. Adjustment, like acceptance, seems to be a fluid, ongoing process. Debilitation, too, exists on a spectrum, I've learned. Some parts of me may flail while others improve, and some maybe even attain a kind of superhuman strength, like my amygdala.

The amygdala is the part of our brain in charge of security and safety. It protects us by controlling the fight or flight reflex. When I think about the roiling sea of chaos, terror, and uncertainty I tumbled into following that workplace incident, I find it amazing that I survived.

I suspect that my amygdala must be made of something indestructible, like titanium, because it is so strong, it powered me through that time and, to this day, it keeps on fighting and protecting me, even when there is no real threat. My titanium amygdala never gives up. So neither can I.

I am Titan Amy.

(Do you hear dramatic music when I say that? Sometimes I do, and suddenly, I am no longer reclining in a beat-up poang chair in my basement apartment kitchen while my calico cheshires at me from her windowsill perch. Instantly, I see myself dancing atop a high mountain, singing out loud like Julie Andrews in the hills of Austria, with the dawn of a new day breaking across the distant horizon, and a long, dramatic cape whipping in the wind behind me. Not a flimsy superhero cape. Something stylish yet warm, like cashmere, or alpaca. Yep, that's the stuff, and it feels *awesome*!)

It was a tough road to get to my sweet spot on that mountain, and I know countless others are traveling a similar path. I don't want anyone to have to go it alone, so I've written this book for people with CS and CSS, and for those who love or provide services to them.

This is the book I wish someone had given me when I first got sick. Part handbook, it contains easy-to-understand facts about CS and CSS as well as an in-depth look at life with these conditions. I detail step-by-step strategies to aid in managing symptoms, getting out of crisis mode and regaining stability, and working towards long-term healing. I break down each topic into brief, informative pieces, for easier digestion by those with CS and CSS (who often have limited concentration or feel easily overwhelmed). I've created an extensive index for ease of referencing by topic, and I've included a segment near the end specifically for those who are not ill but who love someone with these conditions and want to learn how to help and how to cope. (If you are one of those readers, a special *Welcome!* I encourage you to read the book as a whole to aid your understanding and inform your decisions and expectations.)

This book is also part companion, a compassionate resource for folks with CS and CSS to pick up when they're having a rough time, to find hope or comfort, and feel less alone. I include personal essays, literary snippets, and ancient mystic poems throughout to enable readers to connect on an emotional level and understand better what it's like to live with these conditions, what kind of losses one may suffer and grieve, and how recovery is possible. *What's a revelatory book without stories and poetry, I ask you?*

Make no mistake, this is a revelatory book. A chronic, relatively unknown, and potentially incurable illness demands a transformation. Thrust into uncertainty and change, the person with CS and CSS has loads to learn and a bunch of decisions to make. Big ones. Some are easier than others. Who do you want on your medical team? Should you stay or go? What do you do when support falters? Should you keep working? How will you survive without working? What treatments are right for you? Yep, CS and CSS can turn your life upside down and inside out. This can be a blessing and curse. You have the opportunity to re-envision and recreate your life (blessing) but you have to do it while accommodating a chronic illness that has some pretty steep tolls (curse). How you look at it is up to you. What you do about it is up to you.

I also present the findings from my own experiments regarding coping with, managing, and healing from CS and CSS. Yep, I said experiments. Nothing like doctors Frankenstein or Jekyll, mind you—those two were in way over their heads—but I have found that developing practical ways to make life with CS and CSS manageable requires the frequent posing and testing of hypotheses. In fact, my experience with these conditions has led me to believe that life is an experiment. You may find it helpful to adopt a similar philosophy. You know you have this illness, and you know it can be triggered anytime, anywhere. That's enough to make most people hide in a Himalayan cave for all eternity, but acceptance takes the pressure right off. And experimenting, well, it enables me to make my life better. I hope that the strategies I've developed through trial and error can save you from having to start from square one. Think of me as a scout who went ahead and left some anchors and flags that may aid you as you learn the ropes and rigors of this new territory.

I don't know if everything I do will work for you. I don't know if what I've experienced is always going to be relevant to you, but I do know that CS and CSS all have one thing in common: a central nervous system that's gone a little haywire. I know ways to address that, and I know how to live with these conditions without suffering. I want to share that knowledge with you.

Perhaps most important, I know what it's like to hear a friendly voice amidst all the external challenges and internal noise, the voice of someone who understands what it's like to suddenly be facing and forced to live with a mysterious and treacherous chronic illness, to lose employment and income and have to fight a bureaucratic insurance corporation for compensation, to lose friends, home and hearth and keep on going. A friendly voice kept me going when I had nothing to hold on to, and still keeps me going to this day. At the most basic level this book is for you. You aren't alone, though it sure may feel like it, and I'm right here, talking to you.

1. Sensitization
and Syndrome Basics

What Is Central Sensitization?

Dr. Muhammad B. Yunus, a Rheumatologist specializing in Fibromyalgia in Peoria, Illinois, encapsulates Central Sensitization, or CS, "as an amplified response of the central nervous system to peripheral input."[1] For those of you who don't speak scientist, this basically means that the brain and spinal cord aren't responding to the body's incoming sensory signals appropriately. I'll explain further in a moment.

The first thing to note is that CS is a challenging and relatively new field and is considered *idiopathic*, which means scientists don't yet know for certain what causes CS.[2] We know many of its symptoms, and we understand some aspects of its *pathology* (or typical behavior). It is known that different factors can participate in its *pathophysiology* (functional changes associated with CS), including genetic predisposition, infection, inflammation, physical injury/trauma, poor sleep, psychological stress, environmental/chemical exposures, and autonomic nervous system dysfunction.[3] While increasing numbers of researchers are turning their focus to CS, they are still deep in the process of discovery. Currently we make sense of CS, in great part, by applying what is known about the pain pathway system, that is, how pain is perceived and managed by our brains and bodies. So please note, what I'm about to say is well-supported scientific assumption yet definitely not 100 percent verified facts.

It is understood that CS involves two processes:

1. The sensory nerves that initially pick up an irritation, whatever it might be—for example, in my case, a toxic chemical irritating my throat and lungs—send a sensory alert signal to the brain. This signal could be alerting the brain to anything on the sensory spectrum—from touch to pressure to pain. Our biological response to such a signal involves nerves and chemicals. In someone who doesn't have CS, the chemicals and nerves report accurately to the brain, but with CS, the sensory alert signal is amplified by the nerves, causing a distorted signal. When I say the nerves *amplify* the signal, I mean that the chemicals involved in the biological response are recruiting more nerves than necessary, which results in a signal far more urgent or intense than appropriate. It's like calling in the entire fire department to put out a dwindling BBQ.

2. When sensory nerves send a signal *to* the brain, the brain should send a response via "descending pathways" which basically says, "Stop sending signals. I got it." As you can guess, this message is supposed to be received by the sensory

nerves that are sending the pain alerts, to inhibit them from sending any more alerts to the brain. When CS occurs, that response from the brain never arrives, and the sensory nerves keep on sending alerts, louder and stronger with time. (Hence, amplification of signal.)

Do you know what the amygdala is? It's the part of the brain that controls the fight or flight reflex. The amygdala plays a role in how pain alerts are interpreted in the brain and it also interferes in the descending pathways trying to inhibit the signal. When the body reacts with an "Uh-oh, I smell toxic stuff and can't breathe," the amygdala then leaps into danger mode and activates the fight or flight response. So, if the sensory nerves keep sending signals, what do you think happens next? Yep, the amygdala remains in danger mode for prolonged periods of time.

A basic way to look at CS is to consider what would happen if your central nervous system got stuck on red alert. The senses of smell, hearing, touch, and sight become more sensitive, the nerves become more taut, stuff like that. This may cause someone to become sensitive to chemicals and odors that other folks don't even perceive. One's ability to deal with stress may decrease. One's energy level may drop. One may feel anxious or panicked much of the time. One's skin might become so sensitive to the touch that it aches or burns. Yep, your central nervous system and the amygdala are powerful. They are working for you, but if your system gets sensitized and your amygdala is working overtime, doing all it can to protect you 24/7, it's not always helping you. In fact, CS underlies several health problems—"including neuropathic pain … whiplash … some forms of osteo-arthritis,"[4] rheumatoid arthritis, and post-operative pain—and serves as the primary mechanism behind a group of disorders called Central Sensitivity Syndromes.[5]

What Are Central Sensitivity Syndromes?

In 2000, Dr. Yunus coined the term "Central Sensitivity Syndromes (CSS)" to classify a group of overlapping conditions such as Fibromyalgia, Irritable Bowel Syndrome, Multiple Chemical Sensitivities, and Chronic Fatigue Syndrome—all of which lack a structural or functional disease that could otherwise explain their symptoms, and all of which share a common primary mechanism: CS.[6] In his studies, Yunus found common features among the various CSS, including unrefreshing and/or poor sleep, fatigue, social and/or psychological challenges, pain, and sensitivity to unpleasant and/or toxic stimuli.[7] In 2011, researchers at the University of Florida Center for Comprehensive Pain Research in Gainesville supported Yunus' theory, stating that his classification and concept of CSS would improve communication and "cross-fertilization" among researchers engaged in studying the syndromes as well as understanding and treatment of the syndromes "through an appreciation of their shared pathophysiology."[8]

While the name and theory behind CSS has seen increased recognition and acceptance in the 17 years since its inception, the cause(s) and mechanism(s) behind CSS remain "incompletely understood."[9] Although experts haven't yet figured everything out, sensitization of the central nervous system "has emerged as one of the significant mechanisms" of CSS.[10] It's known that far more women than men have CSS, and that folks with CSS commonly present, or develop, more than one of the syndromes. Recent research has also expanded the list of common CSS features to include "persistent pain as a predominant feature, along with multiple and numerous comorbid symptoms such as fatigue, sleep problems, dizziness, cognitive problems (e.g., difficulties with attention, memory, concentration), depression, anxiety, and irritability."[11] To be clear, not everyone with Central Sensitization has a CSS; however, Yunus states in his 2007 report that someone who has CS may develop CSS in future.[12] This outcome is not a proven inevitability; strategies and treatments (including those in this book) may help prevent it.

Dr. Ric Arseneau, Director of Program Planning and a clinician at the Complex Chronic Diseases Program in Vancouver, British Columbia, explains CSS as a "family of disorders, an umbrella term to capture the overlapping relationship these syndromes and the pathophysiological mechanism (e.g., CS) that is common to them."[13] While several similarities exist among the syndromes, there are also countless differences. "Individuals presenting with identical CSS diagnoses exhibit a great deal of variability in the degree of pain, number and nature of physical symptoms, and psychological distress that they experience."[14] Yep, psychological distress. CSS are *not* mental illnesses; however, they can and often do lead to conditions such as depression and anxiety. (They don't *have to*, though. More on that in the chapter on coping.)

Because the scientific realm of CS and CSS is so new, the list of syndromes is still being compiled. Currently, proposed members of the CSS family include the following, in no particular order:

- Chronic Fatigue Syndrome aka Myalgic Encephalomyelitis aka Systemic Exertion Intolerance Disease—"a complicated disorder characterized by extreme fatigue that can't be explained by any underlying medical condition. The fatigue may worsen with physical or mental activity, but doesn't improve with rest."[15] Key features are post-exertional malaise and crashing. (If you aren't familiar with these terms, don't worry. I'll explain them soon.) Cognitive impairment and pain are other common symptoms.
- Irritable Larynx Syndrome—a disorder in which the muscles around the larynx overreact to normal sensory stimuli, causing chronic cough, speaking and breathing difficulties, and related issues.
- Myofascial Pain Syndrome—a chronic pain disorder in which "pressure on sensitive points in [the] muscles (trigger points) causes pain in seemingly unrelated parts of [the] body,"[16] or referred pain.
- Regional Soft Tissue Pain Syndrome—a chronic localized pain disorder.
- Tension-type Headaches—"the most common headache … it has been discussed for years without reaching consensus on its pathophysiology, or proper rationale management."[17]
- Migraine Headache—a type of headache that "can cause intense throbbing or a pulsing sensation in one area of the head and is commonly accompanied by nausea, vomiting, and extreme sensitivity to light and sound."[18]
- Restless Legs Syndrome (RLS)—"a disorder that causes a strong urge to move [the] legs. This urge to move often occurs with strange and unpleasant feelings in [the] legs."[19] Because it often disrupts sleep, RLS is also considered a sleep disorder.
- Periodic Limb Movements in Sleep (PLMS)—"repetitive movements, most typically in the lower limbs, that occur about every 20–40 seconds, … brief muscle twitches, jerking movements or an upward flexing of the feet. They cluster into episodes lasting anywhere from a few minutes to several hours."[20]

- Pelvic Pain Syndrome and related disorders—chronic pain in pelvic region.
- Temporomandibular (TMJ) disorders—chronic pain in jaw joint and related muscles.
- Postural Orthostatic Tachycardia Syndrome (POTS)—a disorder closely related to Orthostatic Intolerance, a condition in which a body can't adjust properly to an upright posture. POTS is characterized by a heart rate increasing excessively when one sits or stands up, and often includes autonomic nervous system issues and thus abnormalities in many organs and functions, including digestive problems.
- Non-cardiac Chest Pain (Costochondritis)—a chronic pain disorder due to inflamed cartilage between breastbone and rib(s).
- Female Urethral Syndrome—chronic frequent urination, painful urination, and/ or discomfort above the pubis.
- Primary Dysmenorrhea—a disorder involving chronic menstrual cramps, or cramping/pain in a woman's lower abdomen before or during her menstrual period, and an absence of pelvic disease that could cause these symptoms.
- Interstitial Cystitis (aka painful bladder syndrome)—chronic pressure and/or pain in the bladder.
- Multiple Chemical Sensitivities, aka Environmental Illness aka Environmental Sensitivities aka Environmental Intolerance aka Toxicant-Induced Loss of Tolerance—"a chronic state of ill health characterized by the triggering of symptoms in various body systems. A person becomes intolerant of foreign chemicals that are present at low levels in modern environments…. Most patients experience symptoms of reduced ability to concentrate (mentally), to multitask, to remember and retrieve information."[21] Other common symptoms include fatigue, nausea, headache, skin rash, and more.
- Irritable Bowel Syndrome (IBS)—"a common disorder that affects the large intestine (colon) … [IBS] commonly causes cramping, abdominal pain, bloating, gas, diarrhea and constipation."[22] The majority of those with IBS do not experience severe symptoms.[23]
- Fibromyalgia—a disorder whose main symptom "is body pain that is felt in all parts of the body and has been present for at least 3 months." Other common symptoms are "fatigue, poor (non-restorative) sleep, cognitive dysfunction … mood disorder (this includes depression and/or anxiety)…"[24]
- Post Traumatic Stress Disorder (PTSD)—"a mental health condition that's triggered by a terrifying event—either experiencing it or witnessing it. Symptoms may include flashbacks, nightmares and severe anxiety, as well as uncontrollable thoughts about the event."[25] Note that the classification of PTSD as a CSS is under debate because PTSD is considered a psychological, rather than physiological, condition. However, some people with PTSD have other CSS, or CS alone, so it remains on the list for now.

Recent studies have suggested that additional syndromes be classified as CSS, such as these:

- "Centrally Mediated Abdominal Pain Syndrome (CAPS)—formerly known as Functional Abdominal Pain Syndrome … [CAPS] is a result of central sensitization with disinhibition of [unrestrained] pain signals…"[26]

- *Some* Chronic Low Back Pain—"Central sensitization … may be a contributory factor for a sub-group of patients with chronic low back pain."[27]
- *Some* Osteoarthritis (OA) Pain—While [OA] is not being classified as a CSS at this time, a 2016 review states, "Clinicians should be aware of [CS] in patients with chronic OA pain, especially in patients presenting with severe pain with unusual features."[28]
- Joint Hypermobility Syndrome/Ehlers Danlos Syndrome, Hypermobility Type (JHS/EDS-HT)—Findings of a 2016 study "imply that pain in JHS/EDS-HT might arise through central sensitization…. In patients with JHS/EDS-HT, the persistent nociceptive [sensory nerve] input due to joint abnormalities probably triggers central sensitization in the dorsal horn neurons [nerves in the posterior spinal column] and causes widespread pain."[29]
- Sickle Cell Disease—"Recent evidence suggests that [CS] may explain differences in the symptom experience of individuals with sickle cell disease (SCD)…. In general, SCD patients with greater CS had more clinical pain, more crises, worse sleep, and more psychosocial disturbances compared with the low CS group."[30]
- Neurocognitive Disorders (NCD)—Another recent study reveals, "Central sensitization may be a possible risk factor of widespread pain in elderly patients with NCD."[31]
- Overactive Bladder (OAB)—One recent study discovers that "[CS] describes an induced state of spinal hypersensitivity that is associated with a variety of chronic pain disorders that share many attributes with OAB, albeit without the presence of pain," and suggests that CS might play a role in "understanding the mechanisms and clinical manifestations of OAB syndrome."[32]

It's not uncommon for people with CSS to experience symptom overlap. If you have symptoms commonly attributed to a particular syndrome, that doesn't mean you'll be diagnosed with it. For example, I've been diagnosed with three CSS—Irritable Larynx Syndrome, Multiple Chemical Sensitivities, and Chronic Fatigue Syndrome—and experience symptoms common to those syndromes on a daily basis. However, on bad days, I also experience symptoms such as bloating, diarrhea, inflammation, and pain. Does that mean I have Irritable Bowel Syndrome or Fibromyalgia too? Not necessarily. Since those symptoms occur only on bad days, my specialist considers them "overlapping symptoms" rather than cause for additional diagnoses.

It can take months or years to get a diagnosis. Waiting can be an awful limbo, and the trap of self-diagnosing may have some tempting bait, but only a medical professional who understands CS and CSS should diagnose you. Find one as soon as possible. While you're waiting—and even after a recent diagnosis—your body may seem like a stranger to you, or a betrayer, or a foe. You may find yourself distrusting your mind, your senses, and your ability to function well physically or cognitively. When I first developed symptoms, I had no idea what was happening. I would go for a run—even a short 3-kilometer thing—and it wouldn't be a great run, but it would feel ok. The next day, though, I wouldn't be able to walk, my limbs felt like lead, my muscles were inflamed and tender. I would have trouble reading a sentence. The words seemed to swim before my eyes, and I could not comprehend their meaning. I had difficulty constructing sentences, had to speak very slowly, and struggled to access vocabulary. Those symptoms would last for weeks, just because I'd taken a single short run, or walked five blocks to the grocery store and back—things I used to do several times a week without thinking, on top of hour-long workouts three times weekly in the gym. At first I thought I had a flu, but when this experience persisted for months, I came to believe I was dying. Over a year later, I met a doctor who recognized my symptoms. I won't lie—having an invisible, debilitating illness is no joyride—but learning what the problem was and how to manage my symptoms made a huge difference. It allowed me to create healthy expectations and healing goals, and move forward.

We'll look at treatment methods throughout the book, but keep in mind that because CS and CSS are "new" scientific fields, and because everyone's circumstances, responses, level of health, and central nervous system are different, there is no "one-size-fits-all" treatment, and no 100 percent cure.[33] In general, treatment should be patient-centered and tends to go something like this: the doctor assesses what symptoms are most severely diminishing a patient's quality of life and addresses those first. S/he weighs the pros and cons of various ways to decrease those symptoms, and then discusses with the patient and decides how to proceed. In addition to addressing acute symptoms, treatment seeks to normalize whatever biopsychosocial (biological, psychological, and social) factors can be normalized, to make life with CS and CSS manageable and optimize the patient's quality of life. (Medical providers, see Appendix C for treatment approach details.) As I mentioned in the Preface, there's a whole lot more to CS and CSS than symptoms, and these conditions can devastate one's social, home, and financial life and upset one's mental health, especially early on, during what I call the *crisis phase*, when symptoms progressively worsen. My goal is to get you from crisis phase to stability phase (when you start to get the upper hand on CS and CSS) to what lies beyond as quickly and painlessly as possible.

Whether you are dealing with CS alone, or one or more CSS, a major root of the problem is an oversensitive central nervous system. Worrying or feeling anxious about your symptoms and situation can intensify symptoms. It's hard, but keep calm. Don't worry overmuch. Check out the strategies in the chapter on coping. Tell your brain that everything will be all right, and *believe* it.

Remember, you aren't alone, though it sure may feel like it, and I'm right here, talking to you.

Central Sensitization and the Gut

Officially known as the Enteric Nervous System, our guts are a hot topic in health research, with findings showing that they do a whole lot more than process nutrients and dispose of waste. While remaining relatively unassuming and highly underrated (except in hip medical circles) the enteric system influences our mood, mental health, and well-being, and also "plays key roles in certain diseases."[34] How so? Well, for a start, 70 percent or more "of our immune system is aimed at the gut to expel and kill foreign invaders," so if you've got gut problems, how might that affect your immune system?[35] Also, "95 percent of the body's serotonin [a neurotransmitter, or chemical secreted by the brain that is involved in one's sense of well-being and happiness] is found in the bowels," and serotonin leaking from the gut into the bloodstream is suspected to play a part in many conditions, including autism.[36]

By the way, our guts are filled with so many neurotransmitters and lined with such a substantial network of neurons (cells that transmit nerve impulses) that some researchers fondly call the enteric system our "second brain."[37] Formerly thought of as part of the autonomic nervous system, the enteric is now considered one of the main divisions of our peripheral nervous system because it can "control gut behavior independently of the brain."[38] Check out Diagram 1 if you need a visual.

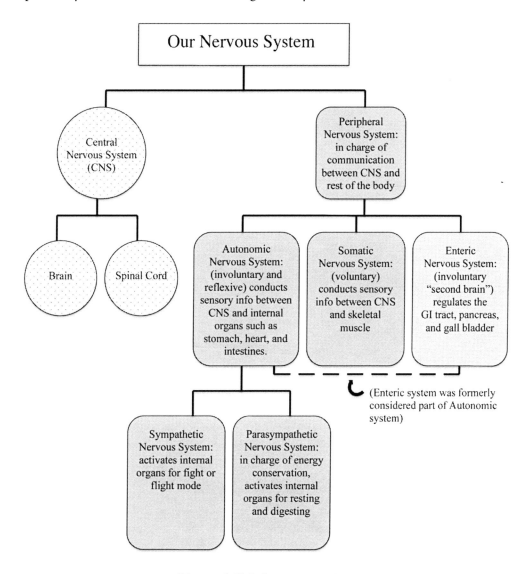

Diagram 1. Enteric nervous system

So, does the enteric system's relative independence from the central nervous system mean the guts won't get unreliable signals from the sensitized brain? This is lucky for people with CS, right? The answer is yes, and no. Basically, while the "second brain" doesn't tend to take orders from the central nervous system, the guts aren't immune to the effects of CS on the body. In fact, many people with CS experience abnormal gut activity—yep, even those without an Irritable Bowel Syndrome (IBS) diagnosis may have issues with bloating, leaky gut, serotonin imbalance, food sensitivities, or more. Because of this, I've developed a pet theory that both the brain and the "second brain" become sensitized when CS develops. I look forward to the time when researchers prove me right (or wrong).

There are still many unknowns amidst the knowns, even with a common condition such as IBS. For example, one recent study proposes that infections that indirectly cause the central nervous system and other physiological functions to be compromised may be one of the causes of IBS, but further research is needed to say for sure.[39] That same study reports, "the presence of small intestinal bowel overgrowth (SIBO) has been documented in patients with IBS," and reducing SIBO resulted in decreased IBS symptoms.[40] When I learned this, I wondered if SIBO might be present in those with CSS other than IBS, or even in CS alone, and how much SIBO might be increasing CS and CSS symptoms. No conclusions, but I came to believe that "it is mandatory to consider SIBO in all cases of complex non-specific dyspeptic complaints (bloating, abdominal discomfort, diarrhoea, abdominal pain), in motility disorders, anatomical abnormalities of the small bowel and in all malassimilation syndromes (malabsorption, maldigestion)."[41] That is, when I realized I was having gut issues, I talked to my doctor about my symptoms and applicable testing, including SIBO.[42]

How do you know if you're having gut issues? Good question. Some symptoms are more obviously gut-related than others. The following may indicate a gut issue:

- Belching, heartburn, acid reflux or GERD
- Food sensitivities, allergies, and/or intolerances
- Iron and/or B12 deficiency
- Hormonal imbalances
- Depression, anxiety
- Skin rashes, eczema, acne/rosacea
- Asthma, COPD
- Fatty stools
- Headaches, brain fog, and/or any other symptoms common to CSS
- Abdominal pain or cramping, a bloated feeling, gas, mucus in the stool, or diarrhea or constipation (these are also common IBS symptoms)
- Rectal bleeding, nighttime abdominal pain, or weight loss (any of these may indicate a more serious condition)

If you experience any of the above, see your doctor. Symptoms might indicate a number of conditions, from heartburn to CS to Celiac Disease.[43] The important thing is to figure it out and treat it and then see how you feel. I can't stress this enough: **gut problems affect one's general health, and they can compound or intensify CS and CSS symptoms.** If your doctor isn't knowledgeable in the fields of gut health and Central Sensitization, find one who is. Identifying the condition(s) affecting the gut will involve testing. Procedures can vary, from a blood, stool, or breath test to an elimination diet to a more invasive procedure like a colonoscopy. Treatments also can vary, from antibiotics to trigger desensitization to meditation and diet. (I'll be discussing these soon.)

Gut issues can cause both physical and mental suffering, yet you may find it difficult to talk about symptoms, even to a doctor. Feelings of fear, shame, or disgust may cause you to choose to suffer in silence. Believe me, not knowing what you're dealing with is far worse than the few minutes of discomfort you may experience while having that conversation with your doctor. It's worth taking that risk and getting an appropriate diagnosis as soon as possible, because once you do, you can start restoring gut health and feeling a whole lot better. Remember, you aren't the only one with CS to experience enteric system issues, and I'm right here, talking to you.

Chronic Fatigue Syndrome aka Myalgic Encephalomyelitis aka Systemic Exertion Intolerance Disease

The Centers for Disease Control and Prevention (CDC) state on their website that Chronic Fatigue Syndrome (CFS) has various "case definitions," all of which list "fatigue" as a symptom.[44] "The 1994 CFS case definition," which is the one the CDC employs, assesses CFS by the following requirements:

1. The patient must have experienced "severe chronic fatigue" for at least six continuous months that is not caused by "ongoing exertion or other medical conditions associated with fatigue."[45] (The definition stipulates that a physician must eliminate such possibilities once diagnostics are taken.)[46]
2. The patient must have fatigue that "significantly interferes with daily activities and work."[47]
3. The patient must have at least four of these symptoms:
   - "post-exertion malaise lasting more than 24 hours
   - unrefreshing sleep
   - significant impairment of short-term memory or concentration
   - muscle pain
   - pain in the joints without swelling or redness
   - headaches of a new type, pattern, or severity
   - tender lymph nodes in the neck or armpit
   - a sore throat that is frequent or recurring."[48]

This definition stipulates that the above symptoms must not have presented prior to the fatigue, and must last (or repeat during) at least six continuous months.[49]

Nutshell, CFS is a debilitating condition involving both physical and cognitive impairment. According to the Institute of Medicine, "ME/CFS affects 836,000 to 2.5 million Americans."[50] Roughly "84 to 91 percent" of those with CFS have yet to be diagnosed; thus, the actual presence of the condition is yet to be determined.[51] More women than men have CFS, and "most patients currently diagnosed with ME/CFS are Caucasian, but some studies suggest that ME/CFS is more common in minority groups. The average age of onset is 33, although ME/CFS has been reported in patients younger than age 10 and older than age 70."[52]

You now know more than most about CFS. I'll delve deep into this condition once we've addressed the basics, starting with this: *Why does this syndrome have so many names, and which is the correct name?*

Myalgic Encephalomyelitis (ME): CFS is often referred to as ME/CFS and/or confused with ME; however, the Institute of Medicine (IOM) reports that "'myalgic encephalomyelitis' is not appropriate to describe Chronic Fatigue Syndrome (CFS) because there is a lack of evidence for encephalomyelitis (brain inflammation) in patients with this disease, and myalgia (muscle pain) is not a core symptom of the disease."[53] This is one of those aspects of living on the edge of medical research—it takes time to get terminology straight. To avoid confusion, I will not be using the abbreviation ME/CFS when referring to Chronic Fatigue Syndrome in this book, nor will I use the term "Myalgic Encephalomyelitis" to refer to Chronic Fatigue Syndrome.

Systemic Exertion Intolerance Disease (SEID): This is a new name for Chronic Fatigue Syndrome, introduced and recommended by the IOM in 2015. Why does this condition, already confused with ME, need *another* name and acronym? Research has proven that "the term 'chronic fatigue syndrome' affects patients' perceptions of their illness as well as the reactions of others ... [and] can trivialize the seriousness of the condition and promote misunderstanding of the illness."[54] The IOM believes that SEID is a more appropriate name because it describes a core element of the condition, "the fact that exertion of any sort—physical, cognitive, or emotional—can adversely affect patients in many organ systems and in many aspects of their lives."[55] I tend to agree with the IOM on this one, but because "Chronic Fatigue Syndrome" is the most widely recognized, accepted, and used name at time of writing, and SEID has yet to be embraced officially by the medical world, I'm going to use the acronym "CFS" when discussing this condition throughout this book.

I'll discuss CFS in detail in Chapter 3. If you are reading this book only for help with CFS, you may feel tempted to skip ahead, but I recommend that you skip nothing, as you'll need the upcoming information regarding how to create and use a bubble for recovery and healing from CS and any CSS.

Multiple Chemical Sensitivities aka Environmental Illness aka Environmental Sensitivities aka Environmental Intolerance aka Toxicant-Induced Loss of Tolerance

This condition's nomenclature, like that of CFS, continues to evolve as researchers move towards consensus. In 1987, Dr. M. R. Cullen from the Yale University School of Medicine, Department of Internal Medicine, published this definition: "Multiple chemical sensitivities (MCS) is an acquired disorder characterized by current symptoms, referable to multiple organ systems, occurring in response to demonstrable exposure to many chemically unrelated compounds at doses far below those established in the general population to cause harmful effects. No single widely accepted test of physiologic function can be shown to correlate with symptoms."[56] This is still considered a valid definition today, although more case definitions have been developed, proposed, and accepted since then.

"Consensus criteria for the definition of multiple chemical sensitivity (MCS) were first identified in a 1989 multidisciplinary survey of 89 clinicians and researchers with extensive experience in, but widely differing views of, MCS."[57] Their top five criteria define MCS as follows:

1. "a chronic condition
2. with symptoms that recur reproducibly
3. in response to low levels of exposure

4. to multiple unrelated chemicals and

5. improve or resolve when incitants are removed."[58]

In 1999, the Environmental Health Association of Nova Scotia proposed the addition of "a 6th criterion," via its own consensus group:

6. "requiring that symptoms occur in multiple organ systems."[59]

The 1999 consensus found that although "these criteria are all commonly encompassed by research definitions of MCS … their standardized use in clinical settings is still lacking, long overdue, and greatly needed—especially in light of government studies in the United States, United Kingdom, and Canada that revealed 2–4 times as many cases of chemical sensitivity among Gulf War veterans than undeployed controls."[60] Basically, due to a lack of a proper diagnostic definition of MCS, medical providers were not diagnosing the condition. This is bad news. Anyone who has had to wait for proper diagnosis knows it is essential to one's quality of life and sense of well-being, primarily on two levels:

1. Physiologically: Diagnosis allows the patient to learn about, manage, and possibly heal from the condition.

2. Psychologically: Diagnosis not only validates the patient's experience, it allows one to understand and predict, to manage expectations. Diagnosis tells the patient what the new playing field looks like, or at least offers a glimpse of the terrain. With an appropriate diagnosis, the illness becomes a tangible thing, and the patient can move forward, even if only one step forward.

Based on the high prevalence of MCS, the Nova Scotia consensus "[recommended] that MCS be formally diagnosed—in addition to any other disorders that may be present—in all cases in which the 6 aforementioned consensus criteria are met and no single other organic disorder (e.g., mastocytosis) can account for all the signs and symptoms associated with chemical exposure. The millions of civilians and tens of thousands of Gulf War veterans who suffer from chemical sensitivity should not be kept waiting any longer for a standardized diagnosis while medical research continues to investigate the etiology of their signs and symptoms."[61]

The additional MCS criteria, "having a stronger sense of smell than others, feeling dull/groggy, feeling 'spacey,' and having difficulty concentrating,"[62] was proposed in 2001 following further epidemiological research.

Meanwhile, the terminology race for this condition seems to be between these two frontrunners: MCS and Toxicant-Induced Loss of Tolerance (TILT). TILT was proposed in 1997 by Dr. Claudia S. Miller, a professor at University of Texas San Antonio's School of Medicine, whose research found that MCS "appears to be the consequence of a two-step process: loss of tolerance in susceptible persons following exposure to various toxicants, and subsequent triggering of symptoms by extremely small quantities of previously tolerated chemicals, drugs, foods, and food and drug combinations including caffeine and alcohol. Although chemical sensitivity may be the consequence of this process," Dr. Miller believes *TILT* most clearly describes said process.[63] I agree, but since TILT is not widely known or accepted at this time, I will refer to this syndrome as "MCS" throughout the book.

How does MCS affect someone's life and lifestyle? As is common with CS and CSS, severity of symptoms and debilitation levels can vary, but a look at my symptoms may give you an idea: After being exposed to unsafe levels of Volatile Organic Compounds (VOCs), particulates, fumes, dust and whatever else at my workplace, my body began to react to people's perfumes, colognes, odors trapped in their clothing from cigarette smoke and scented laundry products. At first I would get burning eyes, a runny nose and sore throat, postnasal drip, and maybe sneeze or cough a little, until I got away from whatever the irritant was. My reactions worsened over the next few months. Strong or synthetic smells triggered an asthma episode, headaches, nausea, and/or coughing severe enough to make me pass out. The minor burning eyes, runny nose and sneezing developed into full-on hay fever episodes. Painful, bulbous skin rashes formed on my hands and feet if they touched fabric or surfaces that had been cleaned with certain chemical products, and a single mosquito bite on my knee developed into hives that covered my leg. Antihistamines provided no relief, and allergy tests showed that I wasn't allergic to *anything*. As time passed, I experienced increasing pain, fear, and confusion.

Meanwhile, the sensitivity of my olfactory system heightened. Within a few months I could smell things that others couldn't detect. Everywhere I went, I could *smell* new products off-gassing (aka outgassing, this is the process in which products release VOCs or other compounds—toxic and/or non-toxic—in the form of a gas). I made jokes that I was going to get a job as a drug sniffer dog, or as the world's most discriminating sommelier, or maybe I could work with the gas company and sniff out leaks and save people....

But in reality, it was terrifying. Why could I smell things other folks couldn't? Why were my reactions increasing in frequency and severity? Why couldn't I go anywhere without having a coughing fit, a dizzy spell, a headache, and feeling sick? My ears felt plugged all the time, as if my whole head were congested. I was constantly clearing my throat against what felt like a softball-sized wad of mucus lodged there. My voice was changing, becoming weak, thin, raspy, and I could no longer sing. I became prey to panic and anxiety, as you can imagine, and even lost my sense of humor for a while. It was a grim time indeed.

Along with the increasing symptoms and sensitivities, and decreasing ability to breathe and manage in public, I was also facing loss of employment, struggling to pay my mortgage, learning the rigmarole of workers compensation, and dealing with the effects of too many medications given to me by doctors who didn't know what the problem was. Don't get me wrong—I have great doctors. They have been amazing and still are. But it took some time to get access to a specialist who understood what was happening, and in the meantime, my doctors tried lots of different remedies, hoping to discover a cure. The medications made me jittery, kept me from sleeping, disrupted my GI tract, made me dopey in the daytime, and gave me incredible mood swings, among other side effects. Suffice to say, it was a horrible time, and it all happened because my central nervous system perceived a threat that wasn't really there. My titanium amygdala did not let me down. Not for a second.

From what I understand, different people react in different ways, and irritants, too, vary. I've developed some strategies to get through life with MCS, and even to desensitize my system and begin healing. We'll get to those in the "Decreasing Trigger Exposure and Impact" chapter and beyond.

RECOVERING FROM AN MCS EPISODE

What happens after an MCS episode, you ask? And how *does* one recover from an acute episode like the ones I just described? Well, if it's real bad, I may pass out for a while, and then pick myself up off the floor with as much dignity as I can muster. After that, I do three things:

1. remove myself from the environment as soon as possible,
2. retreat to my bubble, and
3. stay clear until symptoms subside.

Step 1 is also known as the *CS Scramble*, and there's an art to it. My acute symptoms tend to include gobs of phlegm coating my throat, nose and face, so my scramble involves intensive cleanup along with hacking and gasping. If you venture from your bubble often enough, you'll develop your own style. Hopefully you won't look like a two-year-old with a cold whose parent can't be bothered with nose wipes, but hey, even if you do, you aren't the first and won't be the last. You aren't alone on this odyssey. I'm right here, talking to you.

Irritable Larynx Syndrome

It's probably been years since your 11th grade anatomy and physiology class, so here's a larynx review: Commonly known as the voice box, the larynx is a thick, cartilaginous space in the throat that connects mouth to lungs. It houses the vocal chords and has the power to block food and air from getting into the lungs. Got it? Let's move on.

In 1999, Irritable Larynx Syndrome (ILS) was originally defined by Dr. Murray Morrison, Dr. Linda Rammage, and AJ Emami of the Pacific Voice Clinic at University of British Columbia and Vancouver General Hospital as "hyperkinetic laryngeal dysfunction resulting from an assorted collection of causes in response to a definitive triggering stimulus."[64] That is, ILS causes the muscles around the larynx to overreact to normal sensory stimuli [usually an odor, but can also be an emotion or other stressor] and "trigger an involuntary, often protracted, laryngeal closure reflex that can be bothersome or frightening to the patient. The laryngeal muscle spasm can cause episodes of coughing without apparent cause, a sense of a lump in the throat (globus sensation) and/or a 'laryngospasm.'"[65] A laryngospasm is "characterized by adduction of the true vocal folds" and obstructs the patient's airway, impeding breathing, especially inhaling.[66] Laryngospasms that recur are sometimes referred to as "Vocal Cord Dysfunction (VCD)" or "Paradoxical Vocal Fold Motion (PVFM)."[67] "The laryngeal muscle spasm may lead to muscle misuse voice problems, manifest as episodes of dysphonia [difficulty in speaking] and vocal dysfluencies [rough, nonfluid speech], or a more chronically dysphonic voice, commonly referred to as Muscle Tension Dysphonia (MTD)."[68] Nutshell, ILS occurs when the sensitized central nervous system perceives an airborne threat and tries to (over)protect the lungs by tightening the muscles around the larynx, effectively cutting off the air supply to the lungs and thus saving the day. Only problem is—yep, you guessed it—then the person with ILS has difficulty in talking and, more importantly, breathing.

Over a decade later, in 2010, Doctors Morrison and Rammage added ILS to the growing list of CSS in their report, "The Irritable Larynx Syndrome as a Central Sensitivity Syndrome."[69] Also in 2010, researchers outlined a specific type of ILS, called "Work-Associated Irritable Larynx Syndrome (WILS)."[70] In 2015, researchers proposed a new classification scheme for VCD/PVFM (also known as Paradoxical Vocal Cord Motion, or PVCM) that "divides PVCM into primary, or psychological, and secondary. The secondary form consists of medical disorders divided into irritable larynx syndrome and neurologic disorders."[71] The placement of ILS in a category with neurologic disorders, separate from psychological ones, not only supports the CSS-related findings of Doctors Morrison and Rammage, but it's a big step towards validating the condition and debunking the prejudice that ILS is merely "all in your head."

What does ILS look like in real life? Remember the description of my MCS symptoms in the previous segment? Mixed in there, unbeknownst to me, were ILS symptoms as well. The loss of voice, the coughing, the wad of mucus in my throat, the eventual gasping for breath, and utter darkness of unconsciousness—those are primarily symptoms of ILS, while the runny nose, nausea, headaches, hay fever, rashes and such are technically more common with MCS. For me, they are all one, since I have both conditions. You, however, may not experience all of these symptoms. You may not have full-on ILS, merely some vocal chord dysfunction or periodic laryngospasms due to CS. For example, I have a friend with Fibromyalgia, and on bad days, she also experiences scent sensitivities and an irritable larynx. Remember, you and I may both have CS, we may even have the same CSS, but we can present with different symptoms and/or similar symptoms of differing severities.

Eight months after symptom onset, I got to see an ear, nose and throat specialist I'll call Dr. Y, who specializes in vocal chord dysfunction. Here's what my ILS diagnosis looked like.

Dr. Y ushers me into his exam room, and I sit in the Frankenstein chair. *Be cautious*, I tell myself. *Don't get all excited about finding answers. You might not get any today.* A good-natured, paternal looking guy, the doc settles on a low swivel stool in front of me and stares at my neck so intently I begin to wonder if I've stumbled onto a vampire movie set.

"Can you remove your scarf, please?" he says. "And tell me your story."

My voice is hoarse and powerless, and pitched several tones higher than my real voice. I cough every few words. My nose is starting to run, and I grab a Kleenex from the shelf beside me. His gaze doesn't waver from my neck as I struggle to talk. He takes deep breaths. I try to do the same, but my breath gets caught in my throat and I return to shallow breathing, like a panicked animal. When I'm finished with my story he makes a sound like "hrum" and scribbles in my file.

"Can we have a look at what's happening inside there?" He points at my throat. I nod. He sprays numbing spray up my left nostril and picks up a long, thin tube with a sunflower seed-sized nob on the end. This he attaches to a cable that is connected to his computer.

"Is that going up—?" I indicate my nose.

He nods. "We're going to make a video. There will be some discomfort, I'm afraid."

For once I'm grateful for the largesse of my family nose. His video contraption would never fit into a cute little button nose. When he inserts it into my left nostril my eyes sting and tear. The pain is odd, not sharp or throbbing, just ultra-stimulating. Like when you sniff the air in 40-below and your nose sends a shock that electrifies your body. I feel the camera tube in my nose, up, and down the back of my throat. Then I'm gagging on it.

"Say ah … eee … longer eee … can you sing it? Eee…"

I try to follow his directions, try to make the sounds while not gagging while new shocks tremor through my body every time he moves the tube.

"OK," he withdraws the camera and hands me the box of Kleenex. Tears and phlegm run down my face and throat. I'm coughing, mopping up, shaking.

"The unpleasantness is done now. Let's have a look at those vocal chords."

We watch the journey up my sinuses and down my throat. It's all pink and red and wet and slimy looking—very Jules Verne. Dr. Y seems pleased, pointing out the various anatomical features. I try to learn but have to keep blowing my nose and wiping at the steady flow of tears that must not fall onto the pages of questions in the notepad I hold on my lap.

I check the time. It has been well over ten minutes, the limit to which most doctors strictly adhere. I realize with a jolt of terror that I'd forgotten to ask how much time we get. "Um, doc, I have a bunch of questions." The questions I've had for months that no one else could answer—why were my ears plugged? Was my hearing damaged? Why did I cough and why did my nose run when I ate? Why couldn't I sing? Had my vocal chords been damaged by the months of coughing and clearing my throat? Would I ever sing again? Why did I have post-nasal drip all the time? Why didn't antihistamines work when I got hay fever? Was this permanent? *What was wrong with me?*

. "Well, let's take them one at a time," he says, leaning back in his chair as if he has all the time in the world. In my experience, most doctors do not behave this way. After a stunned pause, I ask the first question. In the next 20 minutes or so, he answers every one. I am beginning to feel like he is the Candy Man or Santa. His eyebrows are bushy enough to be Santa's.

"From what I've seen today," he says, "I feel you will certainly sing again."

More tears. Major floodgate breach. My body shudders, like when you are three and something eternally and catastrophically horrible happens, like your ice cream falling on the ground. That's what my body does. It shudders like that. I even sob a few times before I get control of myself. *I will sing!*

"Your ears are clear, your hearing is not damaged," he says. "I think your ears feel plugged because of acid reflux."

"But I don't have that," I say. "I have no heart-burn or burping … my father has had GERD for as long as I can remember. I don't have that."

"Everyone has *some* reflux," he says. "Yours is out of control right now. And some common though perhaps lesser-known symptoms of acid reflux are runny nose, feeling of plugged ears, post-nasal drip." He pauses and makes a note in my file, then turns back to face me. "You have developed something called Irritable Larynx Syndrome, as a reaction to the incident at work. Your larynx muscles are over-protecting your throat, lungs, and voice. This makes it hard for you to breathe and to speak, laugh, sing, etc. Feel how tight these are?" He taps my neck muscles. They feel solid, like rock.

As he speaks, making sense of the nonsense I've lived with for eight months, I feel increasingly weightless. I feel no resistance. I feel *resonance*, as if he were speaking for the disorder within me, explaining why it has treated me thus, and what it has been trying to tell me all this time. Now it is sounding a long, low tone of agreement.

His diagnosis is the first thing the western doctors have said that makes sense to me, that explains the inconsistency of my symptoms, and why it has been worsening as time goes on, why the asthma puffers can't control it, etc.

"You need to see a psychiatrist and a speech pathologist right away," he says.

"I don't have money for a shrink," I say. "I was referred to outpatient psych at the hospital here but that was months ago and they still haven't called. There's a long waiting list, I guess."

"I can do better than that." He doesn't hand me a candy cane when he says that, but I think he might have winked.

When I left there that day, I felt immense relief. Someone knew what was wrong with me. I wasn't going to get passed off to yet another doctor and get pumped full of trial medications while I waited another three months, only to be told that they had no idea what was wrong with me and I should go see so-and-so. Eight months of questions, fears, and suffering ended. There were new questions, but now I had someone to ask. And best of all, I would sing again. I would sing!

Ah, so triumphant! I love moments like that, don't you? Must savour them, I tell myself. *Savour* them ... mmmm ...

ILS is complex and complicated though, so when you finish savouring, read on for more learnin'.

The Complexity of ILS

A feedback cycle inherent in ILS makes it perhaps more complex than other CSS. There's more to this condition than the body perceiving an odor as a threat and shutting off incoming air. Because the larynx is connected to the sinuses, the lungs, the vocal chords, and the mouth (which is connected to the esophagus and stomach), if one of these areas or connected systems gets irritated or a little out of balance, it can cause an ILS episode.

Can you guess what this means? Strong smells aren't the only things that can trigger ILS. People with ILS also need to watch out for stuff like this:

- An asthma episode
- Post-nasal drip, sinus congestion and/or infection
- Acid reflux (everyone has some, but if you have more than normal, it can be a cause of ILS episodes)
- ILS episodes themselves (I'll explain this in a minute)

In fact, any of the above can contribute to causing any of the above to happen. All it takes is a little irritation or inflammation in the wrong place. Fun times, eh?

ILS episodes often occur when emotions run high, when under stress, and/or dealing with fatigue. Laughing, crying, shouting, singing, speaking for a long duration—these can all cause an ILS uprising. When I am under stress, the muscles around my larynx tend to tighten. When I'm tired, same deal. When I'm having an emotional conversation while under stress and tired, look out! I never thought about how lucky I was that I could laugh when I wanted—talk when I wanted, *sing* when I wanted—without negative physical response. Truth be told, ILS can really take the fun out of emoting and communicating. It can take the fun out of lots of things. The best way to deal with that, I've found, is to work to prevent ILS episodes, and to recover from them as quickly as possible.

Preventing and Recovering from an ILS Episode

Preventing ILS episodes at first seems like an addictive fairway game at the Make-Me-Crazy Carnival. For months, all I could do was reel, gasping and dizzy, from one episode to the next. But once I knew what the condition was, and how it worked, I began to get a grip on some strategies.

The biggest and most effective prevention method is avoiding triggers, which I will discuss in depth in the next chapter. Controlling asthma is another important component of preventing ILS episodes. If I forget to take my asthma medication, I get into serious breathing trouble soon, both lungs and larynx.

According to Dr. Y, decreasing acid reflux is also helpful. I didn't understand reflux prior to my ILS diagnosis, but I quickly learned that there's more to reflux than a few belches after a big meal and popping a Tums or two. Dr. Y says everyone has some acid reflux. The problems start when you get too much. I never had such problems until after the workplace exposure, so I suspect all the stress and random medications I was given in that time of great diagnosisless uncertainty upset my acid balance. The bottom line is, acid reflux overload can irritate the larynx. People with ILS want a calm, non-irritated larynx, so I tried some of the following things to decrease my acid reflux, with mixed results:

- Proton Pump Inhibitors, aka PPIs, are prescription drugs used to inhibit the stomach from generating too much acid. They didn't make a speck of difference for me in terms of my speaking, singing, or breathing issues, but they did have some strong side effects—bloating, diarrhea … it wasn't pretty. That said, Dr. Y assured me they work for lots of folks, so don't discount them because of my response.

- Dr. Y also recommended that I eat smaller meals, eat low-fat meals, stay away from caffeine and chocolate and red peppers, and even prop the head of my bed up six inches higher than the foot. I already ate small, low-fat meals, drank only decaf, and well, I couldn't avoid chocolate because what's the point in living? But I restricted my intake. I loved red peppers but abstained until my ILS got under control and I started getting my voice back. Now I can eat red peppers on good days without triggering ILS. I never tried lifting the head of my bed, but Dr. Y spoke highly of it.

- I tried a hi-alkaline, low-acid diet for several months. I also cut out about 95 percent of the gluten, lactose, and sugar from my diet. This type of diet may seem extreme, but at the time, I had endured major sinus congestion, loss of voice and the sensation of plugged ears 24/7 for six months, and no one seemed to be able to fix those issues, so I figured it was worth a try. After about a year, the congestion began to lessen, my voice started to return, and the sensation in my ears normalized. I don't know what exactly caused my success, but upon reintroducing gluten and sugar and dairy, I learned unequivocally that they cause my body to produce more mucus and increase inflammation.

- Apple cider vinegar is said to nullify stomach acid. In the past year or so, I have slurped a teaspoonful of the stuff following a spicy or high-fat meal and found that I had no runny nose or plugged ear sensations afterwards. Hard cider has produced similar results. If I consume half a cup or so with a big meal or some spicy, fatty, delicious treat that seems bound to cause an overabundance of acid, I experience no reflux symptoms afterwards.

- I know a guy who takes charcoal to deal with his acid reflux overabundance. Works great for him. I haven't tried it so can't say more than that.

Some techniques can be used for both preventing and recovering from ILS episodes, such as muscle-relaxation exercises. If you can keep the muscles around the larynx relaxed most of the time, then any ILS episodes will tend to be less severe, or take longer to become severe, because the muscles have to go all the way from a fully relaxed state to a fully tightened state. But if the muscles around the larynx never relax, they get increasingly tight and more challenging to release, and the ILS episodes will consequently become more and more severe.

My throat muscles were rock-hard for a good year or more, but eventually I got them to loosen up, somewhat. Are they completely relaxed now? Sometimes. Usually on days when I haven't had an episode for a while, when I'm not stressed or overtired, and when I am hanging out in my bubble. Has my ILS gone away completely? Nope. At time of writing, it's been four years, and I still have ILS episodes every day or so, most of them fairly minor and short-lived. Until I find a way to phase out my ILS for good, I do the following to minimize its impact.

Remember, ILS is a condition caused by a sensitized nervous system, resulting in tight muscles around the larynx. So, to prevent or recover from an ILS episode, it makes sense that one should address both the sensitized nervous system and the affected muscles. We care for the nervous system primarily via the bubble, which I'll detail in the next chapter, and we work on affected muscles as follows:

- **Loosening the neck muscles:** After an ILS episode, it becomes very apparent which neck muscles are tight. The goal is to get them loose again. Heat works well for me, like a hot bath or shower, or a hot pack. I take slow, relaxed breaths, let the warmth seep into my neck and then try to work the muscles a little. First I rub the skin over them lightly, and gradually work deeper into the muscles. Sometimes they don't budge. That's ok, I tell myself, rubbing the skin softly, I'll try again in an hour. Sometimes the muscles are so inflamed, I get fiery pain when I touch them. I'll use an ice pack then, and maybe take some Ibuprofen, and try again in an hour. Other times I can tug the muscles away from the throat—not enough to cause pain, but enough to help them become more malleable, more muscle-like and less stone-like. Gentle, slow, neck stretches to each side can help soften up these muscles too, I've found. Take special care with this area. If you aren't sure how to do neck stretches properly, ask your physiotherapist or doctor.
- **Back breathing/assume the position:** My vocal therapist—whom I'll call Dr. Z— calls this exercise "back breathing." I call it "assume the position." Sit in a chair and roll forward so your head is between your knees, like they tell you to do when practicing the airplane safety routine before your flight takes off. Now breathe as deeply as possible. Don't force the breath. Relax into it. In that position, it may feel as if you are breathing through your back. That's good. Your breath should be deep, slow, calming and relaxing. This strategy works wonders if you have an ILS episode on a bus or train. People clear away from you when you cough like crazy, gasp for breath and then assume the position.
- **Chin-tuck:** Dr. Z also taught me that if you tuck your chin deep into your chest, your airway physically cannot close all the way. Of course, when you're coughing your head off and gasping for breath, it can be hard to remember to keep your chin down, but practice makes perfect!

Remember, the goal is to loosen these muscles *over time*. They're not going to go back to normal right away. If you have acute ILS episodes daily, they will stay quite tight until you can lessen that frequency and severity. So do what you can to keep them as loose as possible, and when we get into the next chapter, you'll learn how to decrease those episodes, and it will all come together.

- **Visualization:** This is a powerful tool that can be used in countless ways for dealing with ILS, other CSS, and CS alone. I'll present this strategy in greater detail later, but for now, here's a little taste: When working stubborn neck muscles, I relax my breathing as much as possible and imagine a serene place—a safe place—where I can breathe. My vision usually involves a tropical beach, me lying on warm sand, with the sun shining down on me, and several scantily-clad men fanning me with palm fronds …
  Ahem.
  After about 15 minutes of that (or longer, if I get a really good vision going) I try massaging those neck muscles again, or tilting my head side to side, slowly, gently, and see if there's some improvement.

This kind of visualization is hard to do when I'm trapped on a crowded bus, engulfed by fragrances and diesel exhaust, feeling my breath lurch out of me with every cough. In such situations, I tend to rely on a more specific visualization exercise I call "Soldiers." Here's how it began…

"We all have soldiers in our minds," Dr. Z said. "They exist to protect us when we are under threat."

I nodded, trying to hold the chin-tuck posture she'd instructed me to use. It felt forced and awkward. I rolled my shoulders back and settled into the chair. Still felt weird.

"Your soldiers have been working overtime since the chemical exposure," she said. "Every time you smell something that your mind feels has potential to injure your lungs, your soldiers spring into action and tighten the muscles around your larynx to prevent further damage to your lungs."

I nodded again, tried not to want to clear the wad of phlegm from my throat. Tried to distract myself. Stared at the books stacked on top of the water cooler in the corner of her office, stared at the water in the big blue jug. I wondered if I could have a drink. But I didn't want to interrupt Dr. Z. It had taken me months to get this appointment. A drink of water could wait.

"You need to order those soldiers to stand down. Can you picture them in your mind?"

"Like athletes do?" The thinness of my voice startled me out of my posture. I carefully re-tucked my chin before continuing. "you mean mental imagery, or visualization?" I knew about that from playing competitive softball and badminton as a kid, and running long-distance as an adult.

She nodded. "It might help to draw your soldiers resting or retreating, and keep that picture in view."

"Ok." I believed visualization worked. And I was also willing to try anything. I simply *had* to sing again. I grabbed my bag, umbrella, coat, stood and tucked my chin in. Walking in this new posture made me feel like a wooden doll. I turned around halfway through the door. Dr. Z was still in her chair, looking up at me with that same good-natured, intelligent expression. "When do I come back?" Again, the reediness of my voice shocked me. It wasn't my voice. My voice was deep, resonant, and it sang even when speaking. Would I ever hear my real voice again? Focus on the doctor now, I told myself. Freak out later.

"Come back whenever you need to." She smiled. "Try the new vocal exercises a while, think about your soldiers, come back when you need to." Dr. Z had such a light, generous way about her. I wished I could come back every week, or every hour, for that matter. Maybe some of her grace would rub off on me. But I had to take the time off from my new job, then make it up later, and I was exhausted. So I'd give it a month at least.

As I huddled in the corner away from the other elevator occupants, tucking my chin and breathing through my scarf, I thought about my soldiers. I pictured them under the command of Sgt. Shultz from the TV show *Hogan's Heroes*. (This may seem like I don't give my soldiers much credit, I realize, but in truth I believe they have done their work above and beyond what I could ever ask for. Shultz is not a comment on my soldiers' capabilities, merely upon their leadership, which is a little unclear on what actual threats are, for the time being. Shultz was never clear on the actual threats either, in my opinion.)

My soldiers wore the black half helmets that lots of Harley riders wear, with the strap pulled tight under their chins. They all looked like dwarf versions of Green Day's lead singer Billie Joe Armstrong, complete with the eyeliner, charcoal shadow, awesome hair, leather pants and jacket. My soldiers were commanded to sit watch all night and often sprang to my defense at 2 a.m., whenever I had a nightmare about losing my home or all my savings or never singing again. They loved me and I loved them.

But in the next few weeks, whenever I started to feel them spring into action and my throat began to close up, I imagined Shultzie towering above them in his long coat, and I altered his orders. Instead of charging my soldiers to defend, I made him order them back to their barracks for a nap. They retreated with reluctance, spears and swords dragging, guns holstered—yes, my soldiers had spears and swords as well as guns—disappointed to miss the chance to wage battle. They climbed into their bunks and pulled the green grey blankets over themselves. The muscles around my larynx would stop constricting then, though they wouldn't loosen back up. It was as though my soldiers were still holding the line, even from their bunks. I couldn't yet persuade them to remove their boots or helmets when they got into bed either, but maybe one day that would come. For now, they lay in bed, blankets pulled up to chins, helmets and boot tips shining in the dim light. They looked like a bunch of hobbit warriors, with nice boots.

At least I wasn't choking, but beyond that, I didn't know if my visualizations were working. I did find that, the more I imagined my soldiers retreating, the easier it became to picture them in my mind. I had used visualization enough in my running and sports experience to believe that this image of sleeping soldiers would become ingrained in my mind somehow. I wouldn't have to think about them eventually. Shultz would learn the difference between real and perceived threats and automatically command my soldiers appropriately. And then, they would go back to being my Reserve Force, lying in wait until I really needed them.

VOCAL EXERCISES

Before the workplace exposure I was a singer. I had always been a singer. There was not a day when I did not sing. It was part of my identity as well as my occupation. I remember being five years old and singing songs to myself, with the radio, with the albums my father put on the LP player. I remember singing in school choirs—a cappella and accompanied, madrigals, experimental, jazz, pop, show tunes, barbershop—writing songs in my teens and recording and performing my own songs in college and beyond.

I sang to bring joy to others, I sang for money, and I sang for myself, to comfort and keep myself company. When I made sound, the vibration in my chest and bones flooded me with ecstasy and made my body buzz. It was the sensation of vitality and connection. Ultimately, I sang to feel my spirit, to feel free and alive. My singing voice was part of me in the way that my heart is part of me. And when I lost it, I was lost.

I was lost in anger. I had shown up and done the work, but my employers hadn't ensured my safety. I was angry at them for being negligent, and greedy, and for lying about the air quality, making it nearly impossible for me to get compensation. I was angry at myself too, for trusting them in the first place. And why did I even have a day job? I was an artist. Every artist knew the saying: *Day jobs will kill you.* Mine nearly did.

I was lost in grief. Who was I if I couldn't sing? What good was I? How could I exist when severed from my spirit? Maya Angelou knew why the caged bird sang, but what of the voiceless bird? I was silenced, by corporate greed, by my own naiveté, by fate and whatever else. Silenced forever? Would I ever sing again? How could I live without my voice?

Desperate questions, desperate desperation, and despair.

I stayed in that lost, bereft, desolate mindset for the better part of a year, but we won't stay there that long. You already know from the earlier passage that Dr. Y told me I would sing again. And I can tell you right now that my normal speaking voice has returned, except for really bad days, and my singing voice has returned, a little. I can sing for a few minutes at a time on good days, though I lack the intonation, power, and endurance I once had. My instrument is not what it once was, but I can make a joyful squawk now and then, I can engender a wee rumble in my bones and a soothing coo to warm hopes. (And, as you can imagine, even that little bit feels *amazing*!)

So let's talk about ILS and the voice. Losing the voice is bad, devastating, even. How did I get mine back?

Avoiding triggers, first and foremost. I'll examine this in the next chapter.

Secondly, diet. Like I said, I believe that changing my diet constituted at least part of my voice recovery. I'll dig deeper into diet soon.

Thirdly, vocal exercises. Dr. Z encouraged me to *exercise* my voice. I couldn't really do much until the wad of mucus in my throat and postnasal drip receded. They kept my larynx so irritated that any attempt to produce sound caused me to cough. So we started small, with posture and breath work. Gradually, as my phlegm overload ebbed, I could make some sounds—*hmmms* and *bzzzes* mostly. (Is healing *ever* glamorous, I ask you? Must dignity flee with health and drag its feet in returning?) Over years, my *hmmms* and *bzzzes* have progressed to extending my dynamic speaking pitch range, examining how I use my voice in daily life, scheduling daily vocal rest, and rebuilding my singing abilities.

I'm no vocal therapist so this is where I stop. If you have ILS and lose your voice, or you are dealing with any degree of vocal chord dysfunction due to CS or CSS, I encourage you to find a reputable voice therapist and learn how s/he can help you. Mine made a world of difference. Without her I wouldn't be right here, talking to you.

The Olfactory System and Fear

CS can heighten one's sense of smell, touch, taste, sight, and/or hearing. This has to do with the sensitized nervous system. When the natural functioning balance of the nervous system is disrupted, it can have trouble managing a vast range of sensory input.[72]

A small amount of light—even from a flashlight in a dark room—can cause patients to feel distressed or confused.[73] CS patients may commonly experience a hypersensitivity to external sensory input—especially light, sound, or smell—yet few know that one's sense of smell can play an important role in inciting and perpetuating fear, and in increasing symptoms.

Out of our five senses, smell is the only one that is hard-wired with an über-fast connection to our limbic system. What's the limbic system? Good question. The limbic system is the part of the brain that controls our emotions (of which fear is one) and our survival drive. The amygdala, which I discussed earlier in relation to CS, is a key component of the limbic system. So basically, our olfactory system is not only on good terms with the part of the brain that puts us in fight or flight mode and makes us feel afraid, our noses have the amygdala on speed-dial.

The more sensitive one's olfactory system gets, the more messages of danger the amygdala receives, the more fear one experiences, the more fighty or flighty, and the more symptomatic one can become. This is not good for someone with CS. Managing how your sense of smell affects you is the first step in addressing this problem. I'll discuss this throughout the book. Here's an introduction …

What Is That *Smell*?

If your sense of smell becomes heightened, a whole world of smells—most of which you probably never wished to detect or even know existed—opens up to you. It kind of foists itself on you, actually. This new ability enables you to perceive things that about 95 percent of humans on the planet cannot detect. Do you understand the full ramifications of what I'm saying? Let me be clear: You now have a superpower.

In addition to a super sensitive sense of smell, you may find that you continue to notice smells for much longer than you used to. For example, when the olfactory system is operating properly and you walk into a room that smells like ammonia, after a few seconds or minutes, your brain tells your olfactory system, "I got it," and your smell receptors then stop sending the message about ammonia to your brain. At that point, you don't notice the ammonia odor anymore. But often with CS, the brain doesn't get the message, or the sensory receptors dealing with sense of smell ignore the brain's dampening messages and continually send alert messages to your brain, so you keep on smelling scents and odors long after a person with a normal sense of smell stops noticing them. This can be delightfully pleasurable, or nauseating, depending on what scents and odors you run into.

People rely on their sense of smell far more than they realize, for taste and sensing danger, and for general perceptions of reality. When my olfactory system first reached superpower level, I'd ask someone, "Do you smell that?" and s/he would always respond, "No," and give me a look like I was crazy. Yep, *crazy*. When enough people had given me that look, I began to wonder if I *was* in fact going insane. For the record, you are most likely not insane just because you smell something no one else can smell. You have a superpower. There aren't a lot of perks with this particular superpower—not a lot of adoring dudes (or babes), or fame or glory—so I say it a lot, "I have a superpower!" and I revel in saying it as much as I can.

You can detect things like off-gassing in malls, newly painted walls, formaldehyde in kitchen cupboards, the gag-worthy cologne that every teenage boy in town wears, wet concrete down the street, donut shops from miles away (ok, so it's not all bad).... But like any new superpower, your sense of smell can be very difficult to control, and anyone who tries to wield it may experience some intense side effects, such as the following:

- **Loss of appetite:** Distorted sense of smell can influence sense of taste, which can affect appetite. Be sure you continue eating properly, no matter what you smell. If you find you are rapidly losing or gaining weight, see your doctor.
- **Parosmia:** An over-eager sense of smell can cause olfactory confusion. For months, my brain interpreted every strong chemical "high-note" smell as urine. Floor cleaners, window cleaners, new PVC, new car smell, old lady perfume, lilies, new paint, hair spray, gasoline, natural gas and pilot lights—even sweat smelled like urine. Even *my* sweat smelled like urine. I felt like my entire world had been shoved into an NYC subway station in August. This phenomenon, of smells being perceived differently than anticipated, is officially known as the olfactory disorder parosmia. *Oh, great!* you say, *now I have an olfactory disorder?* Yep, I know, but the good news is, our olfactory systems are usually pretty adaptable and if you don't focus on your parosmia with dread, it will probably go away eventually. So, fret not. Nothing good comes of fretting.
- **The body and bodily excretions:** My nose is not as sensitive as it was a couple years ago. It still functions at a superhuman level but not on such a universal scale—more a global scale, I guess. But I still smell bodily excretions in Technicolor, and I want to address this in case you are having a problem with it. (This is not for the faint of heart. Illness can be graphic. Some might consider it a little on the disgusting side. Read at your own risk.) When my sniffer first became a super sniffer, I could smell soap residue (from unscented glycerin soap) on parts of my skin. After washing it off, I could smell just my skin. It smelled pleasant to me—it smelled like me—so it wasn't an offensive odor, but it was unsettling at first because I'd never noticed it before. As my super sniffer increased its power, I began to detect other odors coming from my body that I'd never smelled before. I'm not talking about urine, poop and sweat—those were nothing new—although they did smell different to me now, depending what I had eaten or drunk the day before.

   I'm talking about blood. Blood had always smelled kind of like rust to me. With my new superpower, my blood smelled like a steel mill. The scent was all around me during my periods, even when I used a tampon. I couldn't get away from it. I feared that anyone near could smell the blood on me, that I'd be ostracized and sent to a leper colony someplace really cold, like Tuktoyaktuk, or Pluto. (Actually, I've always wanted to visit those places, you know, just to check them out, but not as a leper.) I had the same problem with ovulatory mucus, semen, and all vaginal discharge. At first I thought something was wrong with my reproductive organs because my bodily excretions suddenly smelled so strong, but my doctor found everything normal. Good news!

The bad news was, I was hyper-aware of these odors and I didn't like them. In fact, I intensely disliked them. Can you see the problem I'm getting at?

My sensitized brain was already overreacting to potential threats, and it determined these threats, in great part, by the strength of unpleasant odors. I had to be sure not to add the scents of my skin and bodily excretions to the list. The last thing I needed was for my brain to raise alarms every time I ovulated, had sex, or had my period. I had to find a way to perceive the odors of my bodily excretions as *benign* and *acceptable* (at the very least), *friendly* and *wonderful* (at best) and above all, *not* scary, gross, or signs of trouble. How do you do that when you can't control your super sniffer and are detecting things you really don't want to smell?

This has to do with neuroplasticity, which I will discuss in detail later on, but for now, I'll give you a nutshell: I *programmed* myself. When I smelled one of the offending smells, I gave it a friendly description (like, "oh, wow, hey, that smells like *dandelions!*") and I'd smile and say something positive about it (like, "Hello, ovulation. Thanks for coming by this month. Way to go, you're right on schedule!"). It sounds hokey, I know.

The thing is, it *works*. Generally speaking, if I grin and put a benign and positive spin on these things, and I truly *believe* they are not threats, then my brain won't perceive them as threats either. If you have to know why right this instant, check out the Neuroplasticity segment. Otherwise, read on, good reader.

Review of CS and CSS Basics

- Central Sensitization (CS) describes a condition in which the central nervous system becomes sensitized and no longer perceives or processes peripheral input appropriately. There is still much to learn about CS, related syndromes, causes and treatments.
- Central Sensitivity Syndromes (CSS) are a group of disorders whose primary mechanism is CS. Symptom overlap is common among these syndromes, and many feature chronic pain. CSS can cause severe debilitation and upheaval in one's life.
- People with CS often have at least one CSS.
- Whether you have Irritable Bowel Syndrome, another CSS, or CS alone, it's important to solve enteric nervous system (aka gut) issues. Problems with the gut may exacerbate your CS or CSS symptoms.
- Chronic Fatigue Syndrome involves both physical and cognitive impairment. Multiple Chemical Sensitivities can cause headaches, nausea, hay fever, rashes and serious issues in several physiological systems. Irritable Larynx Syndrome essentially causes the muscles around the larynx to close off the airway when the sensitized brain perceives a threat.
- Those with CS may experience heightened senses. The sense of smell is closely linked to the limbic system, which processes fear and other emotions and controls our flight-or-flight response.
- Some with CS may experience olfactory-related side effects such as parosmia, abnormal appetite, and prolonged sensation of smell.
- It's important not to add benign scents to the sensitized brain's list of perceived threats.

The memory of odors is very rich.
—John Steinbeck, *East of Eden*[74]

2. Decreasing Trigger Exposure and Impact

What's a Trigger?

Whether you have CS alone, or one or more CSS, you've got triggers. In order to move from *crisis phase* to *stability phase* and beyond, you need to know how to identify your triggers and how to use the bubble to decrease trigger exposure and impact (and thus, decrease symptoms).

First off, are you clear on the term *trigger*? The clearest analogy involves a gun: when the trigger is pulled, a reaction occurs. For our purposes, a trigger is something that causes a symptom to present or flare-up. For example, for most people who have ILS, exposure to a strong scent causes (or triggers) the muscles around the larynx to tighten and restrict the airway. Therefore, a strong scent is a common ILS trigger.

Generally speaking, the stronger the trigger, the more severe and/or more lasting the symptom it provokes. Triggers have a cumulative effect as well; so the more triggers our sensitized nervous system must contend with at once, the more severe and/or prolonged the symptoms tend to be.

While some CSS have triggers of their own, all the syndromes (and CS alone) have some triggers in common. This chart can give you an idea what I mean.

COMMON TRIGGERS, LISTED BY CSS

Central Sensitivity Syndrome	*Triggers*
CFS	Over-exertion, stress/stressors, diet, hormonal flux and/or imbalance, acute illness or injury, lack of sleep
ILS	Stress/stressors, strong scents, synthetic chemicals and off-gassing of new materials, stress, diet, hormonal flux and/or imbalance, expressing strong emotions, singing, speaking, humidity/temperature changes, unidentified airborne triggers, acute illness or injury, lack of sleep
MCS	Synthetic chemicals and off-gassing of new materials, cigarette smoke, food additives/preservatives, stress/stressors, hormonal flux and/or imbalance, unidentified airborne triggers, acute illness or injury, lack of sleep
Fibromyalgia	Over-exertion, stress/stressors, diet, hormonal flux and/or imbalance, acute illness or injury, light, noise, touch, strong smells, weather/humidity or temperature changes, lack of sleep
Irritable Bowel Syndrome	Stress/stressors, diet (especially chocolate, fats and fiber), caffeine, alcohol, fizzy drinks, hormonal flux and/or imbalance, acute illness or injury, lack of sleep

Central Sensitivity Syndrome	*Triggers*
Tension-type Headaches, Migraines	Stress/stressors, exercise, diet, over-exertion, lack of sleep, caffeine, nicotine, hormonal flux and/or imbalance
Restless Legs Syndrome, Periodic Limb Movement in Sleep	Stress/stressors, exercise/over-exertion, diet, nicotine, alcohol, certain medications, caffeine, hormonal flux and/or imbalance, kidney issues, diabetes, anemia, lack of sleep
Myofascial Pain Syndrome, Regional Soft Tissue Pain Syndrome, Pelvic Pain Syndrome and related disorders	Stress/stressors, activity, over-exertion, diet, weather/extreme temperatures, nicotine, caffeine, alcohol, hormonal flux or imbalance, lack of sleep
Temporomandibular (TMJ) disorders	Stress/stressors, clenching/grinding teeth, hormonal flux or imbalance, acute illness or injury, weather/extreme temperatures, diet, nicotine, caffeine, alcohol, lack of sleep
Female Urethral Syndrome, Primary Dysmenorrhea, Interstitial Cystitis	Stress/stressors, diet, medicines/supplements, activity/over-exertion, sex, hormonal flux or imbalance, tight clothes, lack of sleep
PTSD	Stress/stressors, trauma, diet, alcohol, hormonal flux and/or imbalance, anniversaries/memories of trauma, body memories, certain smells/sights/sounds/feelings, acute illness or injury, lack of sleep

The above is not a comprehensive list, partially due to the need for more research, and also because CS manifests differently in different people. For example, you might be triggered by something not listed above or that is considered a trigger in a syndrome you don't have. That's ok. What's important is that you can identify your own triggers, which we'll do in a moment. First, we need to talk about stress and stressors—as you may have guessed from the chart above, these are powerful CS and CSS triggers.

STRESS, STRESSORS AND OTHER INTRINSIC TRIGGERS

People talk about stress daily. They say they feel "stressed" or "stressed out" to indicate an out of control and negative feeling, or "under stress" when they feel pressure to achieve or accomplish something, but what *is* stress? I like this definition: "Stress is a biological and psychological response experienced on encountering a threat that we feel we do not have the resources to deal with."[1] Stress is a *response* to perceived threats (real or not), also known as *stressors,* which can be physiological, physical, mental, and/or emotional events. If the central nervous system deems a particular stressor serious enough, our stress response will engage the amygdala and fight-or-flight mode until the threat has passed. This generally short-lived stress response is known as *acute stress* and can support us through a short-term challenge such as a job interview, kid's birthday party, or college exam. The sensitized nervous system, however, perceives both real and unreal threats and challenges as serious and overreacts to them. Thus, people with CS have more perceived stressors and a higher stress response than normal. This can lead to unnecessarily frequent and prolonged activation of fight-or-flight and, ultimately, chronic stress.

Chronic stress has been proven to cause serious health issues—such as heart disease, obesity, diabetes, depression, asthma, and gastrointestinal issues—even in folks who don't have CS. One study calls stress "an acute threat to homeostasis" (the body's natural balance of healthy functioning) and states that stress leads "to the development of a broad array of gastrointestinal disorders,"[2] which, as we learned in Chapter 1, can have a profound effect upon one's health. One study states, "Chronic stress sensitizes neural (nervous system) processes and this over-activation might lead to fatigue."[3] Another study found that chronic stress disrupts the activity of dopamine.[4] Researchers theorize that this dysfunction might be responsible for some of the cognitive impairment many CFS patients experience.[5]

There's some good news though. Studies have shown that the negative effects of stress on one's health are compounded by one's negative *perception* of stress. Dr. Kelly McGonigal, a health psychologist, lecturer at Stanford University, and leading expert on the mind-body relationship, states, "researchers estimated that over the eight years they were tracking deaths, 182,000 Americans died prematurely, not from stress, but from the belief that stress is bad for you." If you perceive stress as positive instead of negative, however, "you can change your body's response to stress."[6] Want to take a bold and immediate first step towards healing? Stop "stressing out," and instead, choose to "stress in," that is, to *in*clude stress in your life instead of resisting it. Change your perspective so you come to view stress as a necessary and positive response, a source of energy, a friend that can help you do and be all you desire.

The sensitized stress response turns normally benign stressors of all types—physiological, physical, mental, and emotional—into perceived threats. Because stressors are an unavoidable part of daily life, they can greatly impact those with CS and should be treated as significant triggers. This is why one of your primary goals is to learn to identify, manage and reduce the negative impact of stressors and stress on you. You can do this in several ways:

- using your bubble and disengaging your flight-or-flight response, both of which I'll discuss momentarily,
- mastering the coping and pacing strategies in this book, and
- making a conscious, daily choice to view stress as a positive entity, as friend not foe.

The word *intrinsic* means "belonging to the essential nature of a thing, occurring as a natural part of something."[7] I use the term *intrinsic triggers* to indicate stress and certain stressors because we cannot avoid these types of triggers the way we can avoid exposure to *environmental* triggers such as synthetic chemicals or fragrances, or new materials. Several intrinsic triggers impact those with CS through things necessary for survival, such as hormones, food, or our own stress response. We cannot avoid these things, so we seek to manage them as best we can. Here are the most common intrinsic CS triggers:

- hormone fluctuation and/or imbalance (physiological stressors)
- diet (a physiological stressor)
- onset of, or increase in symptoms (yep, some symptoms can trigger other symptoms and thus can be considered physiological stressors)
- onset of an acute illness or injury (physiological and physical stressor)
- behaviors, physical activities/exertion (physical stressors)
- emotions and thoughts (emotional and cognitive stressors)

We'll talk more about these in the upcoming segments, as I discuss how to identify, contend with, and manage triggers.

Identifying Your Triggers

You might find it difficult to pinpoint your triggers at first, and if they seem to shift over time, or on any given day, it's probably not your imagination. One day you walk into the kitchen while the dishwasher is on, and your ILS is triggered by the humidity in that room. Another day you walk into the kitchen while the dishwasher is on, and you feel barely a tickle in your throat. What's the difference? Environmental and intrinsic trigger load (i.e., the cumulative impact of your stress response, all stressors, and any other intrinsic triggers combined with the cumulative intensity, frequency and duration of exposure to any environmental triggers). Trigger load versus the body's natural adaptive abilities and defenses equals fluctuating symptoms and triggers.

What I mean by cumulative is this: if you are exposed to, or impacted by a single trigger in the morning, when you have had no other trigger exposure/impact yet, you'll have a lesser reaction than if you are exposed to that same trigger one afternoon, after a triggerful (that is, full of triggers) morning.

Trigger overlap among CSS can make identifying triggers more of a conundrum. Some of my ILS triggers overlap with my Asthma and/or MCS triggers, an MCS or asthma episode will often trigger an ILS episode, and vice versa. So my triggers for all three conditions are inseparable in that sense. Please bear that in mind when checking out the following table of my most consistent triggers and then creating your own.

Wait, did I just say *creating your own*? Yep. It's the first step towards managing your triggers. Create your own table and use it daily to pinpoint which triggers are affecting you at a specific time. The more accurately you identify your triggers, the more easily you can manage them. Table 1 will give you an idea what you're shooting for.

TABLE 1
MY MOST CONSISTENT TRIGGERS

My Asthma Triggers	*My ILS Triggers*	*My MCS Triggers*	*My CFS Triggers*
Dust, drywall dust, concrete dust			
Dust, drywall dust, concrete dust			
Wet cement or concrete, freshly cut wood	Wet cement or concrete, freshly cut wood		
Air conditioning	Air conditioning		
Hot humid air	Hot humid air		
Scented dish detergent, soaps, laundry detergent and fabric softeners and personal products	Scented dish detergent, soaps, laundry detergent and fabric softeners and personal products	Scented dish detergent, soaps, laundry detergent and fabric softeners and personal products	
Paints, sealants, glues, varnish, chemical cleaners, bleach	Paints, sealants, glues, varnish, chemical cleaners, bleach	Paints, sealants, glues, varnish, chemical cleaners, bleach	
Formaldehyde, MDF, particleboard, PVC, melamine, cupboards, bookshelves, bookcases	Formaldehyde, MDF, particleboard, PVC, melamine, cupboards, bookshelves, bookcases	Formaldehyde, MDF, particleboard, PVC, melamine, cupboards, bookshelves, bookcases	
	Exhaust from gas and diesel	Exhaust from gas and diesel	
	New car smell	New car smell	

My Asthma Triggers	My ILS Triggers	My MCS Triggers	My CFS Triggers
	New carpets, laminate floors, drapes, furniture, vinyl decals, dyed fabrics	New carpets, laminate floors, drapes, furniture, vinyl decals, dyed fabrics	
Old carpets, mildew, mold, damp	Old carpets, mildew, mold, damp		
Old books, newspapers, magazines	New books, newspapers, magazines	New books, newspapers, magazines	
	New DVD and CD cases	New DVD and CD cases	
	Drug stores, grocery stores, malls, parking garages, most public spaces, most people's homes	Drug stores, grocery stores, malls, parking garages, most public spaces, most people's homes	
	Perfume, cologne, hair spray, fabric softened clothing, clothing washed in scented detergent	Perfume, cologne, hair spray, fabric softened clothing, clothing washed in scented detergent	
Lots of pollen in the air	Fertilizer, pesticides, bug spray, lots of pollen in the air	Fertilizer, pesticides, bug spray	
	Eating, laughing, crying, speaking, shouting, speaking for more than a few minutes at a time*		
ILS or MCS episodes*	Asthma or MCS episodes*	ILS or Asthma episodes*	ILS, MCS, or Asthma episodes*
Smoke from a wood fire, a charcoal bbq	Smoke from a wood fire, a charcoal bbq, a propane bbq, singed cookies on a baking sheet, (singed anything, really)	A charcoal bbq, a propane bbq	
Cigarette smoke, fresh or in someone's clothing, hair, skin, walls	Cigarette smoke, fresh or in someone's clothing, hair, skin, walls	Cigarette smoke, fresh or in someone's clothing, hair, skin, walls	
Chlorinated swimming pools	Chlorinated swimming pools		
Scary, emotional or stressful situations*	Scary, emotional or stressful situations*	Scary, emotional or stressful situations*	Scary, emotional or stressful situations*
Hormones*	Hormones*	Hormones*	Hormones*
Poor sleep*	Poor sleep*	Poor sleep*	Poor sleep*
	Acute Illness or Injury*	Acute Illness or Injury*	Acute Illness or Injury*
Fatigue, over-exertion*	Fatigue, over-exertion*	Fatigue, over-exertion*	Fatigue, over-exertion*
	Certain chemicals I haven't pinpointed that are used in some unscented products	Certain chemicals I haven't pinpointed that are used in some unscented products	Exercise/HR over 60% of max
	Certain foods/dietary issues*	Certain foods/ dietary issues*	Certain foods/ dietary issues*

*Intrinsic triggers.

This list is as complete as I can make it right now. Until I find a cure for CS, CSS, and Asthma, it will never be finished, I suppose, because new synthetic products are being developed every day, and because of the fluid nature of CS and CSS. The best thing

I know to do is to control what I can control, and normalize what can be normalized, which means managing the impact of intrinsic triggers, and reducing my exposure to known environmental triggers. Then, all that's left is to manage each unavoidable trigger as best I can when it occurs. But I'll get to that. First, "getting clear."

Getting Clear(er)

"Getting clear" is a term I often came across in my research about MCS. Generally, it requires moving for an undetermined amount of time to a trigger-free haven out in the middle of nowhere. The way I see it, "getting clear" is different from reducing exposure to environmental triggers. Both are about avoiding triggers, which is important because the way CS works is, the more you trigger your sensitized central nervous system, the more your body will react. If you give your central nervous system some trigger-free time, it will have a chance to catch its breath, so to speak, and thus become less reactive. That's the theory. From my experience, it's true enough. When I spend time inside my bubble, my symptoms decrease. We'll talk more about the bubble in a minute. The distinction I want to make here is this: there's reducing exposure to, or impact of triggers, which is not an all-or-nothing deal, and then there's "getting clear."

The remote havens I mentioned above are strictly controlled communities, with a fragrance-free lifestyle and synthetic chemical-free buildings, clothing, furniture—so, essentially environmental-trigger-free—inhabited by people who wouldn't look at me like I was nuts every time I ran into a trigger and succumbed to symptoms. They would understand because they had triggers and symptoms too. Life there would be like living in a big bubble, sealed off from the rest of the synthetic-chemically-saturated world. That lifestyle and environment seemed like it would be heaven for anyone with CS contending with environmental triggers, and if I could have gone to one at the height of my health crisis, I most certainly would have.

I was single, though, with a mortgage. I had undiagnosed medical issues and steadily declining health, and the specialists covered by my medical insurance were in the city. I couldn't work, was living off my savings and didn't have much left, and my battle with workers compensation was starting to look like it would become the next hundred years' war. So, there were several financial and medical reasons for me to remain where I was.

There was also something gnawing at me, a doubt about the concept of "getting clear." When I first got diagnosed, a specialist told me that most people with my conditions ended up "living like a recluse in a bubble" for the rest of their lives, isolated from the rest of the world. I decided that would not be me. A bubble for stability and refuge, for sure, but not for *ever*. I couldn't help wondering, if I went to live in the big bubble community in the high desert and my body got used to an environmental-trigger-free world, would I ever be able to return to my normal urban life, or even a rural one? I'd read that people had "re-set" their central nervous system by getting clear in those places, and then they no longer had any CSS or CS. Myth or fact? Maybe fact, for those individuals, but CS and CSS were different for everyone, so could I even permanently "re-set" my system? At that point, I didn't know.

I did know something, though:

- CS and CSS manifest in different people in different ways, and responses to treatments, too, vary.

- The longer one has CS, with or without CSS, the more efficiently the brain reacts to triggers.
- Our brains have the ability to be "re-wired" to *not* react to triggers. (Go with me on this for now. I'll explain in the Neuroplasticity segment later on.)

Based on those facts, it seemed to me that maybe I *could* get clear of environmental triggers in a remote bubble community, and could manage my intrinsic ones enough to significantly reduce my symptoms. That said, I doubted that I'd be able to maintain that level of "desensitization" when I returned to the environmental triggers of urban life. It seemed to me that if my brain connected urban life with "unsafe" and remote bubble community life with "safe," it didn't matter if I re-set my central nervous system in some far off bubble or not. What I needed to do was find a way to manage, and teach my sensitized brain that it was safe to live and breathe in the city, or on a farm, or wherever I happened to be in the world. I mean, wasn't going someplace to "get clear" about the same as wearing a mask 24/7 that blocked out all environmental triggers? I knew some people did that. I suspected I was lucky that I could manage without having to wear a mask. Still, from all I'd learned about the olfactory system's amazing adaptive abilities, it seemed that complete reliance on masks would have a nasty longer-term side effect of heightening the sensitivity of my olfactory system, making me even more sensitive to scents and odors when I tried to take the mask off.

Like any theory, it would have to be tested. And I, unable to leave the city, was the perfect guinea pig. If I can't go to the bubble, I figured, bring the bubble to me!

Shelter Me

Before I got sick, home always meant permanence to me, permanence outside of me. Like the Rocky Mountains in Colorado, like the waving wheat in Oklahoma, like slippers made of rubies. An oft-touring singer-songwriter, I believed that wherever I hung my guitar or lay my head was home. It took months to learn the truth.

* * *

May. I am awakened by an echoing clank followed by a deep hum. Is the building shaking? Impossible. The 20-story concrete tower was built over half a century ago, the kind of chunky stalwart that even a tornado couldn't bully into a tremble. We don't get tornadoes in Vancouver anyway.

Clank! Hummmm ...

My limbs feel like lead and my brain thumps against my skull like I've just returned from a lost weekend in a poppy field. I roll off the mattress onto the carpeted floor. One of the benefits of having to sell your bedroom furniture, I tell myself, is that you can roll from mattress to living room if necessary. I almost chuckle as I coax my body vertical with the aid of the doorframe.

More clanging, and the hum by now has become a constant. The living room looks the same as I left it the night before, the same since I evacuated my home and moved here five months ago, actually—boxes of books lining the far wall, glass dining table serving as a desk piled with legal papers and bills, and a modern magenta chaise in the middle of the empty space, facing the windows. The vast living and dining areas, with walls in need of a fill and paint and stained carpet clamoring for a steam clean, hold no other furniture. The space is neglected, empty, waiting for something to change but powerless to change anything itself. A lot like me.

Here on the eighth floor, nothing short of an eclipse or a cloud derby can interfere with my morning sun, and yet, the light is flickering on the carpet—disappearing, reappearing. I look out the window, expecting the vasty expanse of English Bay half a block away, but instead I see a kid in a sweatshirt, jeans, and steel-toed boots hovering like a bad fairy at my balcony railing. His fist waves a tube of steel about like a magic wand, then releases it onto my balcony. *Clang!* The hum hums as his motorized stage lowers him down to the ground again. I blink. That was not a kid. Ever since I turned 40, anyone younger than 25 looks 17 to me. He's probably around 20. And he is piling scaffolding on my balcony. Scaffolding. That's what they use for painting and renovations.

With trembling fingers, I dial the building manager's office. "Hi, I'm in 801 and want to know... I see, a major balconies renovation... Eight weeks or more? And what will it entail?" Concrete dust, demolition, paint, sanding—you name it—right outside my window. I hang up, dread grating on my nerves like a belt sander. I grab my laptop and fall back onto the chaise. I have no choice; I'll have to break the lease.

After being exposed to unsafe levels of VOCs and particulates a year ago at my office administration job, I have had to live in a virtual bubble, avoiding irritants such as perfumes, fabric softeners, exhaust, dust, paint, smoke, formaldehyde—an endless list. My own home, a cozy ground floor studio apartment in an older wood building, had become unmanageable, primarily due to a damp parking garage, chain-smoking neighbors, and perfumes and chemical cleaners galore in the common spaces. Even some of my furniture was off-gassing and had to be sold. It wasn't the first big loss I'd experienced. Heck, in the past year, I'd lost my health, my job, my ability to sing, friends I'd thought cared about me, and now, this rental apartment.

I remind myself that this high and dry suite and the sea air have done my lungs good, that five months is better than nothing, but I can feel my illusion of permanence being chipped away. A friend of mine used to say, "You can't go back to Kansas," and now I think I'm beginning to understand his meaning. Nothing is certain—income, health, home—and the new realization fills me with a kind of terror.

My mind creates a list of move-out tasks. Everything is a list these days. First I email Uncle Bob and ask when he can bring a truck and a team. Uncle Bob is a six-foot-tall baby boomer with a beer belly and a foot-long greying goatee who owns a local moving company. He hires young Lollipop Guild rejects, teaches them job skills, work ethics, and builds their confidence. He gives me confidence too, knows every storage place in town, and won't rip me off.

"Ask if he has a 'Frequent Mover' card that will give me my third move free," I tell myself.

Still, it will cost me a few hundred. I have no income and have yet to see any money from workers compensation, but I commit to the expenditure without resistance. Spend the money, get out of here, I tell myself. It's another living accommodation. Can't be helped, don't worry about it. Last year I clung to everything I thought I had—job, home, savings, friends—and fought desperately to keep them, only to lose them eventually. I can't say this kind of decision is ever easy, but it does seem like the more I lose, the less resistance I muster when I have to let the remaining things go.

My email notice blips. Uncle Bob will come on Thursday. What's next? I rub my eyes and wish for a fairy godmother to do everything for me in an instant.

Scaffolding and supplies—cabling, jackhammers, pounders, sanders, adhesives—launch over my balcony's railing and land on the concrete floor with thuds, clanks, and shudders, while I lie on my chaise, eyes scouring Craigslist for a new home. It's early in the month, so not a lot is available, and even less with my specific health and financial needs. I can't commit to another lease, I have no proof of employment, and I am living off savings, which means I need low rent. When I was young I used to play competitive softball and subbed in often to pinch-hit, but in Vancouver's rental market, I've got three strikes on me before I step into the batter's box. At least I don't have a little dog too. Most places don't allow pets.

A keen feeling of displacement settles over me like a scratchy, wool blanket, and a dusty moth of a thought flits from the blanket into my mind: If my chemical sensitivities turn out to be permanent, I might have to keep moving for the rest of my life. All buildings need to be repaired some time, especially with the way they build stuff in Vancouver. It all comes down to the same issues: breathing, safety, and stability. It's beginning to feel like there is no home anywhere anymore. There is no safety. No respite, no solace. There is only the fight to breathe, the fight that never stops, no matter how tired I get.

Anxious questions swarm me like starved mosquitoes. How much money do I have left to live off? When will workers compensation make their decision? My medical team—acupuncturist, psychiatrist, vocal therapist, occupational health specialist, the specialists I am waiting months to see—all work here in Vancouver, one of the most expensive cities in the world. Can I leave town? And go where? Why did I pick this apartment of all places? I should've known better. What if I get worse? I'm only 43—what if I am never able to work again—?

Don't ask that.

I scan the ads... An artist retreat in Atlin, a little town in Northern British Columbia by a huge, pristine lake looks nice. Maybe I should move there to save money. Or maybe go west to one of the Gulf Islands? Maybe, maybe... I bookmark the ads of places I think might work, send out email queries, and close my eyes. As I drift off, another thought flits into my mind and darts about: Thrust into this new nomadic existence, maybe I should think differently about home, about holding some home within me somehow, and stop thinking of home as a place outside of myself.

* * *

June. For the past month, I have been living in an illegal bachelor suite tacked onto the back of a two-story house that the owners, a nice couple in their mid–30s, have renovated over the past few years.

On moving day, Uncle Bob's team tucked everything but some clothes, books, and my guitar into storage. "That other place didn't work out, eh?" Uncle Bob asked.

I shook my head.

"This one looks homey." He shrugged as if one place was the same as any other.

"Sure." I shrugged too, waved goodbye, and shut the door.

The place is furnished with a bed, loveseat, TV and DVD player, kitchenette with a mini-fridge and a two-burner hotplate. There's a full washroom and a closet. Hand-me-down furniture. Nothing matches. Normally I don't care about matching, but this place leaves me feeling bereft. The loveseat is striped blue, fluorescent green and orange, and the tv is one of the old tubular kind. Its back end takes up half the apartment. It's the best I could find, all things considered. Though I fill myself daily with gratitude for what I have, I know this is not a home.

Good people with a major incompatibility, my landlords are compulsive project-doers. This goes beyond house-proud into the realm of obsession. On weekdays, weekends, anytime from 7 a.m. to 10 p.m., I endure sawing, drilling, sanding and/or hammering coming from the shed eight feet from my windows. Sometimes they work in the garden beside the shed, or they hammer or drill inside their house, a wall away. The noise comes right on through. Radio on in the shed. Electric guitar wanking in the house. Constant noise. This is not the quiet bachelor suite as advertised. It's like living next door to Wile E Coyote as he compulsively saws, hammers, welds, and detonates things that go *BOOM!*

Before I moved in, the landlords and I had a conversation about my chemical sensitivities. They were not unsympathetic and even postponed some larger projects out of respect for my health. I think we have all been surprised to discover the chasm between our understandings of acceptable noise levels and work hours. A flying monkey swoops into my mind and drops a thought bomb: Why do I always pick bad places to live? Why am I so bad at taking care of myself—

Don't say that.

I swat it away.

I'm also discovering that the more noise I'm exposed to, the more heightened my sensitivities become. This morning, the hammering started at 9 a.m. and it's almost noon. I tell myself I'm safe, the noise won't hurt me, but every hammer blow makes me start like a deer in a lion-filled glade.

Movies help pass the time and mask the noise. I flee to the library to get one. Driving away from the din, my nerves sizzle and hiss like a fritzed toaster cord. The sun shines a warm welcome, and I try to focus on that. The people I pass saunter about in shorts and t-shirts, while I shiver in my sweatshirt and thick scarf. One day, I tell myself, I will be dressed for summer like everyone else, not bundled up like an invalid.

I score free parking two blocks away and walk at the pace of someone twice my age towards the library, testing the air, holding my breath past freshly cut lawn, a lawnmower chugging diesel, a cigarette-toting dog walker, a toddler in fabric-softened clothes... Where is my mind in all this? A dim haze surrounding objectives of safety and DVD attainment. No poetry, no philosophy, melodies or lyrics—they have become the stuff of extravagance.

I've always felt at home in libraries, their easy silence, their timeless days, their reverent shelves displaying tomes that contain other worlds for me to discover. I used to walk up and down the aisles, browsing, sitting on the dusty floor, thumbing through pages, sampling universes. I'd lose track of time and place, and whisper-chat to anyone who ventured into the aisle. Things are different now. Papers, inks, dusts, personal fragrances—so many triggers for my nervous system and lungs. No loitering here, no socializing. Get in, get out.

I'm scanning dvd titles when a woman surrounded by a Pigpen-like cloud of perfume approaches. I breathe through my scarf and move to the unoccupied DVD row. I can read the print, but my brain isn't registering anything. It's things like this that make me wonder if I've developed some kind of chronic fatigue, but with three more months to wait before I can see a specialist, I dismiss the thought. Wondering only leads to more exhaustion.

I try to prompt myself—What looks interesting? What haven't you seen yet?—like I'm talking to a second-grader who would rather be out playing ball than in the library. My eyes feel hot and vision blurs. I go to the computer in the corner and cling to the counter, breathing deep. My peripherals follow the perfume woman and scout for other potential threats. The rest of me is in stasis. Rest. Calm. Breathe. I type into the computer the name of some of my favorite actresses, get a couple film titles, and write them down. The perfume woman leaves the area. I try to match the dvd titles with those on the paper in my hand. All seemed to be checked out. *Bridesmaids* is in. I've seen it before but I take it and go.

The fatigue is pulling at my body now, as if someone has turned up the gravity dial on Earth. I give myself simple commands, like to a droid. Find a self-checkout stall with no one nearby, hold my breath when the perfumey woman steps up to the stall next to mine, finish checking out and exit, into the sun. Exhale hugely, inhale cautiously. Sit on the upwindmost bench in the area. Breathing. Sitting in the sun. Breathing. Sitting. This is the rhythm of my life right now.

Someone sits on the next bench over, a woman who understands allure. She wears her fragrance subtly, but I'm already overexposed today, so her delicate bouquet drifts upwind and scratches at my throat like a cat at a new sofa. Walk two blocks to the car, I tell myself, and sit inside until your body stops feeling like it's elsewhere. Drive back to your shelter. Ignore the hammering. Sit on the couch. I do, DVD in hand, and stare blankly at the wall. I'm not sure for how long. A sweet hummingbird thought darts in: If the library was once home, then home is not about where you hang your guitar or rest your head. It's more about where you feel like yourself, where you feel connected, perhaps... The thought flits into fog.

After a while, I feel cold. I wrap up in a blanket and drink some water. Then I put on the movie, crank the volume enough to mask the hammering, and lie back on the couch. Everything is a to-do list, and the list never ends. I think I believe that if I do everything on the list, I'll get my life back, or at least find a home. I do as I'm told. I do all I can, I tell myself, I do good. Fall asleep within minutes, a dim reminder in the back of my head to check the apartment listings in Craigslist when I wake.

* * *

July. If you don't take care of your body, where will you live? Qi Gong guru Lee Holden asks that question every time I do this meditation with his *Health & Healing* DVD. I lean back against the striped couch and adjust my lotus position. I cycle my breath. The answer is Nowhere. My legs itch where they meet the industrial grade carpet. I dismiss the sensation and cycle my breath. My body doesn't act or react like it used to. Instead of warning me of dangerous odors, it over-reacts to every little scent. And things that once energized me now drain, like when I try running and end up on the couch for days, limbs too heavy to lift. I feel detached and un-alive.

To me, alive means being able to create, to sing, to manifest ideas. Full of exhaustion, sitting and doing nothing for most of every day, with a condition that strictly limits access to my creative energy and prohibits singing or even speaking loudly, I feel like I'm lying in my open grave, waiting for Death to take me, or at least for someone to dump some dirt on me. I'd love to chat with Descartes about this, actually. I create, therefore I am. Who am I if I cannot create? It is like asking what I am if I cannot sing. Why did I get an illness that strips me of my essential self? Do all illnesses do this? I try to think about this through several breath cycles but the thought disperses into the tulle fog inside my brain and I lose track.

I've been ill long enough to know that the worst thing about my illness changes with time. Three months ago, for example, the worst thing was losing my ability to run. Seven months ago, the worst thing was losing my home. Nine months, my job. At this stage, the worst thing about illness is losing my connection to ecstasy. Singing, creation, these are not things I used to do as much as they were states of being through which I connected to the world.

Too esoteric? Okay, well, how about quantum physics, which says every thing in the universe is energy? From there, assume every person connects to the electricity grid of life somehow, by doing whatever it is that makes them feel alive. It could be trading on Wall Street or riding a luge or slinging arrows. When they do their thing, people are tapping into the energy of the universe and are flooded with vitality, joy, and ecstasy. Their body no longer constrains their spirit somehow. Not like astral projection … more like what the fictional dancer Billy Elliot says—when he's dancing, he feels *electric*. That's how I felt when I could sing, and run, and write. Like I was connecting to some universal energy, channeling energy through me, feeling the vibration in my bones. I'd get high off it and feel alive through it. I felt like I belonged then, like I was home. Now, I am like a short circuit on a stereo system, isolated and numb in the resulting silence.

I cycle my breath, let the thoughts come and go. Adjust my lotus again. Lee Holden teaches that by practicing Qi Gong daily, we can re-connect to our bodies through breath and find where we live. Ecstasy before the mundane, he says, leading my breath. I imagine a golden path and, with a hungry spark of hope in my core, I follow.

* * *

August. I found an apartment today that I think might work. It is in a 50s-era terraced building on the mountainside. The property owners don't require a lease. They don't require proof of employment. They ask for five months' stay at least. That's all I have money left for, so that works out.

"I have some questions, uh—they might seem a little weird," I say, "because of my chemical sensitivities." The office reeks of some gelatinous air freshener, like wilted lilacs and Lysol combined. My throat is tightening involuntarily. I'm sitting by the open door, breathing through my scarf and turning my head to inhale from the doorway. Ruth, the building manager, sits across her desk from me. She's small, with a grey pixie cut, and she doesn't look harried like most property managers do. In fact, she has a Buddha-like unflappability about her. I cycle my breath. It's almost a reflex now, to breathe deep, to feel the breath flood me with energy.

"The complex is non-smoking," Ruth says. "What else?" She smiles at me from across her desk, on top of which lies a rental agreement for me to sign. I look at it warily, and then scan the checklist I clutch in my hands.

"Are you planning any building repairs or renovations projects for the next year?" I say.

She shakes her head. "We did balconies two years ago, roof and paint are fine."

"Great." I went down my list. We'd checked the laundry facilities, which consisted of a small room with only two washers and two dryers. I could monopolize them each time I did laundry and thus escape all but the residual fabric softener and detergent fumes. Not ideal, but better than most, and workable. "May I have an assigned parking spot outdoors rather than in the parking garage?" She nods. "When was the laminate flooring installed in the suite? And when was the interior last painted?"

"Flooring two years, paint one year."

Good. That explained why I had detected no off-gassing in the suite. "And you are agreeable to removing the blinds and not painting when the current tenant moves out?" She nods. "The holes in the walls can't even be filled," I say. "I know it sounds weird but that hole filler stuff is really bad for breathing."

"No problem," she says. "I understand."

I doubt that she does, but I like her presence, which is almost serene. I glance at the rental agreement on the desk and go through my whole checklist one more time in my head. The apartment building has exterior corridors and faces south so, even though it's a bachelor suite, it will get sun. If I have to move in a hurry, the penalty for leaving before five months is $200 rather than the full month's rent that other places charge for breaking an agreement. It's the best I've seen since having to leave my home eight months ago.

Time to make a decision. I inhale against resistance—it quivers in my chest—and all I see for a moment are my recent apartment fails. I remind myself I've evaluated all the information I have on hand and can only make a decision based on that. That's all anyone can do, I tell myself. Breathe. I do. I feel the chair under me, solid and strong. I imagine I am the same. What's the worst thing that can happen? I die of asphyxiation from a painter gone postal who breaks into my apartment and flings paint everywhere?—not likely—or some emergency repair comes up, and I move again.

Hard to take a risk when I'm scraping the bottom of the faith barrel. It seems like every time I start to believe in permanence, or certainty, Fate knocks it out of my hands and crunches it beneath her knee-high Doc Marten boots, cackling like the Wicked Witch of the West. Does everyone have that experience? We dream, we believe, we become disillusioned. I guess the choice is, do we allow ourselves to dream again, or do we remain disillusioned forever?

I take a breath and picture myself living in that apartment—my books in the bookcase, my pillows and quilt on my mattress, the smells of soup that I make from scratch wafting from the kitchen, a *Carpenters* song on the stereo, chestnuts by the humble fire—

Don't.

Is this home? Could it become home? I shake my head and take a breath.

There is something primal about home. It vibrates in your gut like a song. Home is permanent, sure, indestructible, yes, but it is *within* me. And any shelter I occupy is made to feel more comfortable, more nurturing and safe, more home-like, by what I bring to it from within me. Not the other way around.

I take a breath, feel it fan the flames of hope at the hearth I have not lost. What I need is a place to live, and this apartment best suits my needs. For now. I click my heels three times, sign the agreement, and begin making a list of move-in tasks.

Building Your Bubble

Before I go into all things bubble-related, I need to make this blanket statement: If you have CS, you need a bubble. Even if you don't have a CSS, or any environmental triggers, you need a bubble. Why? Because even without environmental triggers, you still have intrinsic ones, and the bubble helps to reduce the impact of some of them and to restore balance to your nervous system.

In crisis phase (when my conditions were consistently worsening and death seemed not only imminent but inescapable), the most important step towards stability was finding a safe place, a place where I could breathe and rest. A place with virtually no triggers. A trigger-free place. This was harder than it sounds.

Why? you ask, *I mean, aren't there scent-free offices and buildings? How hard can it be?* Good questions. Let's start with terminology.

A scent is a common trigger for those with MCS, ILS, and other CSS, right? Right. But a "scent-free" or "fragrance-free" policy at an office or hospital merely seeks (and rarely succeeds) to eliminate *one* kind of environmental trigger: synthetic fragrances. All the other environmental triggers remain in that space. Plus, folks with CS have intrinsic triggers wherever they go. Therefore, "scent-free" or "fragrance-free" does NOT equal "trigger-free." What you want is a *trigger-free* bubble, and this can be challenging.

Rental apartments or houses have new paint or carpet, or dust or mildew, they want a year's lease and a tenant with a job, and the more affordable rentals have a shared laundry room somewhere in the building that is chock full of detergent, bleach, and fabric softener fumes—known lung irritants and very resilient, smelly stuff. There are other issues, like building repairs, cigarette smoke from neighbors, noisy or aggressive neighbors—lots of stressors and irritants I never considered until my overtaxed nervous system could no longer endure them.

My goal was to "get clear *enough*." That is, not "live-forever-in-a-remote-bubble" clear, but as clear as possible in the urban setting so that I could decrease my symptoms and central nervous system reactivity over time. To begin, I needed a bubble of my very own. My studio apartment was the logical place, and the first step was to get rid of anything inside it that triggered a CSS.

- **Moveable furniture:** If it triggered me, it left the building: anything containing particleboard, melamine, glues, lacquers, PVC, ABS plastic, new vinyl, and certain foams and/or fillers, some fabrics and dyes. I replaced necessary pieces with unstained wood. Even the strong scent of new pine triggered my ILS, so I bought used pieces. (Craigslist was a godsend, although the aesthetic left something to be desired. I promised myself that when I reached *stability phase,* I could take my time in finding nicer stuff. In *crisis phase*, I had bigger problems to focus on.) I made sure the pieces I got were screw-together or pegged, not glued, or steel and glass.

  When buying used furniture, I always start by asking if the furniture was in a smoke-free environment, a pet-free environment, and how old it is. If it's new, I don't buy it, no matter what it is, unless I want to put it outside for an undetermined amount of time to off-gas before I can use it. I think function over form as much as possible. I think of the furniture as a tool for me. Did my bubble look fabulous? No. But everything had a place, and I had a safe bubble, and that was the goal.

- **Fixed furniture:** Some kitchen cupboards were off-gassing formaldehyde and whatever else, so I kept their doors closed. I could still smell the formaldehyde even then, so I pinned a sheet around the cupboards, and washed the sheet whenever the odour seeped through the material. I put a used pine shelving unit in the hall outside the kitchen to hold my dishes and kitchen stuff.

- **Cleaners:** I disposed of all cleaners that triggered me, got a vacuum with HEPA filter for the hardwood floor, and started cleaning with vinegar and baking soda.

- **Bath products:** I cleared my space of scented shampoos and hygiene products, colognes and perfumes, nail polish, shaving cream, etc. I replaced all bath products with unscented glycerin or olive oil soaps until I was out of *crisis phase.* I used olive oil for lotion.

- **Laundry products:** I'd never used fabric softeners, and avoided them like the plague once I got sick. I encourage you to research these products. They are toxic, even to folks without CS or Asthma. Scented detergents as well. Even some of the ones that say "no added fragrance" have triggering stuff in them. I began using only "free and clear" detergent. Laundry products are made to get into the weave of your clothes and linens and stick there, so they smell like that product for days, or longer. Think about what that kind of invasive, long-lasting chemical product does to your skin, respiratory system, and nervous system. Again, if you are resistant to dropping scented laundry products, do the research.

- **Clothing and allergens:** My pillows and comforters were down, which is allergenic for lots of folks. When I got CS, I started to react to down, so I got hypoallergenic instead. I didn't have a down winter jacket, thankfully, but my old wool sweaters and socks started to irritate my nose and skin, so I boxed them up, hoping I could wear them again when I reached my *stability phase.* (I can wear them now, most days, with no issues.)

- **Pets:** I don't have pet allergies, but after I got CS, wet dog smell and some dog dander became problematic. Scented dog poop bags and flea collars also trigger me. More frequent pet washings (with unscented shampoo) and home vacuumings (with a HEPA-filtered vacuum), along with unscented poop bags helped minimize those triggers. The dog had to be trained to sleep in a different room on a material that was easy for me to vacuum or throw into the wash. Pets are a joy and joy is healing. Adjustments to keep them are worth it, thousand-fold. I was able to find very manageable accommodations that allowed me to keep my pet in my bubble. As a backup plan, though, I found someone who agreed to give my pet a foster home until I could reach a point in my recovery when I could welcome her home again. I didn't need this plan, turns out, but CS and CSS can be unpredictable, and I found it helpful to have a backup plan in place for my pet.

- **People:** I lived alone until I could no longer afford it, and then I rented a room in someone's home for the better part of a year. What a challenge! All inhabitants of the living space need to commit to a lifestyle change to support the one who has CS. They need to dispose of their own triggering products and refrain from painting, doing renos, and bringing new products and other triggers into the environment. Don't be afraid to talk with them about this. Be direct. Bring a list of triggering products for them to refer to. You are worth it. And you'll be surprised how good it feels to ask for their support and get it. (More on asking for help coming soon.)

- **HVAC, Allergens, and Neighbors:** Forced air heat or air conditioning vents are problematic for me, as dust can collect in ducts and then be blown into the air. Even without dust, cold or hot air blowing on me sometimes triggers a reaction. Living in an apartment or flat that is connected by HVAC ducts to other apartments or flats in the building allows allergens such as pet dander, cigarette smoke, fragrances and cleaning chemical fumes to waft into my bubble via the ducts.

  It's difficult to control such things. One solution is to ask a friend to tape off the vents using plastic bags and duct tape. Of course, the bags and tape may smell enough to trigger you, so you may have to get creative. I find that only white plastic grocery bags trigger me—I know not why—but clear ones don't. Saran wrap can work if doubled up. When I had the tape installed on the inside of the vents rather than on the side that was in my bubble, it didn't trigger me.

  Cutting off ventilation can cause temperature or air quality problems. You may need to use a radiant space heater or an air filter (if you can't buy one used, get it at least three months before you need it and store it somewhere away from you to off-gas. Better yet, have a friend use it in their relatively trigger-free home—no smoke or scented laundry detergents there, especially.) I prefer to keep a window open, provided that this doesn't invite triggers from a neighbor smoking outdoors, or a nearby garden or laundry vent.

- **Environment around the apartment:** As my sensitivities increased, I found I was being triggered by smells of damp soil and decomposing leaves in my patio garden—I could smell them through the glass windows and sliding door! My chain-smoking next-door neighbour's cigarette smoke, too, permeated that barrier. My apartment front door opened into the building's lobby, which meant that as my olfactory sense became more attuned and my reactions more severe, I could smell and was being triggered by fragrances worn by people passing through the lobby, newspapers and journals stacked in the lobby, and chemical cleaners used on the floor tiles.

Eventually I had to evacuate that apartment. Financially unable to leave it vacant, and believing I'd be able to return one day, I rented it out. The rental market at that time was saturated, and I lost money on it monthly—the first of many financial losses I incurred due to CS and CSS.

I found a drier place with radiant heat on the eighth floor, high enough off the ground that garden-based irritants didn't trigger me most days. It was located half a block from the sea, so I got fresh air off the water, which made breathing in general much easier. Was it perfect? No. I still got occasional fumes from a smoking neighbor somewhere nearby, and if the wind blew just right, I could smell the fabric softener exhaust from the laundry room eight stories below. But that was rare, maybe one day a month. I breathed better there, because I had reduced the amount of environmental triggers I came into contact with, and that was the whole point. I stayed there for five months, until I awoke one morning to find a crew starting balcony renovations right outside my window. We're talking jackhammers, concrete dust, paint, sanding, stucco—the whole deal. I needed a new bubble in a hurry.

Unforeseen Triggers That Can Pop Your Bubble

I've had to move nine times in the past three years because of environmental triggers in my household. Some were obvious, but countless unseen and unexpected popped my bubble time and again: PVC in-floor heating pipes off-gassing under floor tiles, the apartment across the hall suddenly embarking upon a renovation, smokers hanging out beneath my window or moving in next door, diesel trucks idling in the loading zone upwind of my windows, laundry fumes venting near my windows, or into the building's ventilation system and filling the hallways, the tenant downstairs who paints her ceiling with Killz … the list goes on. If I had a bunch of money, I could have bought or rented a fairly isolated house anywhere as a work around, but I was limited by my limited funds, so I took the hard road to getting clearer. What I learned is that bubble building is a process and my ideas about it must remain fluid, like everything else with CS and CSS. I make my bubble as safe as I can for as long as I can, and I also accept that I will most likely have to evacuate at some point, when something unmanageable occurs.

How do you conduct an efficient and fruitful search for that dream bubble? Use the list of triggers you compiled in the last segment to customize "bubble search criteria" based on your own triggers and region. Your criteria will differ from mine, but here's a look to give you an idea. I consider big picture issues first, and then the smaller details.

Big Picture Bubble Search Criteria
- **Neighborhood:** When I need to move, I always start my new bubble search here. Using a map, I look for neighborhoods that would have the cleanest air. I avoid areas downwind of and in close proximity to factories, treatment plants, industrial areas, non-organic farms, freeways and traffic-jammed streets, and cottonwood trees. (Come end of May, that cottonwood fluffstuff flurries about *everywhere!*) Sure, wind changes direction when weather patterns shift, but I base my decisions

on the norm. When I find the areas that have the cleanest air for the majority of the time, I circle them on my map.

- **Altitude:** Does your region have hills or mountainous areas? I've noticed that the higher I go, up to about 5,000 feet, the more easily I can breathe, so I circle these areas on my map.
- **Proximity to large bodies of water:** I also breathe more easily near the ocean and the mouth of rivers, so I circle those areas on my map.

Wherever I have overlapping circles on my map, I start my small picture bubble search there. (If no overlap, then I search within all the circles.) I always give the areas closest to supportive friends, medical help, the library, and/or groceries priority.

Small Picture Bubble Search Criteria
- Does the building have upcoming renovations planned? If there's no work planned for at least two years, I consider the building a contender.
- Did the building undergo recent renovations? If the apartment hasn't been painted, re-carpeted/re-floored or renovated in the past two years, I consider it a contender.
- Are the cupboards off-gassing? Does anything immoveable in the apartment trigger me?
- Is it a non-smoking building? Do people smoke on the grounds?
- Does the building have HVAC or radiant heat? I have lots of trouble with HVAC so tend to steer away from buildings with it.
- Does the apartment have doorway opening to the outside (*not* opening onto a lobby or enclosed, shared hallway that can fill with fragrances, cleaners and other triggers)?
- Ideally, the apartment has in-suite laundry, but that usually jacks up the rent so it may not be feasible. Where is the laundry facility? Where does it vent? Which way does the wind usually blow? (*Oh, yes!* Figure it out. You'll be glad you did!) Can you navigate the laundry room without increasing symptoms? If not, will management allow you to have an apartment-sized washer and dryer inside your apartment? (More on advanced laundry survival techniques coming soon.)
- Is the apartment quiet? Do they have parties, yelling matches, or young children upstairs or next-door? (Remember, this needs to be a peaceful bubble as well as toxin-free. Startling and loud noises can ramp up symptoms.)
- Is there a window from which you can look out onto the world? Bubble life is isolated. You need a window to the world, and daylight.
- Proximity to places you need to get to? Grocery store? Doctor? Pharmacy? Supportive friends?
- Parking garage or street parking? Some parking garages are manageable for me, if well ventilated and clean and my parking spot is close to the exit, but most are not.
- Covered balcony? If you can't find certain necessities used, you may need to purchase new materials, and they may off-gas for a few weeks or months. Covered balconies make perfect "off-gassing stages." (If the object is large or off-gassing enough that I can't sit on the balcony without being triggered, however, I ask a CS-free friend if s/he will store the product at their place until I can tolerate it.

- Riding in an elevator is often like being trapped in a half-empty cologne bottle someone used as an ashtray. I only ride in them as a last resort, and I plan for recovery time before and after. Can you access the apartment without using the elevator? If you need to take the stairs, are they manageable? Stairs often smell musty or reek of chemical floor cleaners, urine, and/or smoke.

As I said, the above list was made from the list of *my* triggers. One size does NOT fit all, so you need to base your own bubble search criteria on *your* triggers. And remember, no matter which CSS you have (or if you have only CS), you need a safe bubble to help you manage environmental and/or *intrinsic* triggers.

For example, those with few environmental triggers may have a trigger list that looks something like this:

- Stress/stressors (stair climbing, underground parking garage/no street parking, an hour's drive to groceries, friends, or doctor, etc.)
- Fatigue
- Feeling unsafe
- Certain foods
- Only on bad days: diesel exhaust, bleach, Sheila's clothing, Bill's cologne, sound, light, and loud noises like yelling and chainsaw motors

Thus, their bubble search criteria list will need information on these issues:

- Stress and stressors: here you'd list what kind of places would be least stressful to you, based on whatever your chief stressors (mental, emotional, or physical) are.
- Fatigue: what kind of place would be restful to you? A dark basement suite? A penthouse looking out over a city? Describe it here.
- Feeling unsafe: here you'd list what kind of places make you feel safe—upstairs, downstairs, five acres of wheat growing around you, a cabin in the woods, a chocolate shop next door, or whatever.
- Certain foods: this doesn't have to do with housing in the grand scheme, but maybe you need to be within a block from the grocery store or a special health foods store. If so, this should go on your list.
- Only on bad days: diesel exhaust, bleach, Sheila's clothing, Bill's cologne, sound, light, and loud noises like yelling and chainsaw motors. Even though you don't experience some triggers everyday, treat them as you would any other triggers and do all you can to select a bubble location without them.

Safety Is Key

Your bubble may be your house, your apartment, a room in your house or apartment, or a closet in a room in your house or apartment. It may be a shed or clubhouse, or even a root cellar, bomb shelter, or cave in your backyard. Whatever you choose, it has to be *yours*. What do I mean by *yours*?

- You control the bubble space. People don't barge in on you (unless there's an emergency). You control what comes in, what goes out, the bubble's temperature, and how it's furnished and decorated.

- You ensure the bubble contains as few of *your* triggers as possible. It's tailored to your specific needs, no one else's.
- You feel *safe* in the bubble. Have you noticed that I keep bringing up safety? That's because with CS, you've not only got a sensitized nervous system, but the limbic system is often involved and working overtime. (You may recall, the limbic system controls our emotions—of which fear is one—and our survival drive.) So if you want to decrease your symptoms and get your body's protective systems back on track, safety is key.

We don't tend to give safety much thought until we lose it. When I got CS, my feeling of safety completely disintegrated. Everywhere I went, even in my home, environmental triggers were "attacking" me—at least that's how my brain interpreted it. And it found other threats too, but these were specific to me as a person, regardless of CS. These were things that I had always avoided or protected myself against without thinking about it. Things like always having a good deadbolt on the front door, steering clear of the drunk person on the street who is toppling cars in a rage, or never taking a ground floor apartment because of perceived intruder risk. Things I'd seen as common sense had become, with my sensitized brain, perceived as *active* threats. So, I had to do some brainstorming and figure out what makes me feel safe in general, in the home, in public, wherever.

You may need to do this too. Besides decreased exposure to, and impact of your triggers, what do you need to feel safe? For me, it was something like this:

- Neighborhood safe enough that I can walk alone at night
- Good deadbolt, window locks
- Distance from angry or volatile people
- Bottomless stash of chocolate
- Stuff like that. Heck, you may want a German Shepard, or a teddy bear, or frolicking puppies and kittens in a field of waist-high cosmos. Whatever you discover about yourself and what you need to feel safe, it needs to be part of your bubble.

Inside the Bubble

Got your bubble sorted for the time being? Great. Now what? How do you use the bubble? What do you put inside it? What do you do in there?

Good questions.

My bubble is currently a tiny room in my apartment. (When I've had a studio apartment, my bubble was a dark, curtained-off corner in that space.) My bubble contains an old, fully off-gassed semi-reclining chair, a warm blanket, and dark curtains on the window. Some LED holiday lights are hung in the shape of a spiral on one wall, and a large picture of the ocean is tacked to another. An old pine table holds a DVD player and small tv, Qi Gong and meditation DVDs, and an old yoga mat and off-gassed resistance bands sit in one corner.

That's it. I like it simple.

How you furnish your bubble depends, of course, on your triggers and personal taste. What you *do* in your bubble also plays a role in defining its contents.

REST

What you do in your bubble is rest.

I cannot write enough about rest, nor sufficiently emphasize its importance.

Even if you experience no extreme fatigue or chronic pain like that associated with CFS, Fibromyalgia, and other CS chronic pain syndromes, rest is *crucial* for people with CS. This is because, in order to decrease reactivity, your central nervous system must have rest. It doesn't matter which syndrome(s) you have—you need to rest, *every* day, probably several times a day, depending on your particular condition and symptoms.

It's important to understand that rest does not necessarily mean sleeping. For our purposes, "rest" means sitting or lying still, with eyes closed, in your bubble or another safe and trigger-free place, in quiet comfort, while taking slow, relaxed breaths. Dim lighting is good, or in sunshine, if you like. If you think you might fall asleep, set a gentle alarm for 30 or 60 minutes, unless your doctor tells you otherwise. Sleeping too much in the daytime can make it harder to sleep properly at night.

You need to carve out time every day to rest in a safe place. This is usually your bubble, but fit rest in wherever you feel safe. When I have to go somewhere, I usually arrive at least ten minutes early and then rest with eyes closed, taking slow, relaxed breaths, in the parked car. Your central nervous system needs to re-normalize. This means don't rush. This means don't over-extend. This means take breaks and move slowly and find lots of time to rest.

This applies to daily living activities—tasks like acquiring, preparing and eating food, paying bills, and maintaining a healthy level of hygiene—no matter how important an errand or some research might be, ask yourself first:

- How important is this? Can it wait for another day?
- What would happen if I waited until … Thursday?
- What would happen if I waited until next month?

I'm not advocating languid procrastination or becoming derelict in your responsibilities. I'm saying it's important to NOT be busy 24/7. It's important to look at your to-do list in the context of CS now and to prioritize based on what your body needs: rest.

This includes taking care of business. If you are working, take a break every hour at least. Download a free timer app for your phone or computer and adhere to it. Sit back with eyes closed each time it signals a break and take relaxed breaths. Even just two minutes can make a difference. If you feel yourself getting frustrated or stressed over a job or someone on the job, take a break. Let your nervous system know that you are safe, there is no threat, and nothing is more important than your well-being.

If you aren't able to work, you still need to make decisions in favour of your health. Disability and employment compensation battles can stretch on for years and take a toll on both energy and spirit. I have to balance the amount of time I spend fighting such battles with the amount of time I spend resting and doing healing things for myself.

The same goes for researching possible treatments. It's tempting to spend every spare moment desperately Googling for solutions and options, to leave no stone unturned in the quest for a cure. And there's a whole wide web out there, but that doesn't mean I should spend all my time and energy on it, every day.

Balance. Prioritize rest. Prioritize me. *So difficult to learn!* But I did, and you can too. Prioritize you and your health first, don't give more than you can afford to, and *rest*.

Rest and Intensive Bubble Time

Note that we will be working with two degrees, or intensities, of rest. Normal rest, as defined in the previous segment, usually satisfies the needs of those with light to moderate symptoms, but people with severe symptoms often need to employ a greater degree of rest I call "intensive bubble time," a strategy I adapted from Greg Charles Fischer's "Aggressive Rest Therapy."[8] Intensive bubble time involves retreating into the bubble, lying down and resting with as little sensory stimulation as possible. No music, no lights, no sounds or scents, no tv, no telephone, no internet or books—just me, relaxed breathing, with eyes closed, thinking happy, peaceful, healing thoughts. Each hour I do a minute or two of muscle stretching to minimize pain or, if even that is too much I'll caress or pat my skin lightly.

I practice intensive bubble time until my severe symptoms subside. Then I shift to regular bubble time, which allows me to sit in the recliner if I want, and intersperse brief, simple activities with my bubble time, provided the activities don't increase symptoms. Depending on symptom severity, intensive bubble time could last hours, days, weeks or months, and this can take a toll on one's mental health as well as one's exertion tolerance threshold and functional capacity. I'll talk more about mitigating these problems soon. For now, know that intensive bubble time is necessary sometimes, and the sooner you surrender to the need for intensive rest, the sooner your symptoms may subside and you can leave the bubble again.

Do Something

My first few years, especially while in crisis phase, my doctors repeatedly said, "Be mindful. Rest. Don't push," but my brain was continually barking out orders, *DO SOMETHING! FIX IT! FIX EVERYTHING! NOW!*

Many experience such a conflict when CS (with or without CSS) occurs, and it's compounded by the facts that when you get sick, you aren't operating at your best and there is a lot to do—financially, legally, medically, personally. The pressure multiplies for single people and others with little to no support. So, the brain is not wrong to be cracking the whip. If I wasn't calling doctors or researching treatments, I was fighting workers compensation or shopping or doing household chores, and… That's all important stuff, and it's tangible stuff, so doing it gave me a sense of accomplishment and control while the rest of my life was this massive cyclone of uncertainty that offered no immediate gratification whatsoever. Me? I like immediate gratification. It makes me feel like I'm on solid ground. Nevertheless, compulsions are like wild animals: the more you feed them, the more they hang around and the more of a nuisance they become. Ignore them and eventually they will go away. Starve that compulsion to *do something*. It's not good for folks with CS, and it doesn't give us what we really need: rest.

Intensive Bubble Time and Entertainment

TV programs, movies, social networking, internet surfing, books, music—there is no limit to entertainment for us these days, even for those doing bubble time. Unfortunately, most of us have grown accustomed to 24/7 entertainment, and downtime can make us feel uncomfortable, disconnected, and lonely. As I've iterated and reiterated, bubble time needs to be quiet rest with minimal sensory stimuli, so you will need to choose to "unplug" whenever you do bubble time. While it may seem preposterous at first, this gets easier with practice.

Folks doing intensive bubble time and/or living alone for long durations, however, may have trouble coping with the longer-term isolation required when tackling severe symptoms. This is normal. Humans are social and inquisitive beings who need a certain amount of stimulus and change, and intensive bubble time deprives us of that. In crisis phase, I did over a year of intensive bubble time, living alone and leaving only once or twice a week for short errands, so I understand boredom and loneliness and feeling pent up and needing entertainment. Some days I thought I would go as loony as the hermit in Tom Stoppard's play *Arcadia*. I'm not suggesting that you go 100 percent without entertainment during intensive bubble time, but you must keep CS in mind when you select the type and duration of entertainment.

Do you mean some entertainment might harm *people with CS?*

Good question.

When you watch a scary movie or a thrilling drama, listen to angsty pop songs, or read an emotion-gripping story, what happens? You get scared, sad, angry, anxious and/or tense. These reactions tax your central nervous system. Bubble time is for *resting*, feeling safe and at ease.

Ask yourself, which is more healing?

- A comedy, a thriller, or an über-drama-filled soap opera? (comedy)
- Peppy pop music, heartbreak ballads, or Mozart? (*not* the ballads)
- Binge-watching a murder mystery for three days straight or watching a half-hour sitcom and then resting without sensory stimuli for an hour? (non-binge-y sitcom and rest)

Note that when you are doing intensive bubble time, you should choose upbeat entertainment *and* limit the amount of your "entertainment time." The central nervous system processes all input—listening to music or concentrating on TV, books, or internet takes energy. The same with talking on the phone or with a friend who comes to visit. You need to limit entertainment and interaction and maximize rest. Don't fall into the trap of thinking, "Well, I might as well cruise the internet all day every day since I can't do anything else," or "I need the TV on all day to keep me company—I'm not really paying attention to it." If you use entertainment that way, you will inhibit your recovery and have to extend your bubble time. Instead, rest all you can and keep entertainment in reserve for those times when you start to go stir crazy or feel super lonely or frustrated and absolutely *need* a break from resting.

Tip: Make a list of entertainment sources—funny or heartwarming youtubes, shows, books, music playlists, etc.—so when you need a break during intensive bubble time, you don't have to expend energy coming up with entertainment ideas.

There is more than one way to do your bubble time and get the rest you need, even if you have young children or live alone. Have patience and give yourself time to figure it out.

Review of What We Do Inside the Bubble

REST.
Get the idea?

Doing Bubble Time When You Have Kids

Parents with CS need to do bubble time and need to give their kids love, support, and care. It may seem impossible to do both, but you can. Many parents with CS do. Here's how:

- Be honest about your condition, as appropriate for your child's age. Let your child know that you have an illness and that your illness sometimes limits your ability to participate in activities.
- Do as much of your bubble time as possible while your kids are at school so you can sit and interact with them when they get home each afternoon.
- If you need to do bubble time in the afternoon and/or evening too, help your children plan activities to keep them occupied while you do your bubble time.
- Tell your kids how they can help. For example, younger kids can get you a cold pack or pick up toys. Older kids can help younger siblings or take on age-appropriate responsibilities around the house such as cooking, cleaning, doing laundry, or taking out garbage, to allow you to conserve energy that you can then spend doing fun activities with your kids.
- Let your kids know that if they need to talk to a counselor or therapist, they can.
- Don't make false promises. Be honest. Make sure they understand that you have to go day by day, see what symptoms arise, before you can decide to attend or do something.
- Find ways to rest while being with your kids. For example, you can rest on the couch while they play a game with a friend, or you can rest on the lawn while they do chalk drawings on the driveway.

If you have kids too young to occupy themselves, arrange for someone to come care for them or to take them out of the house while you rest. Have a list of at least four people you can call anytime to come get your kids or help with the kids if you have a bad day. You may experience some parental guilt here, but you can't give kids all they need while suffering from and being debilitated by symptoms 24/7. You need that bubble time to decrease your symptoms, so you can be present for your kids as much as possible.

Restoring Balance to the Autonomic Nervous System

So far, I've discussed the central, peripheral, and enteric nervous systems as they pertain to CS and CSS. Need a review? Our nervous system is divided into two parts: central and peripheral. The central nervous system, made up of the brain and the spinal cord, is our "control center," while the peripheral is in charge of communication between the central nervous system and the body. The enteric nervous system, also known as the "second brain," is the gut. CS sensitizes the central nervous system, interfering with the brain's interpretation of sensory information and causing it to send out unreliable messages to various parts of our nervous system. One part of the peripheral nervous system in particular tends to be significantly affected by CS: the autonomic nervous system (ANS).

The ANS "influences the function of internal organs. The autonomic nervous system is a control system that acts largely and unconsciously and regulates bodily functions such as the heart rate, digestion, respiratory rate, pupillary response, urination, and sexual arousal."[9] There are two branches of the ANS: sympathetic and parasympathetic. The former controls the fight or flight response, and the latter allows the body to rest, relax, reboot, and heal. People with CS tend to have a dominating sympathetic system and need to find ways to engage the parasympathetic, which should be active most of the time, except when we are under real threat, or perhaps running a marathon. Check out Diagram 2 if you need a visual.

The parasympathetic (aka the rest-digest-repair system) is in charge of conserving energy, increasing sleep, promoting growth, and recharging our cells' powerhouses, the mitochondria. We need all these things for healing; thus, part of decreasing symptoms involves restoring balance to the ANS, so the parasympathetic regains the "upper hand," so to speak, over the sympathetic.

Quiet rest while taking relaxed breaths can help engage the parasympathetic and

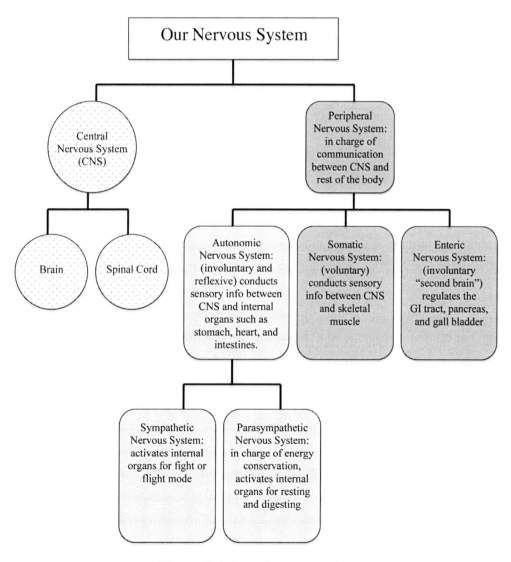

Diagram 2. Autonomic nervous system

increase production of natural serotonin, a neurotransmitter that helps us sleep and relax. When I was in crisis phase, all I could manage was rest, along with these easy parasympathetic-stimulating actions:

- The first requires only that you sit with a relaxed pelvis, your legs uncrossed and spread a little wider than your hips (you know, the way some men do in movie theatres, on transit, and on airplanes? Guys, you know who you are!) I call this "sitting wide." Relaxing the pelvis in this way can engage the parasympathetic.
- Tap lightly on your solar plexis (breast bone) or collarbone, or run your fingers over your lips. These actions stimulate your parasympathetic system, and you can do them anywhere—outside the bubble, in a triggerful place, in the car at a stop-light, etc.

The more you stimulate your parasympathetic system, the better. If you are out of crisis phase and have enough energy, you may try practicing one or all of the following techniques inside your bubble—in addition to plenty of quiet rest, of course—to help encourage and speed the restoration of balance to your ANS.

MEDITATION

I've always believed that anything we lose and find ourselves in (in a blissful way, not a drug- or alcohol-induced, head-in-the-sand, escape-y kind of way) is a meditation. For me, running was a meditation. So were gardening, writing, singing, reading, dancing, and I guess pretty much anything creative that I did pre–CS. I meditated by doing something that fed my spirit and grounded me. Formal Meditation (with a capital "M") however, was different. That kind of Meditation required years of ascetic training, wearing itchy hooded robes, chanting, possible vows of silence and celibacy, no chocolate and, in my case, could only result in utter failure.

Years ago, before I got CS and CSS, I studied hatha yoga. I liked the stretching and postures—I liked *moving*. That made the idea of Meditation more fun, doable. I stopped taking classes when "hot yoga" took over my city. Doing yoga in a steamy room with a profusely sweating crowd and an off-gassing PVC floor didn't appeal to me, but I still practiced yoga on my own at home sometimes. When I got sick, however, the exertion and strength required for yoga postures became too much for me. I took up Qi Gong but as my symptoms worsened I had to stop that too. When I got diagnosed with CFS my specialist told me to Meditate to help engage my parasympathetic system. "Formal Meditation," he said, "every day." Imagine my ecstatic response.

This type of Meditation required that I sit and focus inward. Instead of finding bliss, I found discomfort. I sat and watched my thoughts whiz by while trying to acknowledge and let them go. It was uncomfortable knowing I had that many thoughts about stupid stuff, or that I had the same stupid thoughts over and over again. I didn't want to know that about myself. Who wants to know that?

Yet I tried. And I try. And I'm no Buddha. My mind whizzes all over the place most days, but I no longer judge. I let my thoughts go, one after the next, and I focus instead on relaxing my breath and my body. I imagine that with each breath, I'm generating serotonin, engaging my parasympathetic system, and infusing my body with healing energy and light. And it feels pretty darn good, actually.

Meditation isn't what I'd thought. It's not becoming some masterful monk. It's about paying attention to how I feel, and taking the brain to a happy place—a place free of worry and to-do lists—and feeding the brain and body lots of oxygen and serenity, so it can heal itself as much as possible. It's about letting go of the past and any regrets, and ceasing to feel anxious about what might happen in the future.

Many people get frustrated with their attempts at Meditation. They have unstoppable thoughts, or a busy mind, they can't sit still, or all they do is tell themselves to *stop thinking!* Negative self-criticism isn't helpful and, as I'll discuss in the segment on self-compassion, can be detrimental. Perhaps try thinking about Meditation as a gift you are giving yourself, rather than a chore or something to learn. Think of it as an opportunity for your mind and body to rest and regroup. The aim is to ground you in the present moment and place. Meditation will enable you to *notice* how you're feeling and, over time, to cultivate an inner awareness that can liberate you from automatic, conditioned responses that you've developed. Once you can identify what you're feeling and thinking, you can then *choose* how you want to engage or respond to the challenges life gives you, rather than simply *react*. This new inner awareness and the freedom from automatic responses are two primary gifts of meditation. Other boons include engaging the parasympathetic nervous system, decreasing the central nervous system's reactivity, and increasing self-confidence, for starters.

There is no right way or wrong way to meditate. Sit yourself comfortably on the floor with crossed legs or on a chair with feet firmly planted on the floor, or even lying down. Let your weight sink in, close your eyes, relax your breath, and away you go! Trust that you are doing exactly what you need to be doing, the way it needs to be done, to get you where you want to go. A teacher of mine told me that if, out of 20 minutes of meditation, I get only 3 seconds of serene, thoughtless bliss, then that's great. Once I heard that, all the pressure to Meditate with a capital "M" went away. *Three seconds? I can do that!* And I can. You can too.

It's important to practice meditation regularly; that is, you'll receive more benefit from meditating every day for five minutes at a time than to meditate for 20 minutes once a week. Choose whatever time of day suits your schedule and energy level the best.

There are countless types of Meditation—some focus on an intention or on a rhythmic phrase, others focus on the breath or on different parts of the body, on building compassion for yourself and for others, and so on. As you get into a regular practice, you may wish to explore and discover which kinds of Meditation appeal to you most. Check Appendix F: Recommended Reading and Viewing for places to start.

In time, you'll find that in addition to engaging the parasympathetic system, meditation is a grounding technique, a confidence-builder, a sleep promoter, and a keystone of transformation and healing. And all it takes is a safe bubble and you.

Qi Gong

I first heard about Qi Gong, an ancient Chinese healing practice, when my Acupuncturist suggested that it could help restore my energy. A gentle, moving meditation that cultivates the body's life-force energy, Qi Gong is perfect for people with CS because it requires minimal exertion yet stimulates the parasympathetic system, increases circulation, and strengthens and stretches muscles (which can help decrease pain). And you don't have to be athletic, flexible, or in shape to succeed at Qi Gong. You just need to practice with intention, and *breathe*.

YOGA

Yoga is another meditative practice that stimulates the brain's parasympathetic response, improves circulation, and invites gentle stretching and deep breathing. Attending a yoga class at a studio is anything but relaxing or meditative for those with environmental triggers, or severe fatigue or pain, but there are lots of books and dvds available for learning and practicing yoga at home, in your bubble, at your own pace. My favorite is *Moving Toward Balance: 8 Weeks of Yoga with Rodney Yee* because it teaches yoga in a simple, clear manner and provides bite-sized daily practices so I don't over-exert. (Always check with your doctor before embarking on any new exercise.)

ACUPUNCTURE AND ACUPRESSURE

Both acupuncture and acupressure work to free the flow of energy throughout the body by activating specific points with pressure or with needles and can help restore balance to the autonomic nervous system. Acupuncture uses needles and must be performed by a licensed practitioner. Acupressure, however, works through touch or pressure, and you may perform some simple acupressure on yourself; for example, the tapping technique I mentioned at the beginning of this segment accesses acupressure points on the lips and collarbone. I use both, although I have found that acupuncture yields stronger and more lasting results than acupressure. Acupuncture played a significant part in helping me through crisis phase. Then, I'd feel calm and relaxed for a few hours following a treatment (or until I ran into an environmental trigger). Now, the acupuncture brings my system's reactivity down for 12–24 hours or more, depending on trigger load.

MUSIC

Music is a magical healing thing. It transports, it transforms, and it works wonders on the brain itself. Generally speaking, I use music in two ways.

First, as a balm while outside my bubble: When I'm feeling glum or notice depression nipping at my heels, I listen to what I call "bubble gum pop" music—happy upbeat stuff—Shania Twain's "Up!" and Taylor Swift's "Shake It Off" are perfect examples. As a die-hard melodic rock fan, I never would have ventured into the realm of bubble gum pop pre–CS, but now I find the beats invigorating and the lyrics infectiously optimistic. I created a playlist called "listen on down dayz" and promised myself I would. Keeping that vow never fails to make me smile.

I also use music inside my bubble sometimes to encourage healing changes in my brain (which I'll detail in Neuroplasticity). All kinds of studies have been done about the way music affects the brain, and the results convinced me that folks with CS can benefit from using music as a healing strategy. For example, researchers found that "patients who listened to instrumental music (such as jazz) versus relaxation sounds (such as ocean sounds) during surgery had lower levels of the stress hormone cortisol in their blood during surgery: about 20 percent lower than the group that didn't listen to music."[10] Cortisol, "the primary stress hormone, increases sugars (glucose) in the bloodstream, enhances your brain's use of glucose and increases the availability of substances that repair tissues."[11] Cortisol is released by the sympathetic nervous system to help the body wake up each day, exercise, and survive life-threatening situations. Elevated cortisol over the long term results in elevated glucose levels in the blood and can lead to weight gain.

Can you guess whether folks with CS tend to have elevated or decreased cortisol levels? Yep, elevated, and often for prolonged periods of time. This can wreak havoc on many internal systems, including sleep.

One way to fix this problem is to engage the parasympathetic system as often as possible. And one way to do that is by listening to music. So I listen to classical music and Gregorian chants while resting with my eyes closed. I take relaxed breaths and do my best to imagine that my central nervous system is healing, my soldiers are sleeping, and my sympathetic system is taking a nice long winter's nap …

Review of Triggers, Building the Bubble, Rest and the ANS

- There are two main types of triggers: environmental and intrinsic. You may have only intrinsic triggers, depending on your level of health, your CS and/or CSS.
- Stressors can be physiological, physical, emotional, and/or mental. Stress can cause serious health issues, and stressors can be significant CS and CSS triggers. Rather than believing all stress is negative (aka "stressing out") choose to "stress in" or *in*clude stress in your life as a positive, *friendly* force. "Stressing in" is a healthy choice that can help decrease your symptoms and improve health.
- Those with CS need a safe place that is as trigger-free as possible in which to rest. This is called the bubble.
- Use your bubble to give your nervous system a rest and to decrease overall trigger load. Bubble time can help to decrease severity and frequency of many symptoms.
- There are two degrees of rest: regular bubble time (for light to moderate symptoms) and intensive bubble time (for severe symptoms).
- You can do intensive bubble time without negative effects of prolonged isolation. The right type and duration of entertainment helps with that.
- With communication and planning, parents with CS *can* balance bubble time and good parenting.
- With CS, the sympathetic branch of the ANS tends to dominate over the parasympathetic branch. To decrease the impact of CS and CSS on one's life, this balance must be restored.
- We restore ANS balance by engaging the parasympathetic system via resting in our bubble, yoga, meditation, qi gong, and music.

> *Life is liquid. The Chinese were wrong to believe*
> *that the essential was breath. Perhaps the soul is breath.*
> —John Berger, *Pig Earth*[12]

Foraging

Grocery run mandatory today. No more putting it off. It's been ten days and all I have left is wilted kale and a sesame rice cracker I found lodged in the dark corner of a cupboard. After thoroughly examining the cracker for lint,

I take a nibble. Tastes like sesame and, inexplicably, chocolate. Maybe if I focus on the grocery list, I can get the cracker down my throat without my mind knowing what I'm doing. Another nibble. A little scribble. Nibble. Scribble. Nib—

It doesn't work. My mind senses an intruder in my throat and immediately goes into defense mode, constricting the muscles around my larynx. I cough. Only once. A warning. I hold my breath and imagine my throat as a vast portal, relaxed and welcoming, until the urge to cough diminishes. At the bottom of the list I add tampons and dish soap. Will have to go to the drug store too. Well, what's an expedition without risk?

I wrap my scarf twice around my lips and nose, lock the apartment door and hold my breath while I wait for the elevator. This old concrete tower has a ventilation system that blows air into the halls, elevator and lobby. A nice idea, ventilation, but the intake vent is located near the common laundry room in the basement, so toxic fabric softener fumes pollute the air blown into the building. I breathe through my scarf, get on when the elevator comes, and say a cheerful hello to the old woman already inside. She stares at my scarf wide-eyed, as if fearing I will contaminate her with tuberculosis.

I hurry from the elevator through the lobby and out the door, exhale and pull down the scarf. *Ah ...* the wind blows in from nearby English Bay, and I inhale deeply. The humidity sticks in my throat, not unlike cracker, and my throat muscles tighten. As I cross the street into the community library parking lot, I engage in the "prbprbprbprb" exercise the vocal therapist gave me. She believes I may someday breathe, speak, and sing freely again, although it will probably take at least six years. All through childhood and my professional singing career as an adult, I used this same "prbprbprbprb" exercise as a vocal warm-up before rehearsals and gigs. It's like making a raspberry sound, but without the tongue.

My lips tingle, and I yearn to sing, but I can't. Not since the chemical exposure at my day job a year ago, when I lost my voice and gained Irritable Larynx Syndrome, one of many disorders under the umbrella of Central Sensitization. That's the technical term for a central nervous system that's gone a little haywire and often perceives deadly threats where none exist. Whenever I detect a strong smell or synthetic chemical odor, the muscles around my larynx tighten, effectively closing off my air supply. My brain is just trying to protect me, I know, but this new über-vigilant world-view has thrown me back into caveman days, when gathering food wasn't as easy as sauntering into the nearest grocery store for a bunch of bananas or a pack of grass-fed bison. Stick with me while I forage in the wilderness of civilization. You'll see.

The vocal exercise does its job and loosens my neck muscles some more. I smile at the bitty victory. Small steps. First breathe. Then sing.

I reach Marine Drive, the main strip of West Vancouver, a beach town populated by retirees, Canadian rock stars, and wealthy Middle Eastern immigrants. A young woman is waiting at the bus stop on my left. Her perfume attacks me from a distance, scratching at my nostrils, clawing its way towards my throat. I halt my inhalation. Normally I'd seek refuge at the far edge of the shelter, the upwind spot—my safe spot—but she's standing there. Still holding my breath, I loop my scarf around my nose and mouth and dart past, to stand beneath the dripping trees upwind of her. Better to be wet than breathless.

Three cars pass, then a garbage truck. I hold my breath as the exhaust from each vehicle washes over me like a wave. There is an art to breath-holding, and I've gotten so good at it that very few notice. Sometimes I can even pass as a normal breathing person. I feel a sense of pride about this new skill, as a wounded hunter in the jungle would, I suppose. Breath-holding allows me to hide my weakness and be accepted by others. Most importantly, it enables me to believe that I can still operate autonomously. What would happen if I lost that independence, on the heels of losing so much else? I don't ask that question. It simply cannot happen. The diesel lingers and my neck muscles slowly constrict. I press my thumb against my larynx and nudge it gently to one side until the muscles around it relax.

The bus roars into view, its wide, gaping mouth of a windshield and bright yellow and dark blue stripes remind me of a hungry tiger. The yellow indicates that it's a new bus. Dread settles like a cloak over my shoulders. I could wait until the next bus comes, but West Vancouver got 20 new buses in the past month, and put all 20 into rotation. I waited an hour one day, holding out for an old blue and white bus, before finally giving up and getting on a new one.

The bus is purring and kneeling in front of the perfume girl now, as if it's tame, cuddly even. Keeping as much distance as possible without the bus driver leaving me at the curb, I follow her on and stand with my toes at the red line, nearest the front door. I press my scarf's layers against my nose and lips and breathe shallowly through my mouth.

Mind over smell. Stay calm.

I tell myself these things, as if I possess a disciplined brain, but the truth is, my brain is not the brain I once knew. I can't rely on it. I don't feel I even know it anymore. Its reactions have moved beyond the rational and into the caveman. I know it's trying to help me, but I sure wish it would allow me to manage it, instead of leaping into full limbic red alert, survivalist defense at every scent. The specialist said I could try taking drugs to reset my brain, but I'm not ready for that. I've already lost my voice, and part of my brain—two huge parts of me, of my identity. If medications altered my brain some more, would I still be me? Who would I be? I don't know. No one does. So I work on my breathing exercises and believe that my brain will come back to me, as will my voice, eventually.

The new bus smell—like new car smell but bus-sized—infiltrates my scarf like an evil spirit intent on possession, and my airway begins to close. I focus on breathing and count the bus stops. 18th Street. Old lady with hair spray gets on and looks me up and down like I'm a terrorist. 17th Street. Jock kid with a fabric-softener-saturated hoody brushes against me as he heads for the back of the bus. The high-pitched, floral scent from his hoody sticks in my nostrils the way it's intended to cling to people's clothes. 15th Street. My nose starts to run. 14th Street. There are bus stops nearly every block to accommodate the elderly population in this neighborhood. A cough forces its way out of me. 13th street. Businessman who poured on cologne this morning squeezes in against me. Full bus now. The heater comes on and blows the new bus smell right at my forehead. I can't move away. Trapped. My airway closes more. I cough again and sniffle behind my scarf. My upper body begins to sweat. More coughs come. People are looking now, their expressions a progression from fascination to fear to repulsion, and eventually, dismissal. I don't feel like a person when people look at me like that. I feel like something distinct, disparate, unevolved.

11th Street. I push through the glom of bodies and jump off a stop early, at the edge of the sports green where girls play field hockey most afternoons. I pull down my scarf, gulping in the fresh air, and cut across the corner of the playing field to escape the exhaust from the road. Walking too much tires me, but tired beats suffocation in my book. I dig in my pocket for Kleenex and blow my nose. Then I focus on my throat.

"Bprbprbprbprb." The Canadian geese milling about the field pause to stare at me, but my neck muscles are loosening, so I continue. "Bprbprbprbprb." My heart rate is slowing now and the perspiration has ceased. Panic receding. I put a thumb to my larynx and push it as I walk, but the muscles around it are tightening up again as I approach the footbridge. Fabric softener—if people only knew how resilient and damaging that product could be. It's the greatest marketing hoax of the century, in my opinion—I detect it before I see the source: a young mother with baby in stroller heading across the bridge towards the shops. She's at least 50 feet away. Fifty feet! Note to self: apply for a job as a police drug sniffer dog.

Before crossing, I wait for her toxic trail to disperse, right thumb to larynx, push to the left, then left thumb to larynx, to the right. Breathe deep. Prepare for what's to come. I'm still in the open field and it starts to drizzle. I already feel soggy and weary, as if I've fallen into, and crawled out of a quicksand pit. Maybe I should head home. I remind myself of the barren kitchen there and attempt a pep talk: make it through the grocery store and you can eat a nice meal … no chocolate or bread or coffee, no garlic or cheese or pie, but still …

The pep talk falls flat.

Pep talks never really work because I love food so much and now have all these dietary restrictions. Because the specialist says I have acid reflux complicating things. Because JC, the Traditional Chinese Medicine practitioner, says gluten and lactose increase inflammation and mucous. Because it's been a year and I'm having trouble adjusting. Because, more than anything, I want my life back. All my favorite things. Running. Eating. Singing. Laughing. Being with friends. Even necessary things, like shopping or transit-ing. I want it all back. The drizzle thickens into big drops. I convince myself that the sky cries for everyone. Sustained by the poetic genius we all tap into when we most need it, I trek on with dry eyes.

Pressing the scarf closer to my nostrils, I reach for the door to the mall, beyond which lies the drug store. I hesitate. A mall is nothing more than a big box full of new product effluvium with nowhere to go. A drug store is basically a smaller box with the same issue. New products come in and off-gas, and the odors never disperse. Sure, some are filtered out by ventilation systems eventually, but with the massive number of daily deliveries versus the amount of off-gassing and the time needed to flush those fumes out, having a drug store in a mall is, from breathing perspectives, fatally redundant.

I step aside and let other shoppers pass while I stand in the rain, calculating. There is a weariness within me generated solely by the stress of constantly weighing environmental risks, negotiating energy limits, and bargaining against dwindling finances. It feels heavy and numbs my brain, but I do it all the same. The additional monetary expense of purchasing tampons and dish soap at the grocery store seems the better bargain today when compared to the energy deficit a drug store jungle tour will cost me. I head for the grocery store across the way.

The American company Whole Foods bought out a local grocery chain called *Capers* some years ago. It's the only place in town that carries a wide selection of quality organic vegetables, and their prices reflect the strength of that market position. Since being exposed to chemicals and then laid off by a top-ranking "green" architecture firm, I am no longer an avid believer in companies that claim to be concerned about people and the environment, but here I am, shopping at one. Synthetic chemicals did this to me in the first place so, in my ongoing attempt to detoxify my body, I invest in chemical-free food.

I tie my scarf around my nose and mouth as I enter, grab a basket, and with list in hand, begin the quest that is as much about avoiding customers and certain aisles as it is about acquiring the stuff on the list. Midmorning is not as crowded as late afternoon, but this time of day does seem to attract a high percentage of perfumey women and fabric-softened moms n' babes. At least I have room to maneuver.

In elementary school, I excelled at dodgeball. I had a sixth sense, it seemed, that told me which direction people would move, who they were going to throw the ball at, stuff like that. I rely on my dodgeball sense in situations such as these. I can tell when perfumey lady number one is going towards the broccoli so I pivot away from the kale and head for the spinach. I double back for the kale when she crosses to the tomatoes. That's the idea.

I get trapped while checking sell-by dates on packages of bison. A late-middle–aged woman laden with flowery perfume sidles up beside me, stares at my scarf mask, and then pushes in to examine the chicken in front of me, as if I don't exist. I hold my breath and rifle through the saran-wrapped trays to find something not too big. The problem with hurrying while holding one's breath is the potential for panic. I run out of air, start to sweat, my nose runs and airway begins to close, and then everything gets worse fast. Luckily, I make a good grab and retreat with my meat before that happens.

I'm kneeling now, shoveling gluten-free oats into a bag from a bin. My nose dribbles snot onto my upper lip behind the scarf. I snuffle and focus on my task. A man squats at the bin beside me to bag himself some quick oats. On my inhale I turn towards him and rise—an inhalation error, not uncommon in times of exhaustion and duress—and suck up a criminal amount of cologne fumes. A year ago I might have said something with a wink and a smile in passing like, "You catch more with a lure than a beacon." It would be for his own good, really. But past frivolities like educating men about the allure of a hint of musk now pale in comparison to battles for breath. This one could be game over.

The cologne nips the inside of my windpipe like a fiendish fly. I cough. Once. Then again. My eyes begin to tear. Mucous flows down the back of my throat in a thick sludge. I cough more. Time slows. The man, oblivious, scoops his quick oats. My heart kicks in and I begin to sweat. Panic. Full throttle. I throw the oats in my basket and stagger towards the freezers, coughing uncontrollably now. Liquid from my eyes and nose runs down my face. My head gets fuzzy, and I wonder if I'll make it.

The first freezer aisle is clear. I drop my basket, open a freezer door, tear off my scarf and inhale. The cold air rushes at me in a cloud and stings the wet skin on my face. The coughs come in a long, relentless concatenation, each feeding upon the last, each giving birth to the next. Every portal in my face is blocked. Ears plugged. Throat constricted. Nose full of mucous. Dark vision. Eyes awash in tears. The coughing has to stop. It has to. I try to breathe smoothly, to starve the coughs, tell my belly it has no strength left to cough and should rest. Shallow breaths.

Calme-toi. Ça va. Tout va bien. Calme. C'est rien. Rien ...

Long moments pass. As the coughing slows, the tears stop. Maybe they freeze, leaving crispy trails on my face. Then the rampant perspiration shuts off, leaving me chilled and drained. I pull my head out of the freezer, close the door, and stand, clinging to the handle, for some minutes, talking to myself in bad French. I don't know why French is soothing to me. Maybe I have to access a different part of my brain to think in French, so it distracts me from the terror of imminent asphyxiation. Maybe French is just a healing language.

The darkness brightens. I am facing the glass, not seeing anything really, though there are probably several products in the freezer before me. I feel customers passing, their eyes on me. I look like a housewife in the middle of a nervous breakdown, I tell myself, and find some comfort in that. After all, nervous breakdowns are widely accepted these days, and people don't really consider housewives losing it as scandalous anymore, just a symptom of an unfulfilling marriage, which most everyone can relate to, so really, what's the issue?

When the trembling and dizziness dissipate enough that I can stand without aid of the door handle, I reach into my bag and pull out a small mirror and some Kleenex.

"That wasn't so bad," I murmur, as I dab at my washed-out mascara and wipe snot from my chin. My voice is hoarse and the words come out in a grating whisper. "You didn't puke." I blow my nose. "And you didn't die." I put the things back in my bag and pick up my basket, then hold still while the head rush comes and goes. I put a quivering thumb to my larynx, which is so tight it won't budge. "On to the next jungle, then?"

The checkout gods, traditionally more merciless than the bison and oat bin gods combined, must be on their coffee break. My checkout clerk is fragrance-free, and she closes her aisle as I approach. This relieves me, since no scented people can press up close behind, reach across me for a conveyor belt divider bar, corral their kids and raise a cloud of fabric softener around us all. I am now breathing shallowly, trying to pull my credit card out of my wallet without loosening pressure on my scarf mask. I need another hand. The chemical bouquet in the air isn't as concentrated here as in the rest of the store, but my neck muscles remain clenched from that last episode, no matter how nicely I speak French to myself. So close to freedom, I get antsy and start to sweat. The checkout clerk smiles and reaches over to help. I nod my thanks and look around as she swipes the card.

The other customers checking out appear to be unhurried, unsweaty, unanxious, breathing freely. They wield their own credit cards, bag their own purchases, using both hands. I wonder what they smell. If they detect nothing like I used to, before all this happened. If they whiff some synthetic odor but their brains ignore it, like mine used to. Some of them glance around, look me up and down and up again, taking in my red face, my panicked eyes, my damp hair plastered to forehead, finally focusing on the scarf around my nose and mouth. Always the scarf.

Would I behave any differently if I were breathing fine and watching someone in this condition? I don't know anymore. I don't remember what it was like before. It's as if I crossed some threshold into a different dimension when my central nervous system became sensitized. As if I inhabit a different realm now, a desperate realm where Maslow would have a field day, because my brain perceives everything as a fight for survival, with longshot odds, like caveman against T-Rex.

My cloth shopping bags filled, I pay, grab receipt, and rush out into the pedestrian sidewalk. Sweat dribbles down my back. Snot dribbles out both nostrils. My cheeks burn. The shopping bags tug at my arms. I set them down, lower the scarf and wipe my nose.

I left the apartment an hour ago and have nearly died only once. By some respects, this qualifies as a good day. Still, I feel like I could collapse here on the puddling bricks and sleep for months. I remind myself that I can be back in my apartment within the hour if all goes well enough. *Chez toi.* Dry, warm, scentless, safe. "Bprbprbprbprb."

I trudge to the bus stop, my limbs feeling as though they've been dipped in lead. I have my scarf on, my hood up. I breathe lightly through my mouth, thankful for the rain, which keeps dust and odors down. My nose keeps running and ears remain plugged. I try to loosen my larynx again but it won't be pushed.

The journey to the bus stop is unmemorable. That is, I don't remember it at all. I stand in the center of a three-walled plastic bus shelter, imagining that I'm in an ice-fishing shack on a remote frozen lake, enjoying some respite from the elements and predators. I wish I could stay here, alone, forever, just me and the rain clacking on the bus shelter roof, but I can't. Ice melts. Seasons change. Already, I can see people rushing towards me with their many packages and whatever invisible threats they may bear.

The bus comes, another new one. I pull up my scarf, get on, and stand as close to the front door as the driver will allow. The bus interior is hot, and the heat sucks the last dregs of energy from my body. The engine, the chatter, the smells, the people—all the stimulants blur together and encircle me in a confused barrage, like an unkindness of ravens trying to ascertain if I'm carrion or merely playing possum. Every time the driver opens the door, I sniff a whiff of outside air. Then I hold my breath until the next stop.

Maybe I should become a professional swimmer, since I'm getting better and better at holding my breath. I used to swim for hours, all through my childhood and adult life. I loved the underwater world, the way floating grounded me, the sound of waves and water, the freedom and the feel of water on my skin, the cutting, clean scent of chlorine in my hair—

Chlorine. I can't swim anymore because of the chlorine. I rummage around my brain for a joke or a pep talk but nothing comes, only the void of loss, and the overwhelming, instinctual desire to get someplace safe.

I disembark at my stop and make my way through the library lot, arms throbbing with the weight of the groceries. Holding my breath past idling cars' exhaust pipes, trembling with anxiety, sweat-soaked, I dart past the building's front door, across the fabric-softened lobby, into the elevator, down the hall, to my apartment door. Fumbling with the keys, fingers quivering, scarf slipping down, throat closing when I am forced to let my breath go and then inhale the sickly sweet, rubbery, fabric-softened air—

I lunge inside, shut the door behind me, and fall against it. The bags drop to the floor. I allow tears now but none come.

Why is that last distance the hardest, when my little cave is at last in sight? Any number of tragedies may befall me then, when I'm too tired to defend. It's a wilderness out there, but I, indomitable forager, have returned home with victuals. I do my version of the caveman victory dance, which, instead of chortling, grunting, and swinging my club overhead, involves me pulling off my scarf, cracking a weak smile, and murmuring, "*Ca vas. Tout vas bien. Vous êtes ici, chez toi.* You made it, and you are alive."

Bubble Time: How Much Is Enough? (aka Planning and Pacing 101)

Remember when I said my doctor told me that most people with MCS and/or ILS end up living in a bubble the rest of their lives, and I decided that wouldn't be me? Well, this is a lifestyle decision you will need to make for yourself, because the amount of time you spend in your bubble directly affects your condition, and getting better can involve significant sacrifice. A simple equation:

Minimizing your excursions/adventures outside of the bubble

=

minimizing triggers

=

minimizing symptoms

=

minimizing overall impact of CS (and any CSS) on your life

Conclusion: To get clear(er), you need to rest in your bubble. We seek to do four things with bubble time:

1. to decrease the cumulative effects of triggers by reducing frequency of environmental trigger exposure and impact of certain intrinsic triggers;
2. to reduce the severity of acute symptoms over time by giving our central nervous system rest in a safe environment;
3. to recover from acute symptoms as quickly as possible; and
4. to help the central nervous system to desensitize and re-normalize over time.

In crisis phase, I had very little energy and a whole lot of pain and cognitive and fatigue issues, and every exertion or trigger made everything worse. I had no choice but to huddle in my bubble 24/7—leaving only when I had to go to the doctor, the grocery or drug store, or the unemployment or post office—quite simply, that was all I could do, and I lived that way for nearly a year. I was frightened, isolated, bored, depressed, and my life became this very small thing, so insular, I thought I would go mad.

Once I gained some stability and recovered a little energy and brain function, however, I found that I had a lot of trouble defining a task as "crucial" versus "delayable" or even "negligible." Instead of continuing to ignore tasks and activities that didn't matter, I returned to my old "pre–CS" way of doing things, automatically making a to-do list daily and getting it all done, no matter how taxing, or where it might take me. Of course, this only made me sicker. Eventually I realized that I had to do bubble time everyday, strictly prioritize tasks and errands, and make objective choices about when to rest and for how long, and when to leave the bubble and for how long. I call this process …

…Planning and Pacing 101

Big questions formed, filled my mind and demanded to be answered. How could I live, much less enjoy, such a managed, restricted life? I'd always done everything myself, and I enjoyed and prided myself on my autonomy. Besides that, I had few friends, and most of them were so busy trying to stay afloat in an expensive city that they had little time to spare to help me. What is worth leaving the bubble for, and what isn't? What kind of life can you have with CS and CSS? What are your priorities? What kind of life do you *want* to have?

It took me months to mull over these questions and restructure my life so that I had enough bubble time to keep my conditions from worsening while still getting the things done outside of the bubble that needed to be done and/or were too important to miss. I scribbled down ideas to help me sort it all out and ended up with something like Table 2. I recommend you try this process as well—considering and organizing your ideas on paper is far more manageable than trying to wrangle them in your head.

Table 2
My Bubble Excursion Priorities in Crisis Phase

Absolute Obligations	*Life / Social Events I'd Hate to Miss*	*Stuff That's Out of the Question Now (but I Hope to Do Once I Achieve Stability and, Eventually, Heal)*
Medical appointments that *must* be done in person (otherwise I use Skype)	*Some* (not all) weddings / funerals / milestone birthdays and holiday events	More holiday events / weddings / funerals, and milestone celebrations
Drug store / grocery runs when a friend can't go for me	*Some* (not all) friend or family performances	More friend or family performances, celestial events
Workers compensation faxing and mailing at copy store/post office when a friend can't do it for me	*Some* (not all) celestial events like rare eclipses, aurora borealis sightings, meteor showers, etc. (I really dig this kind of stuff—so sue me)	Meet friends in a café, restaurant, or bar. Go to a movie, rock concert, baseball game or symphony
Disability / Unemployment Office visits		Hiking, running, swimming, going to the gym (and pretty much everything I had to stop doing when I got sick …)
Library runs		

While single and dependent-free people with CS may find it easier to *prioritize* bubble time than someone who has a relationship or dependents, single people often have less support to draw from, making it more challenging for them to *actualize* those priorities. Know that whether you are single or in a relationship, with or without dependents, you can make it work. Be creative, and take the time to consider what absolutely requires your immediate attention or presence and what you can ask others to help with. It's so hard to imagine not doing things that you've always done, like driving the kids to soccer practice, or getting groceries, or posting mail, but once you break out of mindsets like "I must do everything myself" or "this has to happen *now*," or, my personal favorite, "this is the *only* way [to get whatever thing done]," you start to see options that will allow you to get the rest you need in your bubble.

For a while, everything seemed very impossible to me. How could I take care of everything I needed to and still get in enough bubble time so that I didn't get worse? I learned that sometimes I felt things were crucial to do on certain days or in a particular way, but when they didn't get done, the world didn't end. All was ok. And I learned that there are always ways to attend to the things that really were crucial. I got caught up easily in a sense of urgency and "doing things" and it took me months to get the hang of stopping myself, looking at my list of priorities, and seeing where the task belonged. If urgent and crucial, then I tried to get a friend to do it for me. If they could, great, and if they couldn't, then I planned to get it done in a way that allowed me to rest beforehand and recover afterwards.

While adapting to this new lifestyle, I often experienced a downturn in my health, what my doctors called a "setback," because I did too much, or spent too much time outside of the bubble, or had an extra bad ILS or MCS episode during a quick trip to the drugstore. These setbacks both frightened and disheartened me, but over time I learned that even with setbacks, if I did my bubble time, I kept moving in the direction I wanted to go: towards stability and healing. With that knowledge, my confidence grew.

Bubble Excursions

Maybe you live with or near someone who can run errands for you. Great! You won't have to leave the bubble nearly as often as someone who lives alone or has kids to shuttle around. Everyone needs to leave the bubble some time, however, so let's talk about how that works.

After I've prioritized my tasks and activities and deferred anything non-essential, I decide when excursions need to happen and schedule bubble time before and after each one. These mandatory rest periods make leaving the bubble manageable for me. *Manageable* means that the excursion does not cause a setback.

Because different folks have different nervous systems and degrees of sensitization and reactivity, there's a lot of wiggle room in this process. What serves as an appropriate amount of pre- and post-excursion bubble time for one person may be too much or too little for others. For example, I've tried bunching all my errands into one day and staying home the rest of the week, but this caused some very severe symptoms, and I'd be in bed for the next two weeks. Doing only one or two errands at a time, so I'm outside the bubble for short periods two or three times a week, works best for me, both in terms of mental health as well as decreasing severity of symptoms and recovery times.

This process of figuring out the correct amount of rest and activities for your particular condition is quite complicated and can take months or even years to figure out. I'll go into greater detail in the section on advanced planning and pacing later on, so you can fine-tune then. Right now, to get from crisis to stability, the basics will suffice. And you've learned almost all the basics by now. Believe it. Here, I'll put planning and pacing in context with what we've discussed so far:

1. Build your bubble.
2. Maximize your bubble time, resting within it and engaging the parasympathetic nervous system. This bubble time limits your exposure to environmental triggers and/or decreases the impact of certain intrinsic triggers.
3. Plan and pace: mercilessly limit your excursions, prioritize what absolutely must be done, and find ways to achieve that without leaving your bubble unless absolutely necessary. When you must leave the bubble, schedule adequate rest time beforehand and afterwards.
4. Minimize the damage done during excursions.

See? You've learned more than you thought—
Wait, minimize the damage done? How do you do that?

Good question. In crisis mode, the nervous system is so reactive that every excursion from the bubble can send you into a tailspin, back to bed for days, weeks, or months. So how do you manage outside the bubble and minimize the damage? At first, I managed by training my eyes and my breath.

My eyes, first of all, learned to identify triggers in two places: in the environment and on people. I learned to avoid the detergents and fabric softeners aisle in the drug store and grocery store (fragrances), as well as the blue-haired old lady whose hair doesn't move on a windy day (hairspray). The woman with the baby in a stroller—also to be avoided, as most babies, I find, are encased in blankets and clothing that have been fabric-softened (sticky fragrances). The man in the business suit (cologne or aftershave, or hair gel), the bohemian-looking boy (patchouli oil), the person with nicotine-stained fingertips (smoker) … you get the idea. At first, I worked in stereotypes alone—woman with baby = fabric softener, or man with gelled hair = liberal amounts of toxic cologne—but as time passed, I honed my skills at intuiting which people had strong scents about them that would trigger me. I also became adept at avoiding them while moving through a store as quickly as I could, to get whatever it was I needed and get out. I came equipped with shopping lists, memorized the layouts of stores and which aisles were impassable for me, and which were the most benign.

I also learned that some stores had "environmental-trigger-free zones," which I used in case of emergency. My safe zone in the grocery store is the freezer aisle. Whenever a wayward environmental trigger caused a coughing or sneezing fit or a wave of nausea, I'd go stand with my head in the ice cream freezer, focus on breathing, and pray to the toxin gods that I not pass out or throw up.

Sound far from ideal? Yep, crisis phase is the farthest from ideal we folks with CS can get. But if you absolutely must go to the store or office building or wherever in crisis phase, remember, your goal is to get in and out as quickly as possible, with the least amount of trigger exposure and impact. So, find your safe zones, avoid the worst areas, and add some of the following to your toolkit.

Transportation

When you have certain CSS (and sometimes with CS alone), buses, boats, trains, and planes can be traumatic and often harmful environments. My pre–CSS lifestyle depended on my ability to walk and run and take transit everywhere I went. I had no car and didn't need or want one. But when I got sick, I found that as my sensitivities increased, I could tolerate proximity to people's personal products less and less. During this time, brand new buses were assigned to the routes in my neighborhood, and the "new bus smell" made it impossible for me to breathe. Meanwhile, my increasing fatigue symptoms soon prohibited me from walking to and from transit stops and my destinations. I had to find an alternative.

Because of triggers, I couldn't take taxis or the specialized bus service for people with disabilities. I had to use some of my dwindling savings to buy a used car in order to maintain my autonomy. The good news is that this significantly cut my excursion time, stress, exertion, and environmental trigger exposures. The bad news is that I had to go to gas stations to fill up, an olfactory ordeal in itself. That said, the gas station was a once-a-month trigger, whereas I had been taking the bus or train several times a week. Although not perfect, this simple transportation accommodation is necessary and effective, and I have benefitted greatly from it.

I should mention that I struggled on transit for months before it even occurred to me to buy a car. Part of the reason is that I had never thought that I'd be able to afford a car, even when I had a full-time job. Another reason is that I had no idea how sick I was, or how long the illness could last. As I mentioned earlier, it can be very difficult to imagine the changes you need to make to adapt to life with CS and CSS. At the time, I couldn't imagine anything but my old lifestyle and had no concept of how drastically serious and chronic conditions can alter one's life. I thought there were only two ways it could go: I'd either die of whatever was wrong with me, or I'd be cured and back to "life as usual" in no time. Finally—and this is a biggee—I was living off savings and concerned about spending money on things I "really didn't need." I'd never needed a car. I was just being lazy. It really wasn't that bad, almost passing out every time I had to take a bus, choking and coughing and avoiding and …

Yep, that was my thinking back then. I had a very difficult time justifying the need for a car, and yet I needed a transportation accommodation in the worst way. What a blind-spot. I was lacking objectivity and self-compassion, for sure. One day, a friend suggested that I get a car, and I was struck by the obviousness of it. Are there transportation accommodations you can make that will significantly reduce stress and exertion impact, and environmental trigger exposure? If you aren't sure, talk to a friend, or better yet, have them spend a day with you, noting where you have difficulties, and then brainstorm and discuss ideas and options.

Note that defenses, strategies, and accommodations will most likely never make things perfect. They are tools to help you manage in triggerful environments and maintain as much autonomy as possible while keeping the impact of, and exposure to triggers at a minimum. Perfection is an ideal, and although I never say never, I accept that life is rarely the ideal. Defenses, strategies and accommodations can make things as manageable and healing as possible. That's the goal.

VISUALIZATION AND THE ART OF THE SIMPLE EXCURSION PLAN

I find it helpful to mentally review and rehearse my goal prior to entering any triggerful environment. For example, let's say I want to enter the drugstore and get tampons and TP while identifying and avoiding environmental triggers before they get to me.

First I ensure the goal is as simple as possible: Do I have a bunch of inessential things on my list? If so, I trim the list. Am I planning on popping into the pet food store right after the drug store but feeling so poorly that it's a far too ambitious plan for today? If so, I decide to grab some low budget pet food at the drug store, just enough to get by until I can go to the pet food store another time. Once the goal is as simple as I can make it, I usually do the competitive athlete thing and envision my journey before the attempt. I picture myself entering the store and encountering no scented people, no triggering odors. I see aisles without customers, checkouts with no lineups, and me with no symptoms. Quick in and out. Of course, this is not realistic—it's best-case scenario—but we do what we practice, right? Practice calm competence, and reap the same. Practice success and succeed. I still get triggered when I go in, but visualizing beforehand reduces my anxiety, builds confidence, and bolsters courage.

Sometimes, though, when I'm doing the actual errand, I can't avoid an evil aisle, or a person drenched in synthetic fragrances sneaks up on me from behind. What are my defenses?

MENTAL AND SELF-TALK

Positive self-talk works much the same way as positive visualization. You may recall the "Soldiers" exercise, which I detailed in Chapter 1. When I enter a triggerful environment and feel the onset of symptoms, I tell myself, "You're ok. Whatever is in the air is normal. No one else is choking or sick, see? Look around…" stuff like that. Note that it's important to only say things you *believe* to be true. Don't lie to your brain. According to Dr. McGonigal, "it's never helpful to lie to yourself because the brain's not going to buy that."[13] Find something you believe to be true, and stick with that.

For months I did this supportive self-talk with no real results, or none that I could detect. Once my symptoms started coming, they hit me full-bore, and no amount of self-talk could stop them. But as time passed, I found that my self-talk could slow the onslaught of some ILS and MCS symptoms, long enough for me to evacuate the trigger zone and avoid a full-on episode. That was good enough to convince me. Self-talk became an essential part of my bubble excursion toolkit.

BREATH HOLDING/SHALLOW AND STAGGERED BREATHING

This one's both simple and tricky. Simple because all it requires is that I hold my breath when coming in close proximity to a visible environmental trigger. Walking through or near the detergents aisle, I hold my breath. Or, I hold my breath while hurrying through the newly carpeted lobby of my doctor's office building. Or, I take shallow, staggered breaths as I weave my way across a crowded mall concourse. The tricky part is, even a world-class free diver can hold her breath only so long, and I'm no free diver. You probably aren't either. So, you know, don't knock yourself out. Also, if you hold the breath too long, or experience duress or panic while holding the breath, then the muscles around the larynx tend to tighten. Thus, breath-holding should be employed in moderation, only in non-stressful situations, and for short durations.

THE SCARF TECHNIQUE

The scarf—it's not just a fashion accessory anymore. It's a tool and, used properly, a defensive weapon, indispensible for avoiding or reducing contact with environmental triggers. I wrap a long scarf two or three times around my neck and nose and mouth and breathe through the layers while in a triggerful environment. The scarf filters out some smells and particles and takes the edge off of others. It helps me to focus on things other than the irritating smells my super nose picks up, like the rhythm and sound of my breath, the feel of the soft fabric on my cheek, and my calming self-talk.

Surgical masks or oxygen masks are close cousins to the scarf. I can't wear them because they reek like bleach, plastic, or vinyl (to me) and thus trigger certain of my symptoms. Maybe you can tolerate them, which would give you more options. Options are good. The thing about masks though, is they tend to be less permeable than scarves. I'll talk about why this may work against you in the long run in the upcoming scent repertoire segments.

I have found that long turtlenecks can work in a pinch, although some days I can't wear anything tight around my throat without causing an ILS episode. Even a thick hand-kerchief in an easily accessible pocket can work, although scarves are good because, when wrapped properly, I can breathe through them hands-free. Since I'm usually wearing the scarf while in a checkout line or putting things in my cart, this is preferable for me.

OLFACTORY PANIC AND ANXIETY

It's pretty scary going out into the world when you don't know what sort of olfactory obstacles you may run into, or how severely they will affect you. Once you've experienced a killer migraine or lung-wrenching, blackout-causing coughing fit from a chance meeting with a new carpet or a well-perfumed personage, you may become excursion-shy, and the more episodes you have, the more frazzled your nerves, the lower your surprises threshold, and the thinner your faith in your own safety…. These are all natural reactions to terrifying circumstances. It is not uncommon for people with ILS or MCS—or with a CS-heightened sense of smell—to panic and/or feel anxious.

Besides causing an adrenaline rush, thumping heart, and drastic increase in symptoms, panic and anxiety can wreak havoc on your mental state. In my early CS days, they would obliterate my confidence with an avalanche of questions. What if I have to move again? What if workers compensation doesn't pay me anything? What if I can never work again? What if I succumb to anxiety and cower in my bubble forever more like a hermit and let myself go, growing a beard that eventually drags on the floor, wearing musty threadbare clothing, muttering and scribbling dark Poe-like poetry for all eternity…? (Yep, if you start thinking thoughts like that, it's a sign—panic and anxiety have dug their claws into you too.)

It took me over a year after diagnosis to get to the point where I didn't panic with every ILS or MCS episode or CS-related setback. Even now, after four years of dealing with these conditions, I still panic once in a while. It depends on my stress and fatigue levels, trigger load, the environment I'm in and how difficult it is to escape, and the severity of the symptoms.

Just remember that you are braver than most to even get yourself out the door of your bubble. When I was first diagnosed, my doctor felt that I was panicking overmuch when I came into contact with triggers I could smell—"Olfactory Panic," he called it— and yet I know that if he could be me for a day, he'd see the massive calm I wield relative to the amount of scary situations I must face. You too. If you get yourself outside, pat yourself on the back.

The next step is to resist panic. When I am confronted by an environmental trigger and feel panic, anger, anxiety or tears ramping up within me, and I can't remove myself from the situation immediately, I rely on several strategies to help me calm down:

- Breath holding, scarf technique, and/or self-talk—as discussed above.
- Mantra chanting (more on mantras in the chapter on coping).
- Distraction techniques—"Ohhhhh, hey, look at the pretty fire hydrant…" yep, as if I were a toddler. I often pretend I'm trying to distract two-year-old me from a dropped ice cream cone. The goal is to divert my focus from the environmental triggers and my symptoms. I immerse myself in a book, my phone, a song, a bird on a wire outside the window, my shoelace, etc. I force myself to focus on something, *any*thing other than the smell of triggers or how trapped I feel in a toxic place, or my shortness of breath or other symptoms.
- Vocal exercises—Worry not about what others think. Do this for yourself.
- Visualization techniques—I imagine my soldiers standing down, sleeping in barracks, or even sunning on the beach.

Probability of panic is also high when I go someplace advertised as "scent-free"—like a hospital or medical office or government building—but it doesn't turn out that way (I know, never expect *any* place to be scent-free, but sometimes I fall prey to wishful thinking, and my expectations rise. Then when I get there and it's so triggerful I crash and burn, I have even farther to fall. Sigh. *On y va.*)

As I've said, when I first got sick, things were pretty awful. I didn't know what was wrong with me, my world was topsy-turvy, and I became very anxious about breathing and finances and bills and everything. My GP said I had secondary anxiety and referred me to Outpatient Psych for group therapy. After a wait of several months, I got the call. A group was starting up in a few weeks. I had a long talk with the facilitator about the fact that I was sensitive to scents and synthetic chemicals and the group would need to be scent-free as well as chemical-safe. She assured me that they could accommodate me.

So I went to the humming, pressurized basement of the hospital's Outpatient Psych Building, inside a small room with a long table, around which eight or ten people were seated elbow to elbow. So close, I could smell the woman's breath next to me—coffee and stale milk—I think I could even smell her ear wax. The facilitators used white board pens that emitted a thin chemical odor that stung my nostrils and throat, and asked people to write their names on *Hello, My Name Is* … labels using Sharpie pens that made me cough, and handed out brand new vinyl PVC binders that were outgassing and incited a migraine. Everyone sat with their binders in front of them on the table, at chest level, prime smell range. I was surrounded. Even when I leaned back away from the table and breathed through my scarf, I could smell it all. Within the first five minutes, my throat was closing, my head was throbbing, and my nose was running like a river.

The facilitators hadn't told people ahead of time that the group was "scent-free." They didn't even mention it during the first session. I had to pull a facilitator aside. "I was told this group would be scent-free as well as chemical-safe," I said, "but people are wearing fragrances, and you're using materials that off-gas, and it's making me sick."

"Oh," she said, as if this was news. "Well, you are welcome to say something to the group after break, if you want."

"That's putting me in the position where I'm asking people for a personal favor just so I can breathe," I said. "This is very different from what I was assured on the phone."

"Well, we can't enforce a scent-free policy," she said.

"Why not?" I said. "The hospital, officially, is a scent-free zone, and this is part of the hospital."

"Yes, but we can't tell people what to wear," she said. "You know, part of group therapy is that it's your responsibility to behave like an adult and tell your group co-participants how you feel when you can't breathe."

"That's interesting," I said. "Because I thought my responsibility was to show up and participate in a therapy group about anxiety, not lobby my peers for my right to breathe. I thought it was your job to ensure that the group is safe for all participants, and that all participants have equal access. Would you hold sessions in a room accessible by stairs only and tell a person who needs to use a wheelchair that she has to ask the group if they'd be willing to meet in a room that had ramp access?"

"No, of course not," she said, "but everyone can see the wheelchair."

I had to smile. The ADA would be proud to hear how ingrained their decades of lobbying and fighting for rights for people who need wheelchairs, scooters, and walking aids had become. "And I have no wheelchair, so it's ok for you to discriminate against me?" I said. "You don't make someone in a wheelchair ask for favors of the other participants just so she can have a safe place to be in the group, yet you expect me to do that very thing."

Her expression changed, as if she were having a real *a-ha*, the moment all teachers strive for in the classroom. "You'd provide a room with ramp access for someone in a wheelchair," I said. "I need a room with scent-free access, as I told your boss weeks ago when she put me into this group. You need to provide that for me."

"I understand," she said. "I'm sorry, but we can't provide that for you."

"But I was told—" I stopped myself. I was getting nowhere with that one. "What about one-on-one counseling?"

"I'm sorry but we don't provide that."

"What do you provide?"

"This might be helpful for you." She handed me a DVD, brand new, in a black plastic case that was shrink-wrapped, and as the odor of new plastic made its way into my nose and down my throat and I began to cough, I thought, man, she *really* doesn't understand my conditions at all. She's just handed me a trigger with a smile!

I know she meant well, but she was so clueless. I was clueless too. I had expected that health care providers would understand my conditions better than anyone else.

The loss of the group counseling was a hard blow. For months I'd held out hope, believing that the group might help me find strategies to deal with the anxiety I was experiencing everywhere. When it fell through, my hope dispersed like steam into air. I was empty. I'd been trying to find solutions to these problems for nearly a year now, yet every avenue I tried—to get myself help, to get compensation, to heal, to move away from despair—every avenue ended up blocked. Each disappointment seemed more severe than the last. And I was running out of options. I kept wanting things, then losing them, then changing what I wanted, then losing that. What would happen when there was nothing left that I cared about?

(Once such questions besiege you for a long enough time, and no answers appear, anxiety can morph into depression. I'll talk more about that in the chapter on coping.)

Preparing for and Recovery from Excursions (aka Planning and Pacing 102)

I always plan for bubble time before and after each excursion, as I've said. If I go out again before I've recovered from the last excursion, severity of symptoms and recovery times multiply. Depending on your condition(s) and symptoms, you may not need as much bubble time as I do, or you may need more. Unfortunately, there is no standardized guide for this. It will take you time, trials, and errors to find what works for you. To give you an idea, Table 3 shows what a sample week looked like for me when I was extremely ill, in crisis phase.

TABLE 3. MY PLANNING AND PACING IN CRISIS PHASE

	Mon	*Tues*	*Wed*	*Thurs*	*Fri*	*Sat*	*Sun*
a.m.	Bubble time	Bubble time	Bubble time	Bubble time	Bubble time	Bubble time	Bubble time
Mid-Day	Doc appointment	Bubble time	Grocery run	Bubble time	Bubble time	Bubble time	Bubble time
p.m.	Bubble time	Bubble time	Bubble time	Bubble time	Cook soup for week	Work on Workers Compensation stuff	Do one load laundry
Eve	Bubble time	Bubble time	Bubble time	vacuum	Bubble time	Bubble time	Bubble time

Note the amount of bubble time I needed to prepare for and recover from an excursion, or even from doing a daily living activity like vacuuming the apartment. This intensive amount of bubble time can take a huge toll on your mental health, especially if you are single and live alone. I'll talk about how to maintain mental health in the chapter on coping.

I was in really bad shape when I finally figured out what was wrong and how to get out of crisis phase, so I had to live by that first activity/excursion plan for about nine months before seeing improvement. Remember, and I cannot stress this enough—I have *three* CSS, which means a *lot* of system reactivity—you might have a lot less reactivity than me. Or you might be dealing with chronic pain and require more bubble time than I did in crisis phase. Respect that. Plan for what you need now. Just because you need so much bubble time today, it doesn't mean you always will.

Here's proof: Table 4 illustrates how things looked for me a couple years later, when my conditions had stopped worsening and I had reached stability phase.

TABLE 4. MY PLANNING AND PACING IN STABILITY PHASE

	Mon	*Tues*	*Wed*	*Thurs*	*Fri*	*Sat*	*Sun*
a.m.	Bubble time	Bubble time	Bubble time	Bubble time	Bubble time	Bubble time	Bubble time
Mid-Day	Doc appointment and drug store	Work on Workers Compensation stuff	Grocery and library run	Medical scheduling, planning and research	Cook soup, fish & other stuff to freeze & eat next week	Work on Workers Compensation stuff	Do two loads laundry, watch a movie or read
p.m.	Bubble time	Bubble time	Bubble time	Bubble time	Bubble time	Bubble time	Bubble time
Eve	Cook dinner & do dishes	Cook dinner & do dishes	Cook dinner & do dishes	Cook dinner & do dishes	Cook dinner & do dishes	Cook dinner & do dishes	Order dinner, no dishes

Looks a lot more functional than Table 3, eh? For one thing, I'm actually eating a real meal and doing my dishes at least once a day—no more surviving solely off protein bars, soup, and smoothies, or piling up dishes in the sink for days.

Remember, this is merely a basic, big picture plan to show you how things can change in general. Let's look at a more detailed plan so you can see the smaller picture:

TABLE 5. MY STABILITY PHASE PLANNING AND PACING, WITH MORE DETAIL

	Mon	Tues	Wed	Thurs	Fri	Sat	Sun
7 a.m. to noon	Alternate resting in bubble for 20-minute segments with getting dressed and eating breakfast in 10-minute segments	Alternate resting in bubble for 20-minute segments with getting dressed and eating breakfast in 10-minute segments	Alternate resting in bubble for 20-minute segments with getting dressed and eating breakfast in 10-minute segments	Alternate resting in bubble for 20-minute segments with getting dressed and eating breakfast in 10-minute segments	Alternate resting in bubble for 20-minute segments with getting dressed and eating breakfast in 10-minute segments	Alternate resting in bubble for 20-minute segments with getting dressed and eating breakfast in 10-minute segments	Alternate resting in bubble for 20-minute segments with getting dressed and eating breakfast in 10-minute segments
noon to 3ish p.m.	Doc appointment and drug store. Arrive at each place at least 15 minutes early and rest in car before going in. Rest in car afterwards for at least 20 minutes.	Work on Workers Compensation stuff in 10–15-minute segments, taking 30-minute bubble breaks in between	Grocery and library run. Arrive at each place at least 15 minutes early and rest in car before going in. Rest in car afterwards for at least 20 minutes.	Medical scheduling, planning and research in 10–15-minute segments, taking 30-minute bubble breaks in between	Cook soup, fish & other stuff to freeze & eat next week in 10–15-minute segments, taking 30-minute bubble breaks in between	Work on Workers Compensation stuff in 10–15-minute segments, taking 30-minute bubble breaks in between	Do two loads laundry, watch a movie or read in 10–15-minute segments, taking 30-minute bubble breaks in between
3ish p.m. to 5 p.m.	Bubble time	Bubble time	Bubble time	Bubble time	Bubble time	Bubble time	Bubble time
5 p.m. to 8:30 p.m. or so	Cook dinner & do dishes in 10–15-minute segments, taking 20-minute bubble breaks in between	Cook dinner & do dishes in 10–15-minute segments, taking 20-minute bubble breaks in between	Cook dinner & do dishes in 10–15-minute segments, taking 20-minute bubble breaks in between	Cook dinner & do dishes in 10–15-minute segments, taking 20-minute bubble breaks in between	Cook dinner & do dishes in 10–15-minute segments, taking 20-minute bubble breaks in between	Cook dinner & do dishes in 10–15-minute segments, taking 20-minute bubble breaks in between	Order dinner, no dishes in 10–15-minute segments, taking 20-minute bubble breaks in between

Note that I schedule in lots of little breaks when I'm doing anything requiring exertion—mental, emotional, or physical—like research or dishes or laundry. You may need micro rest breaks too. Remember also that CS and CSS are fluid, and so are certain intrinsic triggers. Some days you have symptoms in the morning but not the afternoon, and other days it's the opposite. Some days you're under more stress, or your hormones are in flux, and so your symptoms increase and you need more bubble time than usual. My point is this: just because you have developed a pacing plan that works most of the time, that plan isn't carved in stone. With CS (and CSS) you must deal with what comes in the moment, so your plan can only be a guideline. You need to be prepared mentally for daily shifts.

In addition, once you've spent the time to figure out how much bubble time you need and develop a schedule that works for you most of the time, the work doesn't stop there. It's important to adjust your pacing plan ongoing, as the months pass and your reactivity decreases and you move from crisis to stability. It took me over a year, and several pacing plan adjustments, to get from the first chart to the second one. But it was, and is worth it. This tool will allow you access to the outside world without worsening your symptoms. And eventually, it will help you to move towards healing.

LAUNDRY AND SHOPPING SURVIVAL TIPS

Laundry and shopping are often two of the most challenging chores people with a sensitized nervous system face, simply because they tend to involve leaving the bubble, exposure to environmental triggers and all types of stressors, and strong sensory stimulation—bright lights, loud noises, strong smells—you get the idea. Here are my top tips for getting the tasks done with minimal consequences.

Doing Laundry in a Common Laundry Room or Laundromat

As I've said, scented laundry detergents and fabric softeners are made to "cling," so the scent will stay in clothing after the laundering process, and whatever sticky, tenacious chemicals make up these products can wreak havoc on the skin and respiratory and nervous systems. Laundry rooms in which people use scented products don't just smell toxic, they are toxic spaces. (Fabric softeners don't just emit fragrances, they emit *toxins*. Google it.) To be clear, I recommend that anyone with CS use "free and clear" products and avoid all contact with scented laundry products, whether or not you have environmental triggers, because of what they can do to your nervous system.

If you do not have laundry machines in your suite or house, I suggest you consider investing in an apartment-sized washer/dryer set. If that's not an option, how about asking a scented-laundry-products-free friend to let you come over and do your laundry there? Generally speaking, I don't recommend laundry services. They tend to use bleach and strong detergents, but perhaps you can make a deal with your neighborhood laundry professionals.

If none of the above will work and you must use a common laundry room or laundromat, plan time to rest pre- and post-excursion. The following strategies minimize my exposure and discomfort and may do the same for you.

- First and foremost, limit the amount of laundry you need to do. Whenever you do bubble time, wear the same clothes a few times before pronouncing them dirty. Hand wash undergarments in the sink and dry them on the shower rod or an indoor drying rack in between laundry room runs, or buy extra undergarments to avoid having to hand wash.
- When it's time for a laundry excursion, sort everything in your home so you have a separate pile for each load.
- Have your change sorted and in a pocket for quick access.
- Use hands-free scarf technique.
- Hold your breath as much as possible, and breathe through your mouth when you have to take new breaths.
- Arrive when the laundry room first opens in the morning (if you have 24/7 access, go pre-dawn when it's empty).

- Leave the door wide open when you enter, and turn off any unnecessary lights if they are too bright for you.
- If there are windows, open them all wide.
- Put money and soap in the machines, throw in the clothes, and leave.
- That's the easy part. Each time you return, the harder it gets because folks will have their bleach and scented stuff going by then, and exposures are cumulative, so your reactions will increase in severity each time too.
- When your washers are done, use the scarf and breath-holding technique and throw anything that can be dried in your home into your carrier and flee (with calm and dignity) to your apartment.
- If you must do a dryer load, use the same strategy you did with the washer. Fast in and out. Each time.
- If people ask you why you are covering your nose and mouth while you're in there, hand them an informational printout about the toxins in scented laundry products. A little education can go a long way, and if you have it printed out, you don't have to talk. (While you're at it, post your printout on the laundry room bulletin boards and anywhere else in your building. When you have an unknown and invisible disease, education makes a big difference.)
- As with everything, if you are experiencing high symptoms, do not attempt to do your laundry that day. Wait until you have a day with minimal symptoms and triggers. Your nervous system is taxed enough as it is.

Shopping

I recommend online shopping and making trips to actual stores only when you can't get something online. If you can't find a product used in classified ads/Craigslist, buy it new, preferably at least three months before you need it, and let it off-gas someplace (like an outdoor balcony, or a friend's house) until it doesn't trigger you. For groceries, I recommend asking friends if they will shop *for* you once a week, or whenever they go for themselves. Most of the people I know are incredibly busy, and it is difficult for even my most generous friends to provide a stable schedule, so that doesn't work for me, and it may not work for you either. If you have a large support network, however, you could schedule different people in each week, so each person only shops for you once a month. Another option is to order groceries from a home delivery service, if that is available in your area and not cost-prohibitive. Regardless, at some point, you will likely need to venture into stores. Here are my top survival tactics:

- Use your scarf and breath-holding technique. Take a breath only when you need to, and do so using your mouth, not your nose.
- Go at the end, or very beginning of the day, when crowds are smallest. This can be hard to do if you use transit, unfortunately.
- If someone strongly scented stands near you, walk away immediately, even if you haven't selected what you need from that area. You can come back in a few minutes. Don't let their nonchalance irritate you. Easier said than done sometimes, I know, but if you can accept that "stinky" people are part of the shopping challenge and move on, you will breathe easier, believe me.

- Probably the most important key to a successful shopping outing is to find safe zones in each store. Washrooms don't work for me because they usually house chemical air fresheners, scented soaps, bleach on the floors, and perfume-spritzing patrons. My safe zones at the local grocery store are the freezer aisles. The cold air from a freezer helps me to recover from a coughing fit. (Cold can trigger some people, so this may not work for you. Maybe the chicken roasting area is better for you, because it has heat lamps and yummy chicken smells?) Find places that feel safe for you. Hopefully you will never need them, but if you do, you'll be glad you scouted them out ahead of time.

- Drug Stores stock all kinds of out-gassers and scented stuff: appliances, computers, DVDs, cheap furniture, books and magazines, make-up, plastic bins, cleaning and personal products galore—and they always stock the unscented stuff right beside the scented, which makes no sense when you think about it. (Why not have an *unscented* aisle, you say? Yep, I say that too.) Basically, for someone with environmental triggers, drug stores can be a kind of hell. I have yet to find a safe zone there. All I can say is, know what you need, know where it is, wear your scarf, use your nosegay, have payment at the ready, and may your breath be with you.

I know I've said this before, but I always have to remind myself about this and I have a feeling you might need a reminder too: my health comes first. If I can't get to a store one day because I'm having intense symptoms or am super stressed or fatigued or in pain or whatever, the shopping can wait until tomorrow. Going on a bad day will make me sicker. If I stress out about not deferring my shopping, that also makes me sicker. If I REALLY need something on a bad day, I ask a friend to help, or look at delivery options.

Asking for Help

You may have family surrounding you with love and fixing your meals, church groups bringing cookies and casseroles, a scantily clad, adoring lover at your bedside fanning you with palm fronds and feeding you peeled grapes…. If any or all of the above, you are lucky indeed! But if you are like most people, you may find that the longer you are ill, the more the support coming from others dwindles. This can make life with CS even more painful and challenging. The thing about people is, most respond to novelty. If there's a hurricane on the other side of the world, people send blankets, money, and food to people they don't know—which is generous and compassionate, don't get me wrong—but when their next-door-neighbor has been living with a debilitating illness for years, people become blind to the fact that that person could use some help. (I'll talk more about this in the coping section.) Here are some ways to get what you need:

- **Identify assistance needs.** First, consider what you need help with and what you are comfortable with others doing for you. You may be ok with someone doing your dishes or driving your kids around, but not ok with someone doing your laundry. Figure this out before you ask for help.

- **Ask for help.** *Oh, so difficult!* At first I felt ashamed because I couldn't take care of myself all by myself anymore. I had to separate my feelings of self-worth from the limitations that my illness imposed upon me. This took time and practice.

- **Learn to ask for help without expectation that someone will agree.** This too, took time. At first when someone told me *no*, I felt rejected or angry or so life-or-death desperate that this person or agency *had* to help me because it was the *only* way for me to survive. There are many ways to survive, I've learned. Sometimes I can only see one way, but others eventually become clear. Rather than get angry when one option doesn't pan out, I focus on my remaining options and try one of them.

- **Learn who to ask for help with which issues.** Different people are willing to help in different ways. Some offer money, some cook, some prefer helping with cleaning, or by doing errands, etc. It took me over a year to figure out that someone who says no to one request might be very willing to say yes to another. During that time I received hundreds of negative responses—over 90 percent of the responses I got. It gets easier, the asking and the rejections (which, by the way, make the moments when I get a *yes* that much sweeter).
- **Re-ask friends for help as needed.** Periodically, I find I need to remind friends of my limitations and check in to see if they are still willing and able to help.

Review of Excursions and Planning and Pacing Basics

- The bubble is a safe, trigger-free place. It's one of the primary tools for resting, decreasing severity and duration of CS and CSS symptoms, engaging the parasympathetic nervous system, and moving from crisis to stability to healing.
- Part of moving from crisis to stability involves prioritization and limiting of tasks and activities so you can rest. Planning and pacing are a crucial part of this process.
- The first part of planning and pacing involves learning to identify which tasks and excursions are crucial (or not) and prioritizing accordingly.
- When you must leave the bubble, always schedule adequate bubble time pre- and post-excursion so you avoid setbacks.
- Planning and pacing can be a lengthy process, as it involves a lot of trial and error, and ongoing adjustments. Patience and diligence will pay off.
- Intrinsic triggers and unexpected environmental exposures may render a good plan invalid at times. Put your health first, and get back on your plan when possible.
- Asking for help may be uncomfortable at first, but you can learn how to do so and get the help you need.

> *Vulnerable we are, like an infant.*
> *We need each other's care*
> *or we will*
> *suffer.*
> —St. Catherine of Siena[14]

3. Fatigue, Pain, Relapse and Crash

Soup with a View

This essay portrays a typical day for someone in crisis phase with severe CFS, MCS, and ILS symptoms. It's not so different from a typical day for someone in crisis with any CSS, or with CS alone, in that the degree of symptoms is unpredictable, the limitations and restrictions are new, and the patient must develop and maintain a fluid expectation of what may be achieved at any given time. Daily living activities, excursions, and all other activities must be managed with that same fluidity.

* * *

I've made the bed, pulled on clothes. Now I'm sitting in the middle of my studio apartment with a protein bar in one hand, a glass of water in the other, and the expanse of the universe spread out before me. Some days this is as far as I get. Today demands more, and I'm rallying to the call. The call of the soup.

Not everyone hears the call of the soup, and even fewer heed it. The Soup Nazi and the Swedish Chef are two who could respond without balking. Probably Jamie Oliver. And I'm willing, but my body feels like a mini marshmallow encased in a ton of molded Jell-O. A real ton. Or is it tonne? The words drift into a wall of brain fog and disappear—billowing and blankety—fog like they get at the San Francisco airport in summer. My concentration dissolves. What was I thinking about? I feel certain I was thinking about something, but I cannot access whatever it was.

Dr. A, my Chronic Fatigue specialist, says this is a common symptom. He says not to keep trying to focus, or achieve, when I feel this way. "The more you push through things, the more likely you will go down the drain," he always says. Down the drain means bed-ridden for at least a day or two, my limbs and torso heavy like lead, my body feverish, and my mind on another planet. One with lots of haze. Like Neptune. Or Los Angeles—

Soup! That was it. My heart thumps harder than usual for a few beats, like the tail of a dog whose master just came home from work. I need to make a pot of soup that will feed me for 7–10 days. With brain fog this severe, I shouldn't be doing anything, especially involving knives. Trouble is, I've deferred this task for two days already and have nothing to eat now but frozen chicken or protein bars (and that's all I ate yesterday). Sometimes you gotta push through.

It's not a simple decision to make. There's a whole dynamic at work here among the various voices of me.

The Survivor says *you must do this or you starve. Just get it done.* (That's a peptalk as far as the Survivor is concerned.)

The Philosopher says *how is one supposed to heal if one doesn't have the strength to make food? And if one doesn't have the strength to make food ...* (You can see where that is going, and the Philosopher is just getting warmed up.)

The Caretaker says *you can't push yourself like you used to. It will only make your symptoms worse. Wait another day.*

Another inner voice, a little louder than the others, says *you're all exhausting me. I wish I had some grace.* (I'm not sure what to call that voice.)

Fuel first. A Clif Builder's Bar. I've been experimenting with supplements and foods, looking for the right combination to help me do what I must, and to lessen the recovery time needed afterwards. Dr. A is skeptical about supplements affecting Chronic Fatigue. But sometimes it seems to me that this bar helps me endure a workout. A year ago, a workout was an hour in the gym or a 5k run along the seawall. Now, it's making soup.

My little apartment·sits halfway up a mountain on the northwestern edge of Vancouver. Windows form the southern wall, with a glass sliding door in the middle that opens out onto a large covered balcony. Beyond that, English Bay below, the sky and universe above. I gulp down the view like a trapped mouse and savor small bites of my bar like a free one. The bar's layering of creamy chocolate on top of crunchy nuttiness makes it far more palatable than most of its species. I chew each morsel into gritty mush before I swallow. Then a sip of water. Sipping and eating like this helps reduce my cough, but my nose still runs. Dr. M, my ENT specialist, says the source is too much acid reflux, caused by my body overprotecting itself after the chemical exposure last year. My Traditional Chinese Medicine practitioner J— says the source is my kidneys leaking into my lungs because the kidneys have become so depleted that any digestive activity is a stressor. Two profoundly different explanations from two experts. This disparity was once unsettling, but I've come to believe they are both saying the same thing, in different languages.

Nutshell: the fatigue, the digestion and breathing issues—all were given to me by a careless corporation in exchange for a day's work and are mine now to deal with, to solve if I can, to accept what I can't solve.

I swallow some frustration with the last bit of bar, wipe my nose, and focus my attention outwards. English Bay is a smooth grey slate this morning. The cargo ships seem to be embedded in its surface, like miniature toys stuck in the frosting on a child's birthday cake. The ships are the color of rust and charcoal, some with white lettering along their long, low sides. They all point east, ten of them, anchored from their prows, angled by the current, spaced apart from each other on a grid the scale of which only sea captains know. The expansiveness quietens my inner voices. A disproportionate heaviness in my body begins to tug at my awareness, pulling me like gravity through the chair, down into the floor. I flow down the mountain—past scattered buildings and trees, past trails I used to hike, past the pool where I swam, the seawall where I ran—into the bay, where I will float like a jellyfish for the rest of my existence. The waves undulate beneath me, brackish air stings my nostrils, waves *slosh* and *slap* against the shore. I revel in the weightlessness of my limbs ...

Eventually, I rouse myself from … what? A non-slumber? A reverie? No, something deeper, for which English has no words. I rise and walk the 20 paces across my apartment. Some days, too much sitting is worse than no sitting at all, and my hips complain as if they've carried me for 80 years instead of only 43. I wince and shake my legs out.

The Caretaker says *just be happy you aren't running the marathon next month after all!* The joke falls like a baby's mitten into a puddle of sad, and the Philosopher points out that it's too soon for that kind of humor. Maybe tomorrow.

Galley-style, long and narrow, my kitchen is like a dead end in a lab mouse maze. It has dingy, pocked linoleum, a chipped Formica countertop, and off-white painted cupboard doors above and below. A stainless steel sink to my right, and a three-quarter-size fridge to my left. I lift the crockpot from a lower cabinet and set it on the counter. I pull the veggies from the fridge and dump them beside the crockpot. I work in silence.

Another time, I would be a multi-tasking dervish—boiling rice on the stove, popping home-made bread into the oven, along with some marinated tofu layered with zucchini and onions and thinly sliced fingerling potatoes—the ones that taste buttery when undressed. On a whim, I'd soak the terra-cotta roaster, prepare some garlic bulbs, and stuff them into the oven. Then I would start the soup, pouring in a rich base of homemade stock, followed by some beans I'd soaked overnight and pressure-cooked. I'd sift through my collection of spices and select the ones the recipe of the week called for. I would complete my tasks in the most efficient order and clean as I went, the way my father trained me. I would have music playing and would sing and dance around the kitchen like some illegitimate Von Trapp child whose spirit cannot be broken even though she's doomed to work as a scullery maid for all eternity.

Now, silence. If I listen to music while concentrating on something else, my skull will ache, like an intense sinus pain, but in the bones, not the cavities. I don't know if this is a Chronic Fatigue symptom, or my body displaying yet another intolerance to something I once adored. I try not to think about it.

Maybe it will go away, says the Caretaker.

I nod. That strategy never worked with school bullies, but my brain is reprogrammable. I believe it.

As for multi-tasking, I seem to have misplaced that capability in the past year. Some days it's all I can do to mono-task. I don't bother to sort through the vegetables and order them for simplest cleanup. I don't use recipes or spices other than sea salt. I buy the same veggies every time I shop, and the soup is a chunky broth, its base a store-bought bouillon in a box. What matters is getting nutrients in, not gourmet taste. What matters is getting the job done. I focus on the goal: chop and dump all veggies into the pot. Veg in pot. Chop and dump. Ready, go.

Red onion. Many scents can trigger coughing fits, but onion has an oily pungency sharper than a butcher's knife, so I hold my breath, imagining I hear a stopwatch ticking as I peel and chop. Ticking away the time I have to achieve my goal like I'm on some insane game show. Non-uniform onion bits fly into the crockpot. Wash hands, board, knife. I exhale slowly as I pour in some boxed bouillon and water, put the lid on. Shallow inhale. No coughing.

Good. Eyes only barely stinging, nose running, heart pounding. The stopwatch clicks off. I'm tired already.

Push through, says the Survivor.

I comply without thinking.

The leek goes in without a fight, but the yam and celeriac stand their ground and I back away. My body wants to slide to the floor and lie down.

The Caretaker reminds me of Qi Gong guru Lee Holden's teachings: *energy is breath and breath is energy.*

I take deep breaths now, willing more energy into my body while distracting my mind with musings on celeriac, the magical mystery root. Inhale. Celeriac looks like a brain, it smells like celery when injured, but I don't really know what it is. Exhale. When I eat it, it tingles inside me like pure energy. Inhale. I'd eat it every day if I had the strength to prepare it. Exhale. The breathing is working. I dump the celeriac and yam bits into the pot and don't feel any worse than I did five minutes ago.

A giant parsnip eyes me like an ace pitcher on the mound intimidating a rookie batter. I peel it, wishing the store had had wimpier parsnips. This one has a three-inch diameter at its top.

If one doesn't have the strength to cut through the parsnip, says the Philosopher, *how will one eat the parsnip to build the strength needed to cut—*

Don't think about that, says the Caretaker. *Think about breathing.*

I nod. Inhale. Chop. Exhale. Chop. Inhalechopexhalechopchop …

Ten minutes later, the parsnip enters my vegetable *mélange*. My wrist throbs. Fever sends a chill rippling through my body. A cough rumbles within my lungs. My throat tightens. These are the warning signs. I replace the lid and hit ON. Toss broccoli and cabbage back into the fridge. At least I got the basics done. I have to get used to finding satisfaction in achieving basics, not details. Leaving the counter a mess niggles at me like walking with a tiny pebble in one shoe.

Don't think about it. The Caretaker is working her new mantra like a yogi selling satori on a street corner.

I get a glass of water and return to the bed I made an hour ago.

Lying down, eyes closed, I feel the fever lose interest in me. It's 9 a.m. I've gone back to bed at 9 a.m. This is something I'd never let myself do, ever, unless I had a vicious cold, and during those rare times, the Survivor would say *don't get used to this. Don't get lazy.* I smile a half-smile. Sip my water. No rest for the—

That's the thing. Dr. A says I have to let myself rest, several times a day, every day, and it's difficult for me, because I don't really understand the concept of rest. In my life, I eat, I sleep, I do …

I mean, I *did*.

I did do. I did a lot. I did done. Am I really *done*?

My breath hits some resistance in my throat and stutters its way into my lungs.

Resistance nurtures only suffering, the Philosopher says.

I nod. And I again hear that voice within me longing for grace, which, to me, is the opposite of resistance. I prop up the pillows so I can see the edge of my balcony and the pale firmament beyond. The view that saves me, invites me, offers me solace when nothing and no one else does.

My friend Jana came to visit once, months ago. We sat on the balcony beside the sky. "I really admire how brave you've been through all this," she said, stirring her black coffee.

"You think?" I said, trying to repress a cough. "I feel like I've been kicking and screaming the whole way, ever since I got poisoned, railing against fate and assholes and the corporate-friendly system."

There was survival. And then there was bravery. I survived. But I didn't think of myself as brave. Brave to me implied dignity, pride, heroics. Survival was another thing altogether—messy and riddled with mistakes and fear and desperation. There was no heroism there. Just a mindless scrabbling for purchase while one dangles from a high, crumbling precipice during a 7.0 earthquake.

"It embarrasses me," I said, thinking of the countless times I steeped in bitter self-pity like a re-used tea bag before I found the courage to add some sugar, a splash of cream, or make a new cup. "What I'd give for some grace."

"You never give up," she said. "That's the important thing." Jana and I had been friends for years. During that time, she was often a voice of reason for me. If we'd lived in a Snoopy world, I'd have played a coarse and emotional Peppermint Patty to her circumspect Marcie.

I never give up? I felt unworthy of her esteem. I'd given up a thousand times, on hundreds of days, in millions of ways. The tears of despair that I'd cried could fill another English Bay or two.

The scent of onion broth wafts over to the bed and confers with my stomach. Reclining there, sipping water, after a 30-minute soup-making extravaganza has wiped me out, I think I'm starting to see what Jana meant. I still kick and scream sometimes, and maybe I always will. But I get up each morning. I get dressed, and I sit and stare out into the world beyond my window. Even if that's all I do for the whole day. Often I think, maybe I'll get used to being so alone. Maybe I'll get used to the small amount of energy I have, and the few things I can do on any given day. Maybe …

I give up sometimes, but I still think in maybes. I still look ahead. I don't have to worry about grace, I tell the unnamed voice within me. I've got some.[1]

Central Sensitization and Fatigue and Pain

If you are lucky enough to experience little to no fatigue or pain, you may be thinking that you don't need to read this segment, or that it's only for those with Chronic Fatigue Syndrome, Fibromyalgia (FM), and other chronic pain syndromes.

Nope. You should read it.

While we will look more closely at CFS—covering symptoms and impact on lifestyle, and how to reduce symptoms and move from crisis to stability, the information in this chapter is essential for all those with CS who experience any abnormal amount of fatigue, inflammation, or pain, heart rate surges, post-exertional malaise, sleep issues, and/or cognitive issues. Whether you experience such symptoms regularly, or only on "bad days," this chapter is for you. If you simply find you tire more easily than you did pre–CS, or your memory or thoughts are cloudier than before, this chapter is for you.

If you have CS but have never experienced the above symptoms, that's great! To help keep your CS from worsening and potentially developing into any CSS, I *strongly* encourage you to read this chapter. You'll gain a more comprehensive understanding of how to best care for your sensitized nervous system and prevent increases in sensitivity and symptoms.

Chronic Fatigue Syndrome and Fibromyalgia Symptoms

To understand and learn how to manage fatigue and pain in the context of CS, we need to start with terminology. Remember the definition of CFS (used by the Centers for Disease Control and Prevention) that I gave you in Chapter 1? If not, no problem— it's quite similar to the Institute of Medicine's definition here:

1. "Reduction or impairment in ability to carry out normal daily activities, accompanied by profound fatigue;
2. Post-exertional malaise (worsening of symptoms after physical, cognitive, or emotional effort);
3. Unrefreshing sleep;
4. Cognitive impairment; and
5. Orthostatic intolerance[2] (symptoms that worsen when a person stands upright and improve when the person lies back down).

Other common manifestations of ME/CFS include pain, failure to recover from a prior infection, and abnormal immune function. At least one-quarter of ME/CFS patients are bed- or house-bound at some point in their illness. Symptoms can persist for years, and most patients never regain their pre-disease level of health or functioning. ME/CFS patients experience loss of productivity and high medical costs that contribute to a total economic burden of $17 to $24 billion annually."[3]

According to the Centers for Disease Control and Prevention, "Fibromyalgia is a condition that causes widespread pain, sleep problems, fatigue, and often psychological distress. People with fibromyalgia may also have other symptoms, such as

- Morning stiffness.
- Tingling or numbness in hands and feet.
- Headaches, including migraines.
- Irritable bowel syndrome.
- Sleep disturbances.
- Cognitive problems with thinking and memory (sometimes called "fibro fog").
- Painful menstrual periods and other pain syndromes."[4]

Generally, for diagnosis, the pain needs to have been present for at least three months, and the patient must not have a disorder that would otherwise explain the pain. Other symptoms common to FM patients include low exertion tolerance, and sensitivity to temperature/humidity, light, sound, smells, and touch.

Nutshell, FM is not just "feeling pain," and CFS is not just "feeling tired," as many people who have heard only the syndrome names assume. These conditions, and POTS too, affect patients on a physical as well as cognitive level. They may have trouble reading, writing, concentrating, acquiring vocabulary, and/or they may experience poor short-term memory or brain fog. Their limbs may feel heavy, sore, and/or inflamed. Exerting beyond what their sensitized system will tolerate, or being exposed to/impacted by too many triggers, causes them to experience *Post-Exertional Malaise* (PEM).

PEM is a temporary increase in symptoms that can last for somewhere between an hour (ish) and several months. Basically, there are three levels of PEM:

- If symptom increase is of low severity and lasts only an hour, or half a day or so, it is referred to as plain old *Post-Exertional Malaise.*
- If symptom increase is of moderate severity and lasts for more than a few hours, up to ten days or so, it is referred to as a *relapse* or *flare-up.*
- If symptom increase is severe and/or lasts for a prolonged period from ten days to weeks to months, it is called a *crash.*

In my experience, a crash feels like the worst hangover and most treacherous flu I've ever had, combined with what I imagine I'd feel like after being stomped on by a bellowing Sasquatch and flung over a cliff onto a glacier, where a pack of wild dogs gnawed on my limbs for two days before I got rescued. (Yep, fun times.) My shortest crash lasted a month. The longest, about three. That was before diagnosis and my CS and CSS education, of course. I still have crashes, but they are usually *planned*, and I can take steps beforehand to minimize their effects. (More on planned crashes soon.) If you are single and live alone, you may wish to create a "crash plan" to ensure your safety and the fastest recovery in the event of a crash. See Appendix D: For Singles with CS Who Live Alone—A Crash Plan for more information.

What if you have been diagnosed with CS or a syndrome other than CFS, FM, or POTS, yet you experience some of the above symptoms?

Good question. Remember when I told you about symptom overlap among CSS? This is a great example of that phenomenon. A sensitized nervous system is working too hard, so many people with CS tend to experience some level of fatigue, PEM, cognitive impairment, sleep issues, gut issues, pain, and/or inflammation, no matter which CSS their diagnosis contains (if any). So don't let it worry you. Just keep on reading to find out how to minimize these symptoms.

The CS Crash Cycle

People who have CFS, FM, or POTS but don't know it, or who have been recently diagnosed, can easily get caught "in an endless push-crash cycle in which patients do too much when they feel better, crash, rest, start to feel a little better, do too much again, and so on."[5] Many people with a CSS other than those three (or with CS alone) may fall into a crash cycle too, merely to a lesser degree. For example, they may be experiencing some mild cognitive issues, and/or find that they need a long nap every few days. They don't crash as hard, or for as long, and their symptoms may manifest only as minor inflammation or pain and/or small decreases in functionality or cognitive ability rather than significant impairment, but many folks with only CS (or with other CSS) do, without knowing it, crash.

So, for our purposes, I'll be using the term "crash" to refer to the severe crash someone with CFS, FM, or POTS may have, as well as the lesser crash someone with only CS or with a different CSS may experience. Both types of crash-boom-bust cycles revolve around the same things: over-exertion and/or trigger overload resulting in exacerbation of symptoms and decreased functionality.

Before I got a diagnosis and could wrap my head around how to manage it, CFS was like an evil fairytale giant intent on destroying every aspect of my life in one fell swoop. It snatched away all the things I loved and knew and replaced them with murky, heavy, dimness. It worked a spell on me that made everything—my thoughts, my body, my abilities—muted, almost numb, except for the pain. And the pain was distinct, pulpy, hot and torturous. All was relentless. I suffered in ignorance for over a year. I'd go for a short run or a long walk and end up on the couch, writhing in pain, with diminished cognitive performance, for weeks. Then I'd feel a bit better and go for a walk or run and end up on the couch, again for weeks. (Are you seeing a boom-bust pattern there? Good. It took me a lot longer to perceive it.) I tried and failed to get short-term and then long-term disability. The insurance company basically laughed me out the door. I eventually had to stop working and came to believe my brain and body were packing it in for good.

With diagnosis and education, that all changed; eventually, I escaped the CS crash cycle by working on three key points:

1. Opt out of the cycle. It's hard not to go for the gold on a good day, but you will pay for the over-exertion hundred-fold. Opting out of the cycle requires planning, knowing and respecting your functional capacity and exertion tolerance threshold, and pacing. I introduced basic planning and pacing in *Decreasing Trigger Exposure and Impact*, and will go into further detail momentarily. Depending on your condition and situation, the process of getting out of the boom-bust crash cycle could take weeks, months, or years. Hope for the short path but prepare mentally for the long haul.

2. Trust that your brain is doing the best it can and that if you give it what it needs the cognitive issues may very well decrease, or vanish altogether. (I'll detail what the brain needs in the *Brain Health* segment; meantime, speak nicely to your brain. Encouragement really does help.)

3. Severe symptoms can wreak havoc on your income and finances. I recommend that you create temporary financial stability as soon as possible. A good six to nine months' worth, if you can manage it, will reduce mental and emotional stressors and enable you to focus on getting out of the crash cycle and crisis phase. Depending on your symptoms and circumstances, that may mean quitting work altogether and living off savings, or taking out a personal loan (note: loans are far easier to get *before* you quit your job). Or it may mean getting short-term or long-term disability from your workplace. It may mean working only part-time from home, applying for medical employment insurance or a disability pension. If your finances are already in dire straights, you may wish to skip ahead to *Maintaining Autonomy* for ideas on how to stabilize this aspect of your life. It's a real challenge, figuring out CS (and any CSS) and escaping the crash cycle while solving financial conundrums. You can do it. You may need to ask a trusted friend for help if your cognitive issues are too severe, but you can get it done.

4. There is a fourth step that many folks with CS need to deal with before they can escape the crash cycle, and it has to do with severe debilitation due to intrinsic triggers, psychological issues, and pain. If sleep, stress, diet/gut, acute illness or

injury, and/or hormonal imbalance issues are causing severe debilitation and greatly impacting your quality of life, you may need to skip around to those segments before reading further. Moving from crisis to stability is contingent upon getting enough sleep and nutrients and functioning at a certain level. If any of the above intrinsic triggers is creating significant problems or distress for you in crisis phase, it should be addressed as soon as possible. If the above triggers are causing minimal symptoms, then you may be able to wait until stability phase to find ways to treat them. As always, consult your doctor.

The same applies when dealing with debilitating psychological issues and/or pain. Escaping the crash cycle while enduring severe pain or other seriously debilitating symptoms is next to impossible. Bubble time should help decrease all symptoms, especially over the longer term, but you may need to seek treatment to get severely debilitating symptoms to a manageable level, at least in the short term. Prescription medication is a common solution for this. I encourage you to read the next segment before going that route.

PRESCRIPTION MEDICATION FOR PAIN AND OTHER SEVERE SYMPTOMS

Prescription drugs may help reduce severe physical pain and other CS- or CSS-related symptoms. For example, a 2014 report states that the following drugs have had some success in managing FM pain: "tricyclic antidepressants … SNRIs (duloxetine and milnacipran) … gabapentin and pregabalin … Pramipexole, tramadol, other opioids and cannabinoids (nabilone)."[6] I encourage you to consider prescription medication if your doctor recommends it.

When I say, "*consider* prescription medication," I don't suggest that you take it without question. **Always research any treatment your doctor recommends before trying it.** To research medications, use a reliable website like the U.S. National Library of Medicine, or the Mayo Clinic. At the very least, find out the following:

- What problems does the medication treat? (Ensure this matches what your doctor wants to treat.)
- What are potential side effects and what percentage of patients experience them?
- Is the drug safe to take with any other medication(s) you are already taking?
- Is the drug addictive? How long can one safely take it?

Take notes and write any questions down for a discussion with your doctor, which should include the following:

- Ask about common signs that the drug is working and signs that it's not working. Write them down.
- If you have reservations about a certain medication, express them to your doctor. If you question whether certain risks outweigh potential benefits, say so. Perhaps there is a similar medication that has fewer side effects and can provide similar relief.
- Be sure you're clear on whether this is a long-term drug or temporary, and if temporary, ask when you should stop taking it.

- If you have other questions, ask. If your doctor discourages your questions or discussion regarding treatment options, you may wish to find a doctor who invites your participation in your own treatment. (Doctors certified in Functional Medicine are one such option. I'll talk more about this in Chapter 6.)

Ensure you know all you can about prescription medication options before you make your decision. And remember, it is *your* decision to try a treatment or not, just as it is your decision to stop taking a medication if it is not doing its job or is harming you in some way. No treatment is perfect. All you can do is find a doctor you trust, do your research, discuss with your doctor and then make an informed decision. If the treatment helps, great. If not, then you and your doctor can take the next step—possibly other forms of treatment. I'll discuss these in the upcoming neuroplasticity and chronic pain segments.

Meanwhile, doing bubble time and using strategies from the coping chapter will provide long-term support and bolster your health throughout your lifetime.

Learning Your Functional Capacity and Exertion Tolerance Threshold

Functional Capacity (aka energy limit, or energy envelope) is the total amount of time per day that one can be active without increasing symptoms or decreasing functionality (so, all but bubble time and sleeping). *Exertion Tolerance Threshold* is the point at which one gets symptoms (for any given activity). These terms will make more sense in a moment when I show you how to calculate them.

In order to get out of the crash cycle and crisis phase, I had to learn my functional capacity and exertion tolerance thresholds, which required three things:

1. Stop trying to do what I considered "normal" activities.
2. Identify and heed "warning symptoms" that signaled the onset of acute symptoms (such as an ILS or MCS episode, for example), *Post-Exertional Malaise* (PEM), relapse, or crash.
3. A lot of experimentation (and a bit of math).

Number one was hard. Remember your basic planning and pacing? I had to smother my desire to run, to walk, to challenge my body physically. After 40-some years of fitness, sports and competitiveness, this was terribly difficult for me. I had to content myself with a one-minute-long walk—to a bench frequented by folks twice my age—and a few minutes of sitting there. When pain flared or brain power faded, I would trek back to my bubble for a rest. *Oh, so unsatisfying! I wanted only to fly and be free!* But after months of crash-boom-bust, during which I couldn't enjoy anything, I decided to abstain from what I considered "normal" athletic activities if it meant I could avoid being bedridden for weeks and could sit outdoors and do some limited activities around the bubble each day.

The second step challenged me in a different way. First I made a list of my PEM, relapse, and crash symptoms, which looked something like this:

- Inflammation
- Pain
- Limbs feel like lead
- Chest feels so heavy and thick it is an effort just to breathe
- Migraine headache

- Feverish
- Fluey aches—bones and joints—including eye sockets and brow bones
- Problems with lactic acid, resulting in burning sensations and pulpy muscles
- Can't read or write
- Can't concentrate
- Can't multitask
- Can't single task (generally only during bad crashes)
- Can't acquire vocabulary
- Little to no short-term memory
- Tachycardia with minimal exertion (like sitting up or standing up)
- Bad sleep, tossing and turning all night
- Sensitive to light and/or sound (generally only during bad crashes)

That was about it. Even if your crashes aren't this severe, I suggest you make a list of relevant symptoms here too, to help you identify your warning symptoms.

Next, I started tracking how I felt prior to each PEM episode, relapse, or crash. After a few weeks, I saw some common denominators that occurred prior to every onset:

- My facial bones, especially eye sockets and brow bones, would ache
- I'd feel flushed or feel feverish, with burny eyes and cheeks
- I'd become short-tempered, easily irritated, impatient (more than usual)
- I'd experience moderate word salad; that is, a discrepancy between what I meant to say and what came out of my mouth
- My muscles and/or joints would feel stiff and/or inflamed
- I'd feel dazed or confused
- I became clumsy (more so than usual)

These were my warning symptoms that PEM was coming. After identifying your warning symptoms, you can use them to "predict" and prevent PEM, relapses, or crashes. All it takes is some behavior modification and serious will power. Once I identified mine, I promised myself that whenever one or more of them made an appearance, I would cease and desist from whatever activity I was engaged in and do intensive bubble time until the warning signals retreated. This went against my grain. I like to finish what I'm doing before stopping, despite symptoms raring their heads. (My specialist calls this "pushing through.") Rule #1: Don't push through.

Once the warning symptoms have dispersed, I leave the bubble and investigate the incident. What was I doing before the warning symptoms appeared? Had I exposed myself to environmental triggers, or was my activity too strenuous for me? Or maybe I was doing something within my current abilities, but I needed to break it up into smaller increments of activity, with longer rests in between?

For example, let's say I was sitting upright in a chair, typing an email, for 20 minutes prior to getting warning symptoms. So, was the exertion of sitting upright the cause of those warning symptoms, or typing, or both together? I'd have to perform a controlled experiment:

- I waited for a good day, one with minimal exposure to environmental triggers and minimal impact of intrinsic ones.

- I sat upright for 20 minutes (without typing or doing anything else). If I got warning symptoms, I'd know that was too much.
- Then I'd try typing for 20 minutes while reclining in bed. If I got warning symptoms, I'd know that was too much.
- Next I'd try each of those activities at 15-minute durations. If still too much, then ten minutes, or five.
- Because you can only test yourself until you get symptoms and then must rest until they disappear, this experiment can take days or weeks.
- In the end, I had defined a handful of exertion tolerance thresholds—similar to Table 6.

TABLE 6. EXERTION TOLERANCE THRESHOLD RECORD

Activity	Exertion Tolerance Threshold Without Inciting Symptoms on a Good Day (low symptoms, low trigger exposure/impact)	Exertion Tolerance Threshold Without Inciting Symptoms on a Bad Day (high symptoms and/or trigger exposure/impact)
Sitting up at kitchen table	15 minutes	1 minute
Sitting up and typing	10 minutes	0 minutes
Typing while reclining in bed	20 minutes	2 minutes
Sitting up and chopping veggies	5 minutes	0 minutes
Standing and chopping veggies	1 minute	0 minutes

Note that the above example is from my crisis phase. At that time, I worked on making soup for five to 15 minutes, whatever I could do until developing warning symptoms, and then I did intensive bubble time, usually for 20 to 60 minutes until those symptoms disappeared. Then I got up and worked on the soup, or doing dishes or whatever—again, I could usually work for about five to 15 minutes before I had to rest. My whole day was like that—start then stop and rest, then pick up where I left off, then stop and rest, etc.— and yep, it can be maddening and insanely tedious and really, REALLY unsatisfying to do things that way. But that was the deal at that time. If I wanted to avoid relapses and crashes and maximize what I could do, then I had to operate within my exertion tolerance threshold, and I had to be sure not to exceed my functional capacity.

The planning and pacing 101 techniques I introduced back in Chapter 2 hold the key to learning your functional capacity. Once you have an accurate weekly plan, you can total your active time for each day and then calculate your weekly average. For example, Table 7 details the first three days from one of my weekly charts in crisis phase.

TABLE 7. MY DETAILED CRISIS PHASE PLAN

Time	Monday	Tuesday	Wednesday
7:00–7:10	Get up, robe on	Get up, robe on	Severe symptoms. Intensive bubble time/stay in bed
7:10–7:30	Bubble time	Bubble time	Intensive bubble time
7:30–7:45	Get dressed (while sitting as much as possible)	Get dressed (while sitting as much as possible)	Intensive bubble time
7:45–8:10	Bubble time	Bubble time	Intensive bubble time
8:10–8:20	Finish dressing	Finish dressing	Intensive bubble time
8:20–8:40	Bubble time	Bubble time	Intensive bubble time

Time	Monday	Tuesday	Wednesday
8:40–8:55	Feed cat /scoop litter/ put kettle on	Feed cat /scoop litter/ put kettle on	Intensive bubble time
8:55–9:15	Bubble time	Bubble time	Intensive bubble time
9:15–9:30	Sit up and eat protein bar/drink tea	Sit up and eat protein bar/drink tea	Get up, robe on, kettle on
9:30–9:50	Bubble time	Bubble time	Intensive bubble time
9:50–10:05	Sit up and finish eating	Sit up and finish eating	Bring tea and protein bar to bed and eat in recline
10:05–11:05	Bubble time	Bubble time	Intensive bubble time then nap
11:05–11:15	Make bed	Make bed	Nap
11:15–11:30	Bubble time	Bubble time	Nap
11:30–11:40	Brush teeth and hair	Brush teeth and hair	Feed cat /scoop litter
11:40-noon	Bubble time	Bubble time	Bubble time
Noon-12:15	Drive to doc appointment	Work on workers compensation stuff	Order grocery delivery, ask friend to pick up any immediate needs, or defer grocery trip until better. Reschedule library trip.
12:15–12:30	Rest in car once parked	Bubble time	Bubble time
12:30–12:45	Attend doc appointment	Work on workers compensation stuff	Bubble time
12:45–1:00	Rest in car	Bubble Time	Bubble time
1:00–1:15	Drive to drug store	Work on workers compensation stuff	Bubble time
1:15–1:30	Rest in car	Bubble time	Bubble time
1:30–1:45	Go in drug store	Work on workers compensation stuff	Eat soup
1:45–2:00	Rest in car	Bubble time	Bubble time
2:00–2:15	Drive home	Bubble time	Bubble time
2:15–3:00	Bubble time	Bubble time	Bubble time
3:00–3:15	Bubble time	Bubble time	Make/drink smoothie
3:15–5:00	Bubble time	Bubble time	Bubble time
5:00–5:15	Sit and eat protein bar for dinner	Cook dinner	Eat another protein bar, drink water
5:15–5:30	Bubble time	Sit and eat	Rest in hot bath
5:30–5:45	Bubble time	Bubble time	Rest in hot bath
5:45- 6:00	Bubble time	Do dishes	To bed and to sleep
6:00–6:15	Bubble time	Bubble Time	Sleep
6:15–6:30	Bubble time	Watch TV or check email	Sleep
6:30-on	Bubble Time and to bed	Bubble Time and to bed	Sleep
Total Active Time	190 minutes, so about 3 hours	220 minutes, so about 3.5 hours	100 minutes, so about 1.5 hours

Did you notice what happened there on Wednesday? Looks like PEM from the doctor and drug store on Monday. PEM often will arise after a 24- to 48-hour delay. We only looked at the first three days above, but my functional capacity for that week was less than 2.5 *non-consecutive* hours per day. As my health improved, of course, that number grew. My charts served me well. Putting my restrictions and limitations in black and white helped me respect them. It also helped me develop a sense of control and provided tangible proof of my progress as I began to regain some functionality.

As you can see, determining functional capacity and defining exertion tolerance threshold for every activity is extensive work. It took me over a year to get a grip on how little activity my body would tolerate each day, and how much of which activities I could do before getting warning symptoms, and I still have to remind myself that these thresholds are not carved in stone. They fluctuate, depending upon overall trigger load, on any given day. Even with that wild card, they are your key out of the boom-bust crash cycle.

And once you're out, life starts to look a lot different. Daily living activities—and fun stuff—can get done without inciting PEM, relapse, or crash. But exceeding functional capacity or pushing through exertion tolerance thresholds on any given day exacts a price, in energy, cognitive function, pain, or other symptoms. So, you have to plan and you have to pace, and do some math and, like anyone else with CS, you have to do bubble time.

Can I Avoid Relapses and Crashes Altogether?

According to my specialist, the short answer is no. Based on my experience, I tend to agree, although I believe that eventually I will heal my CSS and CS, and then experience relapses and crashes never more. In the meantime, I need to be prepared for PEM, relapses and crashes because (a) life is full of surprises and sometimes dumps more on me than my current functional capacity can manage—unavoidable environmental and intrinsic triggers, deadlines for workers compensation, a broken refrigerator causing unplanned emergency ice run, etc., can result in unplanned relapse or crash; and (b) I will always want to participate in certain amazing life events and adventures which will require me to exceed my functional capacity and, consequently incite what is called a *planned* relapse or crash. (I will discuss this strategy in Appendix E: Travel and Vacations with CS and CSS.)

I'm going to address *unplanned* relapses and crashes here. The deal is, although I can't prevent an unplanned relapse or crash, I can minimize its severity and duration. (And yep, you guessed it, this strategy revolves around intensive bubble time.)

When my warning symptoms hit hard enough to signal imminent relapse or crash, I do the following:

- Cancel any appointments for the next week to month, depending on anticipated severity of symptoms.
- Check the fridge and freezer and order grocery delivery, as needed.
- Put all daily living activities on hold until symptoms move from crash severity to relapse level, or from relapse to mild PEM level, and then do only what absolutely must be done (REST, eat, hydrate, relieve myself, etc.).
- Ask friends for help if something absolutely must be done while I'm in crash or relapse.
- Intensive bubble time, every day, until symptoms disperse.

I used to resist unexpected crashes and relapses no end. *I had all these plans for the week* (you know, relatively speaking) *and now I'm crashing and it's really messed up! I hate this! Rage against the fates and the machine and all corporate enterprises, etc.!*

That's where I went anyway …

It took over two years before I got to the point where I could drop whatever I was doing and duck and cover in my bubble for as long as it took to get rid of the crash symptoms, without resistance. I encourage you to find your Zen on this sooner rather than later. The more you resist, the more symptoms you get and the more energy you expend, energy that could be helping you get out of crash mode and back in the saddle, so to speak. Surrender. I never knew the word intimately until I got CS and three syndromes.

Remember, the goal is to stay within your functional capacity. If a relapse or crash foists itself upon you, get out from under as soon as possible. Setbacks are scary and disheartening, especially the first few times you encounter them, but if you keep your focus and do your intensive bubble time, those setbacks will become shorter, fewer, and farther between.

Review on Fatigue, Relapse and Crash

- Although patients with CFS, FM, and POTS generally exhibit symptoms like fatigue, cognitive impairment, unrefreshing sleep, pain, and/or *Post-Exertional Malaise* (PEM), many people with other CSS, or with CS alone, find themselves dealing with varying degrees of any or all of these symptoms.
- PEM has three levels: *Post-Exertional Malaise, Relapse/Flare-Up,* and *Crash.*
- It's not uncommon for folks with CFS, FM, or POTS to fall into a boom-bust crash cycle. Folks with other CSS, or with CS alone, can also develop that pattern (usually to lesser degree) with regards to fatigue issues, physical and cognitive impairment, and other symptoms.
- Escaping this debilitating cycle is crucial for moving from crisis phase to stability. Strategies include opting out, trusting your brain, establishing temporary financial stability, and addressing severely debilitating intrinsic triggers, and pain and other symptoms as soon as possible.
- It is important to thoroughly research and discuss treatments with your doctor prior to trying them.
- Functional capacity is the amount of time one can be active per day (not including resting or sleeping).
- Exertion tolerance threshold is the point at which an activity incites warning symptoms, that is symptoms that serve as pre-cursors to PEM, relapse, or crash. Determining exertion tolerance thresholds for your activities is a consuming process but will pay back in spades as you continue to decrease flare-ups and crashes and eventually escape the crash cycle.
- Pushing through one's exertion tolerance threshold or exceeding one's functional capacity will cause PEM, relapse, and/or crash.
- Decreasing frequency, severity, and duration of unplanned PEM, relapses, and crashes is an important part of moving from crisis to stability phase.

> *… becoming healthy means not looking upon being sick as the only possible condition.*
> —Christa Wolf, *In the Flesh*[7]

4. Beyond Crisis—
Advanced Symptom
Management Strategies

Beyond the Abutment

He took my hand beside the train bridge abutment and helped me up the last steps to the top of the dyke. His hand was warm and strong. I used to dream of that hand caressing my face and body, tracing messages of love upon my skin. I dreamt of that hand holding mine as he and I wandered the world, adventuring and exploring, through the years. Those dreams were from another day, another life, but I was glad for his hand on this day as I conquered the dyke at turtle pace.

We emerged from the shadow of the abutment into the bright sun. A single train track at our feet ran north and around a bend to the east, out of sight. Old cottonwood trees had grown so tall on either side of the dyke that they seemed to connect the ground to the thin strip of azure sky above us, like columns in a great cathedral with a vast firmament painted upon its ceiling. My heart had been thudding triple time since we started the climb. I dropped his hand and reached for a nearby post. Red letters loomed above my head on a dirty white background: *No Trespassing*.

"There, see?" he said.

I nodded. A distance beyond the signpost, the train track ended at the edge of the abutment as if severed from its destiny. Mid-river, a single-track swing bridge sat open at 90 degrees. There was no one in the control booth. Made of dark, aged wood, the swing-span section looked as though it hadn't moved for months, maybe longer. I looked up again at the sign, then turned my back to it.

"What did I tell you?" he said. He was facing the trees on the west side of the dyke, arms flung wide, as if embracing the world.

Sure enough, interspersed among the cottonwoods, there was a different kind of tree, its leaves glossy and oblong, its branches laden with brilliant maroon and scarlet fruits. I'd never seen cherry trees anywhere but in an orchard, and I certainly had never expected to find them growing wild along a dis-used train track on the fringes of the city's industrial zone. Very tall, these would tower over orchard trees.

"Awesome," I said, meaning it literally. "Thank you." He was the only person I knew who could find a place like this and think to bring me here, besides my father, perhaps, who used to take me to pick cherries when I was young. This was more magical though. Train track, river, swing bridge, no orchard, no trespassing. No one else knew about this place—boughs and branches burdened with clumps of cherries could attest—not even the birds.

I couldn't ignore my racing heart any longer. "I have to rest now," I said, dropping onto a track rail. The metal burned through my jeans, so I slid down to the gravel between the track ties. The bitter smell of creosote stung my throat. "You pick awhile."

A confused half-grin replaced his smile. Here we were, in secret wild cherry paradise, how could I sit on the tracks instead of indulging? His tan forearms showed no sign of chill. His chest didn't heave. His heart probably *tump tumped* softly at resting rate. We'd only walked a short distance at old-ster pace and ascended a dyke—what was that? Five yards of gentle slope? Yet I was shivering, at high noon, in about 29 degrees. I pulled on my jacket and rubbed my clammy hands together. His expression almost shamed me into action, but I had learned the limits of my body.

"I need a few minutes," I said.

He nodded, the disturbing look fading as the nearest cherry tree absorbed his attention.

A minute later, he was filling my cupped hands with the smallest cherries I'd ever seen—half the size of those I used to pick long ago with my father. "Enjoy them now," he said, a smear of magenta visible on his lips, and teeth, when he smiled.

"Mmm," I said, "Thank you." I placed a cherry between my lips and felt its hot skin against mine before I rolled the fruit into my mouth and bit into it. I had imagined that wild cherries would taste tart, have a tough skin, and a mere droplet of juice. I was wrong. This cherry had an intensely sweet flavor. Its juice burst from a delicate skin and made a purple puddle on my palm when I spit out the stone. I popped another into my mouth and dropped the rest into a plastic bag I'd brought along.

"Enjoy now," he said. "That's what today is for. These won't be the same tomorrow."

"I am enjoying, believe me!" I hadn't felt so alive in months. I gulped in the air and made like a lizard, absorbing heat from the rocks below, the metal rail near my back, and the sun above. He offered me another handful and I dumped the cherries into my bag. "I want to save some for another day too." I held up the bag. "I'll need your help filling it."

He scoffed. "Come back tomorrow," he said. "Come back and pick more."

I'd told him several times, but he didn't understand that I couldn't come back tomorrow, or any day this week. That I had just walked farther than I'd walked in several months. That the ten minutes' journey along a flat dirt path had made me feel feverish. That the slow progress up the dyke had made my heart thump and leg muscles quake. That tomorrow I wouldn't be able to get up off the couch, because my limbs would feel like lead. Maybe not the day after either.

I'd explained everything, but he didn't understand why, a year ago, I refused his invitation to a romantic weekend camping trip on the coast. I found myself getting sicker day by day but could get no answers from the doctors.

"You like me, I like you, we're a good match, two free spirits," he had said. "Why don't we go out?"

How could I tell him, "I think I might be dying?" I couldn't even form the words. It was incomprehensible to me that in the span of a few weeks, I went from running 5–10k without a second thought, to being unable to move for days following a run, or even a walk, around the block. How could I explain that to someone with five years on me, nearly 50 years old, who routinely kayaked 100k a week and biked 30k a day? Free spirit means nothing in a body that's shutting down. How could I say, "I want to go everywhere, do everything with you, but I can't keep up—I'm not your match anymore?" How could I say *yes*, knowing that I would suffer and hide my illness that weekend, and that camping trip would be a lie?

"Maybe another time," I had said. "I want you in my life as my friend, though. Are you into that?"

"Absolutely," he said. I think he meant it, but in the following months, we didn't talk or meet up unless I took the initiative. It wounded me at first, but he wasn't the only friend who had moved on. He had never gotten close to chronic illness. I suspected he also didn't know how to be friends with a woman he didn't sleep with. He'd never had to understand those kinds of relationships.

So, after rejecting him romantically last year for reasons he could not understand, I was now trying to—what? Teach him how to be friends with the chronically-fatigued me? Or glean from him a reminder that my spirit remained as big and free as it had been before I got sick? Maybe both. Or maybe I was trespassing where I shouldn't.

"It's all in your mind," he said, leaping from the dyke onto a low, thick cherry branch and plucking more fruit. I was standing again by then, picking two, eating one, picking two, eating three. I managed to fill the bag about a third of the way before I got a head rush and sank back down to the tracks. I had juice all over my hands, sticky fingertips. It all felt delightfully real and rich. "Just be positive," he said, swinging up to a higher branch. Another day I would have imagined him topless like George of the Jungle, no—I mean like Tarzan. I would have summoned him to me with some chortling jungle mating call and made wild, cherry-slathered love to him on the railroad tracks, like an 80s music video, creosote in the air, gravel in our hair—

That was another day.

Today I marveled at his agility and verve, knowing I used to move that way. I tried to leap and fly vicariously through his movements, but it didn't work. Still, I felt a little buzz within me. Air passed with less resistance in and out of my lungs, and I could raise my limbs more easily, as if he could disarm gravity.

"I *am* positive," I said, trying not to think of how many times someone had told me that. It always brought out my residual 15-year-old snark: Gee, if it were that easy, don't you think I would have just "thought positive" and cured myself already?

"What's that?" He couldn't hear me.

My will had gotten me this far, kept me alive through a year and a half of mysteriously declining health, to a diagnosis of an enigmatic disorder called Chronic Fatigue Syndrome, through the loss of employment, my home, plans, dreams, friends who made empty promises or simply disappeared; through countless days, weeks and months of lying in bed, feeling severed from the world, from the body I knew and the life I led in another day. There was only so much the will could do, I'd learned. It could keep me alive, but it couldn't cure me outright. At least not yet. I barely understood this myself, and I was the one who was ill.

"I'll tell you another time," I said, sucking on a cherry stone. I closed my eyes to rest.

* * *

This had been my first good day in a long while. I'd awakened with a clear head, limbs that moved as they should, and a spirit starved by isolation. He worked at a river-view office near the room I was renting, so I took a chance.

"Hey, it's me," I had said. My voice cut in and out although we had a clear cell connection. "Do you want to eat lunch by the river?"

"How about picking cherries?" he said. I could hear his smile through the phone.

"Tempting," I weighed the physical toll versus spiritual benefit, "but I can't drive to·the valley orchards. It's too far."

"You won't have to." He laughed.

I drove from apartments to shopping center to industrial warehouses to trailhead. When I pulled myself out of the car, drained by the ten-minute drive, his embrace shot energy through me—not a sexual jolt, as it would have been another day—like his well-charged internal battery was trying to recharge mine. I clung like the pincher clamps on jumper cables as long as I decently could. He didn't seem to notice that I was doing my best to suck the life out of him. He had lots to spare.

As we walked towards the dyke, he slowed his pace to match mine. We laughed and chatted about anything, everything, through shadows and filtered sunlight. My words and laughter came slowly, like my thoughts, but surrounded by nature, walking beside him, I almost felt like I was myself again, sun-kissed and indomitable.

"My kids are doing great," he was saying, "but I can't seem to keep a family together." I stumbled on an exposed root and he caught me before I face-planted. His arms crooked at a sturdy right angle under my back. I fit snugly against his chest as if built to belong there, but I didn't. Not on this day. His eyelashes tickled my cheek. He smelled of sweat and chai tea, and he seemed to be looking at *me*, the way I was looking at him. I mean, the way I had once looked at him. Like I was for him, and he for me. That moment lasted longer than the average moment.

It was like that time last year when he'd asked me out and every part of me but a tiny stone certainty at my core was screaming *"yes!,"* wanting only to stomp on my compass and lead him over barbed wire fencing, blatantly ignoring a *No Trespassing* sign, taking a wrong path and getting turned around in the cottonwoods, losing sight of the sun and stars. That moment was a portal to a place one may never move out of, from which one may never return. Chronic illness feels like that. He could have gotten stuck there with me. He could have, but we never went.

"Keep a family together?" I said. "Don't worry. You will." I pressed my lips together, found my footing, and swung out of his embrace. It wasn't safe to say more, but I could wonder: Who would he meet? When would I get better, and who would I meet? Few found comfort in uncertainty, but I was becoming accustomed to it. We walked on towards the dyke.

* * *

When I was too tired to pick more of the tiny ruby fruits, I left my bag with him and sat in the concrete niche of the abutment, my feet dangling over the edge. I ate a handful of cherries, pretending they had magical healing powers, and spit the stones towards the derelict swing bridge. They fell short. The bridge never flinched. From that distance, its giant gears seemed locked in place by rust and grime. Perhaps it would never move again. If it did, I wondered, would the single train track on its deck still match the one here on land after months, maybe years of separation, or would something have shifted irreversibly?

"Didn't you see the sign back there?" he said, offering me a smile and a hand. A leaf stuck in his hair. He'd probably climbed a whole tree, or all the trees. His other hand clutched his shirt and my cherry bag. His bronze skin glistened with sweat. "Living dangerously, eh?"

"You have no idea," I said. Another day I would have taken his hand, tugged him down and finger-painted on his skin for hours. Instead I let him lift and steady me through another head rush.

"I expected to find a pile of clothes here," he pointed at the abutment, "and you sunning yourself on that train bridge over there after a little swim. You know, we're here. Why not take a dip?"

I chuckled. I could, sure, especially with his help. He was a strong swimmer and could likely tow me across the river and back more than once, but with my deficient energy reserves, the cold water would turn me blue in seconds and I'd be paying for that skinny dip for up to a month. This outing had already pushed my energy envelope enough for one day.

"Another time," I said.

That look of confusion flickered across his face again. Couldn't he feel the clamminess of my hand, the icy fingers, held in his? Couldn't he see the red fever in my eyes, or my body trembling because his vitality and the sun's heat could not bolster me any further today? He never paid attention to danger signs. I never had either, but now I saw them everywhere. I couldn't afford not to.

Our brains see what they want to see. It occurred to me that maybe I wasn't in a limbo, left alone in the uncertainty of chronic illness while he had moved on without me. Maybe my illness had pushed me beyond a proscribed boundary, across a swing bridge on its final rotation, down some overgrown and disconnected track and into a wilderness, full of new challenges and hidden bits of sweetness to be discovered. Maybe I had left him behind, and he had stayed where he was, long after he'd lost sight of me. With illness comes a severance from our foundations, like the swing bridge that never returns to this abutment.

* * *

"Thanks for today," I said, sinking into the driver's seat. I took the bag from him and set it beside me. It held a few handfuls of cherries, all I'd had the strength to collect. I had hoped for more, but this would have to do.

"You should eat them now," he said, flashing the grin that had first attracted me to him. He shut the door and rested his forearms along the windowsill, his chin on his arms, lips inches from mine. Too close.

The line between another day and this day was blurring. It was dangerous and confusing. He didn't believe in saving some for later, I told myself. He knew only how to live for today, he didn't understand chronic illness, he didn't see me anymore; and yet, I could picture him swimming across the river, against the current, past the old swing bridge, to the opposite shore where the train track started again. I could see him searching for a set of footprints there and tracking them at a run. My footprints.

I could fantasize forever, imagine him as the person I wanted him to be. One who would follow me anywhere if I let him, even into the wilderness of chronic illness, or who would call me up of his own volition once in a while to say hello. The hard part was seeing what was real, like the bag on the seat beside me. The bag I had wanted to fill but couldn't. The bag he had the energy to fill, but didn't.

"We'll come back and get more later." He said it like a plan or a promise. "Those won't be the same tomorrow." He indicated the bagged cherries.

"No, they won't be the same," I said, as he gave me a cherry chai kiss on the cheek. "They'll be better."

* * *

Today I can't walk outside, along a forested path, with a gentle man. I lie on my bed and look out the window, place a cherry between my lips, feel skin on skin, and bite.

Bite into sunlight, smells of hot dust and creosote, rustling leaves. Our laughter. His low voice. My thin one. His quick wit. My slow one. Taste every flowery breath of wind, each lap of water, every sugary bite of the world outside my bedroom walls, outside of my body. Delight in sucking every stone clean of its sweet, wild flesh and spitting it free to take root on some faraway shore. Relish every moment I sat at the edge of the abutment and stared at the track beyond the swing bridge, wondering where it led, and if it ever looped back. I savor it all in the cherries from another day.

Advanced Planning and Pacing

So you've been doing your bubble time, reducing environmental trigger exposure and decreasing impact of some intrinsic triggers, and you've been planning limited excursions, figuring out your functional capacity and exertion tolerance thresholds and pacing, pacing, pacing, and all this has brought you out of the *crisis phase*? No more of the relentless boom-bust downward grind of increasing symptoms and decreasing functionality?

Congrats! Reaching stability is no easy feat. Some people give up and never get this far. I mean it: take a moment to bask in your accomplishment and commitment to your health and to yourself. Take several moments. Take an hour, or a day. Make yourself a t-shirt that says I AM TITAN AMY and wear it proudly as you parade around your bubble!

I always imagine warmth and bright light infusing my being when I reach a healing plateau like this one, and a choir of angels singing a dense harmonic wall of *AH!* all around me—

No, I envision myself as a teabag steeping in water of sublime temperature, and it brings out all the best in me—

No, wait, I'm not the teabag. I drink the tea of my highest potential and it suffuses me with—

Hrm.... Well, no matter what image you use to shower gratitude and love upon yourself, this is a moment to cherish. Make a memory that you can hold onto as you begin blazing your trail across the *stability phase* of CS and CSS.

First I'll introduce advanced planning and pacing concepts, the goal of which is primarily to help you find the most energy-efficient ways to complete your daily living activities so you can make the most of your limited functional capacity and do things other than chores. We'll also look at working with an Occupational Therapist, Graded Exercise Therapy, how to avoid shrinkage of functional capacity, and how to expand both it and your exertion tolerance thresholds. After planning and pacing, I'll move into advanced techniques and strategies for contending with environmental triggers, including how to build a scent repertoire and use the nosegay technique to gain access to triggerful places (and, eventually, *the world!*)

Please note, if you have yet to master basic planning and pacing, or haven't yet figured out your functional capacity or exertion tolerance thresholds for daily living activities, I strongly encourage you to go back and work on those concepts before trying anything in this chapter. If you don't know your current abilities and limits, this advanced information won't do much good and may cause harm. If you have done that work yet found that your functional capacity is about three non-consecutive hours per day or less, the strategies that follow may be too much for you at this time. Read and consider, but please think carefully before trying them, start slow and back off immediately if symptoms worsen, and always check with your doctor before changing your routine or embarking on any strategy or treatment.

On a Good Day

Some days I wake up with virtually no symptoms, or at least dramatically reduced symptoms. I feel like I could tackle anything. "I'm healed! I'm *healed!*" I cry to the heavens, beaming like a sun. I decide to take a long walk down by the bay, followed by a trip to the grocery and drug stores, the pet food store and—why not?—the liquor store. I haven't had a sip of cider for two weeks. Maybe I'll visit a friend too, or go see a movie? Oh, and when I get home I'll do the bills, dishes, laundry, and vacuum. My place will be just the way I like it. Then I'll have a pint of cider with lime and read a novel all afternoon.

"On a good day," I sing to myself as I dress, imagining I sound just like Streisand or Lea Michele, "On a good day," I sing, putting out of my mind the memory of yesterday, when my symptoms were so bad it took me all morning just to pull on socks, "I can do whatever, for ever more—!" My heart thumps in double time, warning me that all is not well, but I pretend not to notice. I sit on the edge of the bed and tell myself it's merely to put on my socks with greater ease, and has nothing to do with giving my heartbeat a chance to simmer down.

The truth is, on a good day, I can see forever. I feel like I can do *any* thing. My energy seems to be boundless. *I have this whole list of stuff I've been waiting to do, and pacing or being cautious seems like nothing more than a big waste of life. I might never feel this good again, and I'll be damned if I'm going to squander it.* Those are the kind of thoughts that run through my head on a good day. For about the first year or so of my hard-earned stability phase I gave in to those thoughts, and I enjoyed that good day to the hilt. But I wound up in a severe crash afterwards, stuck in bed for the next month or so, miserable and unable to manage anything but my most basic daily living activities. Eventually I decided that was a horrible way to live, and that I'd rather be able to function each day for three hours than function for eight hours only one day out of every 30 or more.

This led to the development of my "On a Good Day" list, which contains things that I'd really like to do but are not necessities—things that always get back-burnered by higher priorities. Things like going to the liquor store or chocolatier for a treat, or spending extra time down by the water, walking in sunshine, comforting animals at a shelter, or sitting in a café reading or people watching. I put things on the list that will enrich my life, feed my spirit, and carry me through until the next good day. When a good day arrives, I look at my normal, daily to-do list first and defer anything that absolutely cannot wait until tomorrow, or later. After that, if I still feel good, I do one thing on my "On a Good Day" list. And then, I savor every moment and tell myself, "You will have more good days like this. Lots more. Forever more..."

Minimizing Functional Capacity Shrinkage

One of the great challenges inherent in the way CS and CSS work is that when you crash or relapse, or if you get depressed and stay in bed for days on end (yep, it can happen) your functional capacity can shrink and your exertion tolerance thresholds decrease. For example, let's say you are currently operating with a functional capacity of about five hours per day, and you can sit at the kitchen table and chop veggies for up to 30 minutes prior to getting any warning symptoms. One day, an unplanned crash hits and you must do intensive bubble time for three weeks, rarely leaving your bed. When the crash subsides and you try to resume your usual activities, you find that you can only sit up and chop veggies for five minutes at a time, and your functional capacity has shrunk to about three hours per day.

This phenomenon, known as "deconditioning" or "functional capacity shrinkage" has to do with the level and duration of inactivity. The less active you are, the less physical, mental, and/or emotional exertion your sensitized nervous system wants to tolerate. Why is that? Your body should be rested and raring to go, and your functional capacity should have *increased* after prolonged bubble time, right? Well, have you ever heard "use it or lose it" with regards to a level of fitness? If we don't use muscles, they get smaller. And remember what I said about the ideal of getting 100 percent clear and then trying to adapt back into regular life? Our bodies are wonderful and skillful adapters, so if you remove 100 percent of environmental triggers for a prolonged time, it's very likely your sensitized nervous system will happily accept that level of null triggers as normal and safe. And if you stay in bed for a prolonged time, the sensitized nervous system will happily accept that minimal level of exertion as its functional capacity. Then, when you try to exert, the sensitized nervous system ramps up your symptoms, doing all it can to shut your body down and save the day, or save you anyway.

Functional capacity shrinkage can be frustrating, even demoralizing. After all, you took care of yourself the best you could, honoring your symptoms and doing intensive bubble time, only to make things worse! You were actually *increasing* your functional capacity and exertion tolerance thresholds prior to that crash, and now you're starting five steps back? This type of setback can cause deep depression, especially if you don't know what's wrong or why. I fell prey to it for months before finally learning what the deal was.

First, I had to accept that the more I crashed, the more my functional capacity was likely to shrink. In some cases shrinkage would be unavoidable. I suffered and struggled with the unfairness of it all. Acceptance took time. I'll talk more about this in the coping chapter, but nutshell, I finally realized that CS and CSS had the upper hand and there was nothing I could do to change that, in the short-term at least. At that point, I was able to resign my resistance.

Secondly, I had to find a way to minimize the shrinkage as much as possible. *How could I possibly do my intensive bubble time, yet maintain my pre-crash functional capacity*, you ask?

Good question. I asked a Physiotherapist experienced with CS and CSS, and she told me to do the following while in a relapse or crash:

- Gently stretch my muscles while in bed, at least three times a day.
- Sit up (at least to a partial recline) once every hour—more often if I can—and take slow, relaxed breaths, self-talking my heart to stop racing and resume its normal rate.
- Cut my normal graded exercise therapy in half. So if I normally take three slow 3-minute walks up and down my hallway each day, then when I'm in relapse or crash I should do only three slow 1.5-minute walks up and down my hallway (provided this does not exacerbate symptoms).
- Soak in an Epsom salt bath at least once a day (hot enough to be soothing but not so hot that it makes me feel faint).
- Rest outside in the sunshine as much as possible (with appropriate sun protection).

Remember, symptoms and responses vary with each individual, so what I did might not work for you. Find a Physiotherapist who knows her/his stuff with regards to CS and CSS. Also, remember, this kind of work doesn't altogether prevent one's functional capacity from shrinking during inactive periods. It merely reduces the amount of shrinkage. There is no perfect remedy, not yet.

Increasing Functional Capacity and Raising Exertion Tolerance

As I've said, CS causes fatigue issues and decreases the body's functional capacity and exertion tolerance, regardless of which CSS is present (if any), although the problem tends to be more severe in folks with CFS, POTS, FM, and other chronic pain syndromes. At time of writing, the medical jury is still out regarding increasing functional capacity. I've read about folks who have managed to do so. Some claim to have cured themselves of their CS and CSS altogether. I've also read about doctors who say it's hopeless, and patients who say there is no way to improve their level of functionality, that their level of debilitation will forever remain at the same level they're currently at. I tend not to let that kind of negativity break into my mindset. I want to do all I can to increase my functional capacity, no matter how long it takes.

My CFS specialist told me that the ability to increase functional capacity varies from person to person and, generally speaking, depends on three factors:

- the length of time one has had CSS, or CS alone (the longer one has had the condition, the less likely one is to improve),
- the level of health and fitness prior to getting CSS, or CS alone (the more healthy and fit one was prior to getting the condition, the more likely one is to regain some if not all functionality),
- and the degree of CSS, or CS alone (the lesser the degree of debilitation one experiences, the more likely one is to improve functional capacity).

My specialist's suppositions seem logical to me, yet if you have had severe CSS, or CS alone, for years and weren't particularly healthy or sporty prior to getting sick, the above is not reason enough for you to lose hope about healing. Medical professionals simply don't know enough about these conditions at this point for anyone to say with certainty, "You absolutely cannot beat this thing." (Actually, even if they said that, I'd probably keep looking for a cure, but that's just me.)

I have a few suggestions for increasing exertion tolerance thresholds and functional capacity: engaging the parasympathetic system (which I discussed in the section on decreasing trigger exposure and impact), Occupational Therapy, and Graded Exercise Therapy.

Occupational Therapy

Prior to getting sick, I thought Occupational Therapy was for fitting people properly for wheelchairs, or walking aids, period. I truly had no idea the impact a CS- and CSS-knowledgeable Occupational Therapist (OT) can have on one's life. My OT—I'll call her Brie—first looked at ways to save me energy, decrease inflammation, and improve my physical safety with regards to all my daily living activities. We talked about stuff like this:

- Showering: Would it save me energy if I had a shower stool and didn't have to stand while showering?
- Shower safety: Do I need a rail in the shower for those times I get light-headed, or for getting in and out of the tub?
- Grocery shopping: Can I order grocery delivery instead of over-exerting at the store? If I have to go to the store, can I organize my shopping list by aisle, so I need only make one trip through the store? Can I stock up on certain items so I go to the store less often?
- Cooking: Can someone come in to help me cook? Can I cook extra on cooking days and freeze the rest in meal-sized portions?
- Prepping food: Can I prep food one day and cook another day? Can I sit while chopping vegetables, or better yet buy a food processor that slices and dices?
- Sitting: Do I need a higher chair? A back cushion? A footstool?

I'm a pretty efficiency-minded individual to begin with, and I'd been living alone with CS and three CSS for a few years before meeting Brie, so I had that daily living activity stuff pretty much down to a science by then, but Brie had more to offer.

She addressed ways to decrease my mental and emotional energy expenditures (two powerful intrinsic triggers). I had never thought about this. I mean, I knew that my symptoms increased markedly when I was under duress, and I had been working on decreasing stressors and negative perception of stress, but I guess I had figured that all the strategies I list in the chapter on coping would take care of that. Maybe they would have, eventually, but Brie suggested another idea that not only worked quickly, it appealed to my practical nature. Through various discussions, we determined that dealing with the biased and oft-demoralizing process of workers compensation was taking an enormous toll on me, cognitively and emotionally. Reducing that toll became the goal. The action plan went something like this:

1. For the first week, whenever I caught myself thinking about something related to workers compensation, I had to make a note of it. Then I had to try to push those thoughts aside or somehow distract my brain from them. At the end of the week I discovered, to my surprise and chagrin, that I spent about 60 percent of my waking hours thinking thoughts related to workers compensation.

2. Next, I created a place to make notes about important things I needed to remember to do for my workers compensation claim. Once I wrote something down, I did not allow myself to think more about it.

3. I planned times during the week when I would focus only on workers compensation stuff. These had to be fluid, of course, because sometimes symptoms prohibited any activity, but the designated times allowed me to tell my brain at any other time, "Don't worry about that. It's on the list and will be taken care of in my next workers compensation session."

4. I did a lot of self-talk then too, to deal with my anger, fear, and worry surrounding my compensation claim, and my health issues in general. Around the time I started working with Brie I felt a lot of anger towards my brain, for malfunctioning and causing brain fog and other issues. Brie told me that most major injuries or traumas caused brain fog—not just CS or CSS—often only temporarily. She said my brain hadn't stopped working—it was busy *healing*. She told me to work on trusting it again. So I did self-talk, stuff like, "Hey, I know you're busy. Thanks for all the hard work. You're doing a good job. I know this brain fog is only temporary while you focus on healing...." And yep, like with any self-talk, I felt hokey doing it at first, but not so much now. We all need support, trust and encouragement, so why not massage a little of that into our own brains?

5. I did the above steps for months. It's been six months at time of writing, and I only think about workers compensation a couple times a day now, and it's usually a fleeting reminder to meet some deadline or include something in a review packet. I sleep better and have less compensation-related nightmares. And, best of all, I have more energy and time to do things I'd rather be doing.

If you suspect you may be increasing symptoms and/or wasting an inordinate amount of your already limited energy on emotional or cognitive stressors, try Brie's method and discover what most of your thoughts are about. You have nothing to lose, and only energy and serenity to gain.

GRADED EXERCISE THERAPY (GET)

Graded Exercise Therapy (GET) "is a type of physical activity therapy that starts very slowly and gradually increases over time."[1] There are entire books on GET, and this is not one of them, but I want to share my findings so if you decide to pursue this therapy you'll know what you're looking for and won't waste time or money on unqualified folks proclaiming they can cure you with GET.[2]

Nutshell, GET relies on the premise that if someone with CS or CSS—usually CFS, FM, or POTS—does daily aerobic exercise *within her functional capacity*, starting with a non-taxing level and brief periods (one to two minutes, generally) and incrementally boosting the amount and duration of exertion over time, the sensitized nervous system won't perceive the exertion escalations as a threat or issue and will tolerate them. This therapy may raise the exertion tolerance threshold, and the person doing GET may eventually increase her functional capacity.[3]

I started working with GET in autumn of 2013. I was a runner and workout fiend pre–CS and CSS—an adrenalin junkie, I suppose—all about *ACTION*, both for fun and for a sense of accomplishment. Having to stop running and working out when I got sick was a difficult and significant lifestyle shift, and when I heard that there was a graded exercise therapy that helped some folks with CSS regain functionality, I was all over that. My doctor warned me that I had to start small and go slow with GET, but I had started running years prior as an avid *non*-runner and managed to train for, and complete a half marathon. I knew how to take baby steps and reach what at first seems an insurmountable goal. *Bring it!* I said.

And I crashed and burned. *(Oh, the agony ...)* There were reasons for this.

A general rule that applies to most folks with CSS working with GET is that one's heart rate needs to remain 60 percent below maximum to avoid increasing symptoms, relapsing or crashing. Managing my heart rate was a piece of cake, but GET only has a chance of success if one starts at a level one's sensitized nervous system registers as negligible *and* the exertion is increased in increments the sensitized nervous system registers as negligible. I was used to running several miles at a time, so my idea of "negligible" was nowhere near that of my sensitized nervous system's idea of "negligible." I started out way too high, trying to walk 15 minutes a day, and I crashed. Then I tried ten minutes, then five. Every wee walk caused a big crash.

"When beginning a GET program, it is important for patients to avoid extremes and instead balance physical activity and rest…. Appropriate rest is an important element of GET, and patients should learn to stop activity before illness and fatigue are worsened."[4] Everyone's starting level for GET will differ. Some may start with simple stretching or strengthening exercises, while others may start with a five-minute walk. It's very important to start small and build slowly, increasing by no more than 10 percent at a time, and ensure you plan adequate bubble time pre- and post–GET. Note that you may find you need more rest than usual.

Another reason why GET didn't work for me at first is because I wasn't counting my daily living activities as aerobic "exercise" or "exertion," but anyone with CSS (or CS alone) using GET needs to understand that aerobic exercise doesn't have to be done in a gym or make you break a sweat. It "includes any physical activity that uses large muscle groups and increases your heart rate."[5] Once you start using that definition, you'll find that most activities should be taken into account as part of GET. For example, if I vacuum the hall for three minutes on Tuesday, I count that on my GET log, and it cancels out one of my three-minute walks that day because, in theory, I've expended that energy on vacuuming. This goes for cooking, laundry, cleaning, showering—any physical exertion that raises my heart rate and employs large muscle groups.

This is why it's important to first be sure you are managing your daily living activities as efficiently as possible and have energy to spare *before* attempting GET. This is also why it's crucial that you be out of *crisis phase* and have a solid understanding of your functional capacity and exertion tolerance thresholds prior to attempting GET. You don't want to relapse or crash and end up shrinking your functional capacity. So be sure you are very clear on how much energy you need for your daily living activities and whatever else, versus how much energy you actually *have,* before you try GET. Then, add your GET *within* that functional capacity.

GET and the Heart Rate

What does "maximum heart rate" mean, and why is it that most people with CSS relapse or crash if their heart rate rises above 60 percent of it? Good question. Maximum heart rate is the maximum number of times someone's heart should beat per minute while exercising. "For moderate-intensity physical activity, a person's target heart rate should be 50 to 70 percent of his or her maximum heart rate."[6] At this point, the body engages in "aerobic" metabolism, using oxygen and carbohydrates to fuel the muscles. Generally, when the heart rate rises above 70 percent, the cardiovascular system can't provide enough oxygen to muscles and so switches to "anaerobic" metabolism (using glucose and glycogen for fuel), a process that can result in lactic acid. When lactic acid builds up, it causes inflammation and pain. Combine that with any other symptoms a person with CSS (or CS alone) normally gets from intense over-exertion, and you see the problem with venturing beyond that 60 percent of maximum heart rate threshold: relapse and/or crash.

To estimate your maximum heart rate, subtract your age from 220. Then multiply your result by .60 to calculate 60 percent of your maximum heart rate. Here's an example for a 40-year-old:

220–40 = 180 beats per minute (max heart rate)
180 × .60 = 108 beats per minute (60 percent of max heart rate)

Please note, "maximum heart rate is just a guide. You may have a higher or lower maximum heart rate, sometimes by as much as 15 to 20 beats per minute."[7] Also, some medications can "lower your maximum heart rate and, therefore, lower your target heart rate zone," so be sure to consult your medical provider.[8] The 60 percent is also a guideline. You may find that you can exert up to 65 percent of your max heart rate with no problem. Or you may not be able to go past 50 percent. Pay attention to how you feel after each GET session and make detailed notes as to duration, intensity, and your heart rate. You may find that on days when you feel more fatigued or have dealt with more triggers, you must do your GET at a lower heart rate than on better days. This is common. You may find you feel fine the day you do the exercise but then get warning symptoms, or relapse or crash, 24–48 hours later. This delay is also common. If this happens, then try using a lower maximum heart rate until you find the percentage that allows you to do your GET without this "exertion hangover" effect.

How do you measure heart rate?

Good question. Monitoring the heart rate does not require any special equipment. You can place two fingers to the inside of one wrist and count pulse beats for six seconds. Then multiply by ten to get the number of heart beats per minute. However, once you reach stability phase and start paying close attention to your activities, exertion thresholds and heart rate, you'll probably find that stopping to take your pulse countless times a day is inconvenient and tiring. I found that investing in a heart rate monitor (HRM) benefitted me multi-fold: it increased accuracy of monitoring, saved time and energy, showed me clearly which activities were the most or least taxing, and gave me peace of mind. Many folks with CSS (or CS alone) experience abnormal heart rate surges from relatively low exertion, and this can be alarming. But after getting my HRM, whenever my heart lurched or thumped, I could check its rate and often, I'd discover that although my pulse was higher than it should be, it wasn't anywhere near the soaring rate I'd feared. So the HRM can provide an instant reality check, which is invaluable for those with CS, who need to reduce stressors.

There are lots of HRMs out there. Search Amazon and you'll see what I mean. Most HRMs worth a darn require that you wear a "chest strap," which is just what it sounds like. A tiny receiver in the strap measures the beat straight from the heart and beams it to a wrist-watch-like component you can check easily. I used this a lot as a runner and it worked great, but as a slow walker with CS, I found that my chest strap monitor lost accuracy because my heart rate remained below 105 beats per minute much of the time. I think the chest strap was tuned for higher heart rates.

After extensive research, I found that the Fitbit Charge HR best suited my purposes. A wristwatch-size unit, it doesn't require a chest strap and monitors my sub-105 heart rates with no problem. I can program it to show me only the parameters I need—such as time, date, heart rate, and sleep—and it has a software component that enables me to monitor progress on my computer. The learning curve is nil, which is important for folks who have limited cognitive function and energy.

If you're thinking about investing in an HRM, things to consider are:

- What's your budget? These run from $15 into the hundreds of dollars.
- Size, weight—and can you tolerate the materials?
- Do you need it to be waterproof?
- Chest strap or strapless heart rate monitoring?
- Does it read lower heart rates or is it made for intense exercise only? Check reviews.
- Quality—will it last? Does it measure heart rate accurately? Check reviews.
- Can you return it if it doesn't do what you need? What's the warranty?
- Does it require batteries? How long does the charge last?
- Do you want one that measures other parameters, like sleep, distance or steps?
- Is it easy to read the heart rate or do you have to push three different buttons to get to that screen? Is it backlit or does it have a night light?

GET and Walking

I didn't make any progress with GET until about nine months ago, when I met a Physiotherapist who was experienced with CS and CSS. I'll call her Lu. Lu helped me figure out a reasonable starting point for my GET work. It was a one-minute-long walk on flat ground, three times a day. Yep, a one-minute-long walk. As you can imagine, I had to really rein in my expectations to do the work. I used my HRM to ensure I stayed below 60 percent of my maximum heart rate. I didn't even go outside, I just paced in my hall. Within a month, I could walk one minute, four times a day, without triggering my warning symptoms. (Yep, it took a whole month, simply because I am single and live alone and thus have a lot of daily living activities to take care of—plus workers compensation—so most of the time I had no extra energy to spare to do my walking. I ended up making some of my less-urgent chores, like laundry and cleaning the toilet, a lower priority than walking. Maybe that's cheating, but that's what I did.)

Then Lu allowed me to try two-minute-long walks four times a day. After three weeks, she let me move to four-minute-long walks. After six weeks I moved up to five-minute-long walks—I was making progress! And I still am. I'm up to six-minute-long walks, four times a day, and one of those walks is up the hill in my back alley. I've been at this level for two months. At first my heart raced once I got three steps up the hill. Now I can reach its crest and come down again within my six minutes, stopping only three times on my way up so my heart rate can adjust. It's like sprint training for a marathon but in slow motion. I'm all over that. *Bring it!*

GET and Biking

Dr. Cortez has had some success in treating Orthostatic Intolerance by using tilt tables and GET: She starts the patient with a tolerable amount of exercise in a near-horizontal position on the tilt table and incrementally increases the incline of the table over time; gradually, the patient's postural tolerance threshold increases.[9] This got me thinking about how much energy it takes for us to remain upright and walk or do other exercise, and that my sensitized nervous system might be less agitated about exercise if I were to do it sitting down. It works for chopping veggies, after all! I theorized that if I did my GET in a semi-reclined position, I would tax my sensitized system less than I do with walking and increase my functional capacity even more than I can with walking.

To test my theory, I got a recumbent exercise bike (in some cities you can rent these, which is ideal, in my opinion. You may find used bikes on Craigslist, but delivery can be an issue, and these bikes are *heavy*. I ended up buying a Nautilus 614—nothing fancy—floor model from a gym equipment store (pre-outgassed as well as discounted, and they delivered and installed for a small fee) and started out by biking for one minute, three times a day, at the lowest level of intensity. I had to pedal like a snail to keep my heart rate below 60 percent of max, especially on bad days. I kept at that level for a week and, having experienced no warning symptoms I bumped up to one minute, six seconds (that's a 10 percent increase), three times a day, at lowest intensity. At time of writing, I'm at one minute, 19 seconds, three times a day. Stay tuned …

Review of Advanced Exertion-Related Strategies

- Good days can tempt you to throw planning and pacing to the wind—and pay for it with a relapse or crash—but your "On a Good Day" list can help you enjoy your good days and keep moving toward your healing goals.

- Functional capacity shrinkage (aka deconditioning) can occur following prolonged inactivity due to relapses and crashes.
- Functional capacity and exertion tolerance thresholds may be increased with advanced planning and pacing.
- Occupational therapy can increase functional capacity by streamlining energy efficiencies and improving safety and stress management.
- Graded exercise therapy involves monitoring heart rate during exercise and gradually increasing exertion frequency, duration, and intensity over time without exerting beyond one's functional capacity.

> *Such love does*
> *the sky now pour*
> *that whenever I stand in a field,*
>
> *I have to wring out the light*
> *when I get*
> *home.*
> —St. Francis of Assisi[10]

Minimizing Bubble Dependency (aka Bubble as Refuge, Not Prison)

This segment introduces what lies beyond "getting clearer." In my four years of life with CS and CSS, I can delineate two stages of reactivity to environmental triggers: *ultra-reactive*—during which my central nervous system applied a Chernobyl-like response to the minutest trigger—and, well, what shall I call the next stage? My health had stopped freefalling, and I'd escaped the crash cycle, moved beyond crisis phase and regained some stability, yet CS still captained my ship, so what exactly had shifted? Symptoms. While maintaining their severity, my responses to many environmental triggers had become more selective about when they came out to play, to what degree they exhibited themselves, and how long they stuck around. This is the stage that comes after the ultra-reactive stage. This stage inspired me to experiment with certain environmental triggers and convinced me that, while I may have to play the CS game (for now at least) that doesn't mean I can't bend some of the rules. I'll call it the *desensitization stage*. This is how it happened …

In my third year of life with CS and CSS, I had a big revelation while washing my hair. My shampoo, a blue fruity smelling thing that I rarely gave much thought to suddenly gave me a thought: it wasn't making me cough. (I know you're probably wondering why I, someone with myriad environmental triggers, was using scented shampoo and the answer is, simply enough, money. I'd been fighting workers compensation for three years and gotten pretty much nowhere and meanwhile had depleted my savings. Unscented shampoo was expensive, so I used the cheapest shampoo I could find that triggered only minor symptoms (and didn't give me eczema). Remember, trigger avoidance is about getting clear *enough,* not 100 percent. There is no perfection in this exercise. Now that I thought about it, the shampoo hadn't made me cough for about a month. That was the first part of the revelation.

Part two was, I realized that despite countless coughing fits in countless venues, I had never coughed myself to death. If I hadn't died from coughing yet, even when I was working at GAS and things were at their worst, odds were that now, when I wasn't trapped in a triggerful environment, I wouldn't die from a coughing fit. This gave me some confidence.

Part three (I told you this was a big revelation) was that a few strong smells had stopped triggering me altogether. This revelation—henceforth known as the *Great Desensitization Revelation*—caused me to change up what I was doing. It's easier to explain in a story …

"I've started experimenting with scents," I say. Dr. H had invited me to her office more frequently lately, about every three to four weeks. Maybe her schedule had opened up because she was curing people left, right and center with her psychiatric genius, or maybe I was just becoming a more interesting case study.

"Experiments?" Did her eyebrows just raise up like a mad scientist's or is that my imagination?

"Yep, I was thinking that maybe I could trick myself into believing that a strong smell is not a threat, so my throat won't close up on me. I think it's possible. I've thought so ever since I noticed that there were one or two strong smelling things that I could tolerate with no reaction whatsoever most of the time."

"What things?" Dr. H asks.

"Well, my shampoo is one. It hardly ever triggers me anymore. Also, amber. I used to wear amber oil on my pulse points, but after getting sick, amber triggered me—until recently, that is. I can wear a little of it, even sniff it sometimes now, although sometimes it smells weird, like soap, or rancid oil, or urine. Sometimes everything smells like urine. Oh, and I can tolerate lavender too. *Real* lavender, not some Febreze-y synthetic stuff. I always had bouquets of it in my closets, and I had to bag it up after getting CS. But it hardly ever triggers me now."

"Interesting," Dr. H leans forward in her chair. "So what do you mean by experiments?"

"First I sniffed a sachet of lavender in the drug store, thinking it might mask the off-gassing fumes and prevent ILS or MCS symptoms." Dr. H raises her eyebrows in anticipation, for real this time. "It didn't work. The lavender wasn't strong enough. But the idea was right, I think. If I can distract my sensitized brain from triggering smells with something my sniffer feels is safe, then my throat won't close up, right? I need to generate an olfactory focus, like a police dog sniffing for cocaine instead of a bone," Dr. H jots something down, "metaphorically speaking, of course. Do other CS and CSS patients do this?"

"Well, everyone develops strategies that work for them. Some have less sensitivities, some have more."

It was her stock line. I got it, everyone was different, but it seemed like they should have a handbook for CS and CSS patients by now, called "How to Avoid Living the Rest of Your Life in a Bubble." The situation was maddening and liberating in its own way. I was ok with using my bubble as a temporary refuge, but I was not ok with the "bubble as prison and me serving life sentence" scenario.

Problem was, I'm an artist not a scientist—I have an abundance of emotion and a deficit in cold clinical rationality. I see potential everywhere and resist the confines of reality—so I found it hard to test hypothesis after next in an objective, detached manner. Especially when each failed experiment meant that my quality of life remained on the disabled list. Frustrated or not, I had no other option. If I didn't experiment, then I was doomed to hermit at home in my bubble, waiting for a miracle. I would forge ahead, perhaps where no CS or CSS patient had ventured before! Cue theme music …

SENSORY DEPRIVATION TANKS

This is just what it sounds like: a tank in which the senses are deprived (for the most part). Generally, tanks resemble a Jacuzzi tub (without the air jets) with a roof on it and contain knee-high warm water in which you lie back and float, buoyed by the high salt content in the water. As with any unfamiliar place, you may encounter environmental triggers at the tank place, so before booking a session, go and check it out. Be sure to sniff inside the tanks too. The sessions, in my city at least, are costly, but I found an hour in the tank very beneficial. I felt incredibly relaxed afterwards, as if my parasympathetic system had knocked the sympathetic out of the park. This state slowly dissipated over the next couple days, but it was such a significant improvement—however temporary—that I encourage you to consider tank sessions for both short- and long-term healing.

DETOXIFICATION

We hear a lot about detoxification these days—from the beneficial antioxidant properties of pomegranates and blueberries to cleanses and salt lamps and all kinds of stuff—fiber, IR saunas, mud treatments, iodine, antioxidant teas and foods, and the list goes on…. How much is marketing hype and how much is truth? Good question. If you suspect that toxic chemical exposure has affected your health, talk to your medical professional about tests for traces of chemicals and minerals in the body. It's important to note, however, that the external world isn't the only source of an unhealthy accumulation and/or imbalance of toxins in the body. For example, elevated levels of nitric oxide (a free radical, or chemically reactive by-product of certain physiological processes) can cause and/or support serious health problems.

One such is *oxidative stress*,[11] a term that reflects the body's ability to repair and detoxify itself. Dr. Martin L. Pall, Professor Emeritus of Biochemistry & Basic Medical Science at Washington State University, and several other researchers, has linked elevated nitric oxide levels and oxidative stress to some CSS.[12] I'll talk more about these correlations in the Neuroplasticity segment; for now, I want to point out that Dr. Pall's findings suggest that CSS patients may benefit greatly from certain detoxification strategies. First step, consult your doctor before embarking on a detox plan. Next, keep in mind that detox doesn't necessarily have to be a big, one-time super-treatment. It can be a serious of small dietary changes that will benefit you for the rest of your life.

When I started looking at detox, I was short on energy and cash, so I created a program based on minimal research and expense, like this:

- Eating only organic foods and grass-fed, free-range or wild, GMO- and hormone-free meats and fish (excepting tuna and other fish suspected to have high mercury content), plenty of dark leafy greens.
- Taking Vitamin D, Omega 3 and 6 fatty acids, and vitamin C supplements daily.
- Drinking organic, old-growth, ripened Pu'erh Tea.
- Adding turmeric to my tea or taking "curcumin, a polyphenolic [micronutrient] compound derived from turmeric, [that] protects against myocardial injury by alleviating oxidative stress, inflammation, apoptosis, and fibrosis"[13]

- Soaking in hot Epsom salt baths daily
- Taking a fiber supplement (I highly recommend Nutracleanse)
- Deep inhalations of fresh air daily (and sitting in sunshine when available)
- Eating dulse and seaweed for iodine
- Taking an alpha lipoic acid supplement[14]

Always select and use supplements with caution. Everyone's body, genetics, and circumstances differ, so supplements that help one person may not help another. It's also important to note that the supplement industry is poorly regulated, which makes supplement potency and/or quality evaluation a challenge. In addition, some supplements may be addictive, even those derived from natural sources, so they should be researched fully, just as you would a prescription medication.

The best place to get necessary nutrients is from your food, of course, but if you feel you aren't getting enough of something, or you wish to try antioxidant supplements, find a qualified health professional who is familiar with CS and CSS, takes into account your whole health, and doesn't just treat one symptom.

Desensitization, the Nosegay Technique and the Scent Repertoire

After years of planning and pacing and bubble time passed, my sensitivity to some environmental triggers was decreasing. I could use my cheap shampoo and it rarely made me cough. I could stand at a crowded intersection and, while the exhaust fumes still caused symptoms, the reactions didn't floor me like they used to. Paradoxically, my sensitized nervous system continued to recruit new environmental triggers. I couldn't control the rate of desensitization, nor the accumulation of new triggers, but the sensitivities *were* shifting, and if they were shifting, I figured, they could still disperse entirely. Meanwhile, I would take full advantage of any and all desensitization. Heck, I'd even encourage it to happen! Thus I developed the nosegay technique and set about compiling my scent repertoire.

THE THEORY BEHIND THE SCENT REPERTOIRE

My *Great Desensitization Revelation* sparked a supposition that went something like this: if I could gradually introduce my sniffer to certain scents in the safety of my bubble, then my body might become less likely to react to said scents over time; after all, when I felt safe, my sensitized nervous system was less inclined to express alarm. I extrapolated from there, as follows:

- If my sensitized nervous system doesn't react to a certain scent in my safe bubble, maybe my sensitized nervous system can actually come to *enjoy* that scent again.
- And if my sensitized nervous system *enjoys* that scent in the safety of my bubble, then my sensitized nervous system might also enjoy that scent somewhere triggerful.
- And if so, then maybe my sensitized nervous system won't react to whatever triggers are encountered there because my brain is focusing on the scent that I enjoy.

- And if so, then maybe I can build up a whole repertoire, or collection, of safe and enjoyable scents and gradually reclaim scents as sensual pleasures rather than warning signs of imminent peril.

This theory involved one of the primary assumptions I'd proven in the early days of using my bubble, that if I was in a safe place, my reactions to triggers would be less severe. (Generally this is true. Of course, if I was impacted by intrinsic triggers and/or had been exposed to environmental triggers already that day, then it didn't matter if I was in a safe place or not—I'd have severe reactions. But generally speaking, true.)

When I got CS and my olfactory system became heightened, I lost one of my great sensual pleasures of life—sniffing glorious scents. I didn't think about it at the time, with all the chaos my illness caused, but now I was thinking about it. What scents, pre–CS, had made me feel happy, safe, calm, or grounded? And what scents, if any, could I still enjoy now? After much brainstorming, I developed Table 8, which became the basis for my scent repertoire experiments.

TABLE 8. BASIC SCENT ANALYSIS

Scent	Note Type	Emotion or Sensation the Scent Provoked
Amber	Low	Safe, grounded, warm
Lilac	High	Reminds me of childhood
Roses	High	Reminds me of childhood
Lavender	Medium	Clean, restful, soothing
Strawberry	Medium	Summer, heat, sunshine, fresh, natural, delightful
Chocolate	Low	Calm, safe, sweet, heavy, slow
Coffee	Low	Home, safe, warm
Coconut	Medium	Sea breeze, vacation, warm sand under my feet, relax

COMPILING THE SCENT REPERTOIRE AND USING A NOSEGAY

The following is not for anyone in crisis phase with an ultra-reactive system. Trying to compile a scent repertoire in that state will make you worse. Once you reach stability and have noticed your system becoming less reactive, then you may wish to try this.

I started amassing my repertoire by working with a single natural scent. Since my high-note environmental triggers such as perfumes and colognes, laundry products, and chemical cleaners hadn't budged from their places at the top of my *Most Evil Triggers* list, while some of the low-note triggers, such as exhaust, were shifting, I decided to begin with a low-note natural scent: amber.

I found it relatively easy to convince my brain that amber was safe, actually, perhaps because I had loved it so dearly prior to getting CS. Though I hadn't realized it way back when, amber had served as a grounding scent for me for many years. When I dabbed some onto my pulse points, I felt beautiful, grounded, and confident. I had to stop wearing it when I got CS, of course, but it seemed the logical inaugural scent for my "recruiting safe scents" experiment.

I began by putting a dab of amber essential oil on Q-tip in my bubble, farthest corner from my chair. Whenever I entered the bubble and detected the amber I would intentionally think positive thoughts and induce pleasant memories—how lovely the scent was, how beautiful it had made me feel in years past, how strong and grounded—sappy nostalgia at its best. My nose would run when I detected the amber, but that was my body's only reaction. I did this for weeks, until my nose didn't run anymore, until all that happened when I detected amber in my bubble was that I enjoyed its aroma. Next, I put a bigger dab of amber on the Q-tip, at closer range. I repeated this process for several weeks until I could hold a small scent diffuser filled with amber oil right up to my nostrils, and inhale deeply, as one would do with a nosegay. *What's a nosegay, you ask?* Good question.

The term *nosegay* originates from Medieval times, when civilization was a stinkier place. There was horse dung in the streets, human sewage in the gutters, and people bathed less frequently than nowadays—you get the idea. Folks commonly held small bouquets of sweet smelling flowers, called nosegays, to their nostrils when navigating crowded places and streets to cover the less pleasant odors. Over time the term came to represent larger bouquets used more for ornamentation than smell masking, but some people still use nosegays today. I am one of them. If you experience scent-triggered symptoms, you might benefit from a nosegay too. Please note, for our purposes, a nosegay does more than merely mask one smell with another.

Once I could inhale my newly acquired safe scent from a nosegay at close range and elicit no symptoms, it was time to test in a triggerful place. I went to one of the worst stores I know for off-gassing and trigger scents—a big box store that sells vehicle tires and home furnishings. Normally, as soon as I entered that store, it was "game over" and I was forced to flee, breathless and ill, back to my bubble. But with my amber nosegay, I could actually manage for about ten minutes inside before I had to evacuate. I had to concentrate on that amber scent and self-talk my soldiers down the entire time, but it worked. Now that's what I call progress!

Let me be clear, the nosegay gets me in and out of that store—an environment I couldn't access prior to recruiting amber as the first scent in my repertoire—with far less symptoms, but it doesn't fix my life or get rid of my symptoms. It gives me access to a triggerful place for a limited time, which helps me to maintain my autonomy. After a quick trip like that, I still have to recover in my bubble until symptoms disperse. Remember, my bubble life is not about perfection or getting 100 percent clear, it's about finding ways to live as normally and joyfully as possible with CS and CSS, and using any strategies that increase access and decrease symptoms, while reducing sensitivity over the long term.

I added strawberries as the second scent in my repertoire. I would wait for a good day, with low fatigue, low stress, low exposure, relatively stable hormones, and then sit in front of a bowl of strawberries. Some days, I couldn't put it too close, but other days I could hold a berry right up to my sniffer and inhale deeply. The important thing was to reach the point at which the strong sweet smell didn't trigger symptoms—no neck muscles tightening, no post-nasal drip, no runny nose, no nothing—no response, period. Then I worked to get to the point at which the strong sweet smell of the berries smelled kinda yummy. Then I worked to get to the point at which the strong sweet smell was what it used to be pre–CS—a memory, of hot sunshine and vast farmland, a roadside stand selling fresh strawberries so ripe they almost melted in my fingers. I pop one in my mouth and it all but dissolves on my tongue. Mmmm. Yes, dear Reader, that is what I call reclaiming a scent and adding it to my scent repertoire.

Next? I'm thinking maybe coconut, or chocolate …

Why the Scent Repertoire Is Necessary

I dearly miss sensual olfactory delights and have come to believe that reclaiming my sense of smell for pleasure is reason enough to compile a scent repertoire, but that's not my only reason. I also believe that the more scents I can add to my repertoire, the more my brain will come to re-learn that the majority of scents in the world are safe. Ultimately, my goal is to re-educate my brain so that it finds *enjoyment* in most scents, not cause for alarm. Eventually, I won't need to carry around a nosegay of some essential oil that I've gradually acclimated myself to. I will be able to sniff most everything to my heart's content with nary a symptom, and all the scents in the world will once again comprise my scent repertoire!

Yep, that's the ideal. And until I get there, I'll continue compiling my scent repertoire one scent at a time. The more scents my brain interprets as friendly, the more triggerful places I can go without being triggered. That means less symptoms and more freedom from the bubble. That means reclaiming my life from the effects of CS and CSS.

I should clarify what I mean when I say my brain will *re-learn* that most scents are safe. Sniffing a nosegay is not re-learning. It's sniffing a tolerable, perhaps even enjoyable scent to help you focus on feeling safe rather than threatened while you gain temporary access to a triggerful place. The re-learning happens during the process of acclimating to that scent. The safe and positive thoughts and memories you conjure and focus on while acclimating to that scent in your bubble may, over time, re-educate your brain to react differently. I'll talk more about this process in the upcoming Neuroplasticity segment.

About Scentless Environmental Triggers

There are infinite environmental triggers with no perceivable odor (yep, undetectable, even by a CS super-sniffer). For example, a room that was painted 100 or so days ago will trigger MCS symptoms even though I can't smell the paint off-gassing. Bed linens or towels washed in unscented laundry products (that contain some triggering chemical) will give me a skin rash, eczema, or other symptoms. A café or restaurant floor mopped with an unscented yet strong chemical cleaner can cut an excursion short and cause a relapse or crash.

If I notice warning symptoms appearing while I'm in an unknown environment and smell nothing that could trigger those symptoms, I leave immediately. While leaving, I employ the use of my nosegay and encouraging, calming self-talk. In my experience, this can make a world of difference in mitigating symptom severity and duration.

About the Nosegay aka Scent Diffuser

You can dab essential oil on a handkerchief and call it a nosegay, but I don't recommend doing so. It's messy. The oil gets on your fingers or soaks through the handkerchief fabric and ends up on your shirt, your furniture, or your cat.... I prefer to use a pendant made to hold essential oil inside while allowing the scent to pass through "vent holes." When I enter a triggerful place, I loop de loop the necklace chain around my wrist, hold the pendant up to my nostrils like a nosegay and inhale deeply, so the only thing I can smell is that essential oil. I use this tool to gain temporary access to triggerful places while decreasing (or at least delaying the onset of) odor-triggered symptoms. A few thoughts about nosegay devices (also known as scent diffuser amulet thingies):

- You will find many styles and designs of diffusers for sale on Etsy.com—necklaces, bracelets, even rings that diffuse essential oil. Be aware that essential oils can corrode metals and stain clothing. If you buy a scent diffuser with an open back, or made of silver or gold, check to ensure the compartment that holds the oil cannot leak or spill onto your clothing or corrode the silver or gold you just paid a bunch of money for.

- My favorite diffuser is made of handcrafted pottery. It was given to me by a friend and unfortunately I haven't been able to find another like it, but Etsy does carry some similar models. Pottery diffusers become more fragrant when warmed by the body's heat. They also absorb the oil over time, so you need to add less oil and thus get more bang for your buck. These diffusers also tend to be cheaper than silver or gold. Downside, they are fragile.
- If you want something less breakable, I recommend stainless steel. Diffusingmamas.com makes quality models—mine are a few years old and have yet to leak. My only druther is that I wish they'd make bigger models, with more "vent holes," as their diffusers are all too small to hold enough oil to divert my brain from the super odiferous triggerful environments I sometimes need access to.

Advanced Scent Repertoire and Nosegay Techniques

And I mean ADVANCED. If you are not yet able to use a single scent as a distraction/grounding tool without triggering any symptoms, DO NOT TRY THIS. Odds are, these advanced ideas will only make you more reactive, and then you'll have to do a bunch of bubble time—I mean weeks to months—before you can try this again. I know it's tempting to rush this process of acclimating yourself to scents, but rushing can set you back. Give your central nervous system the time it needs to determine the scent is safe and that you are safe whenever you smell it. Slow, consistent, forward progress, that's the goal.

If you can comfortably work with at least one scent (preferably more) in all kinds of triggerful environments without triggering any of your symptoms, then you may wish to try expanding on that with the following techniques or tools.

Add Another Scent to Your Repertoire and Then Another …

(This is an advanced scent strategy. If you haven't yet read the intro to this segment on advanced techniques, please go back and read that now before reading further. It's for your own good, really.)

As I said earlier, the goal is to experience the whole world as your scent repertoire once again, like you used to, pre–CS. The more scents your brain recognizes as "safe," the more it will accept outside the bubble. So keep introducing and practicing with scents, one at a time, in your bubble, the way I explained earlier. I try to add a new scent every three months, but sometimes it moves more quickly, or slowly, depending on how well I'm managing my intrinsic triggers, my planning and pacing, and bubble time. Be patient. Be kind to your central nervous system. It's working for you, but the process of healing takes time.

Working with Room Diffusers

(This is another advanced scent strategy. If you haven't yet read the intro to this segment on advanced techniques, please read that now, before reading further. It's for your own good, really.)

A friend gave me a "scent-ball" to try out. Ever seen one? It's a baseball-sized plastic sphere with a plug jutting out at 90 degrees. When you place a drop of essential oil on the little cotton pad thingie in front, and then plug the sphere into a wall outlet, the oil is heated (very low temperature) and its aroma suffuses the room.

I have some issues with this: First, if you tend to be triggered by new plastic and buy this product new, it will need time to off-gas before you try it. Second, heating plastic is never a good idea in my opinion, even at the low temperature this device creates. Even if you give it a year to off-gas before using it, who knows what it will release into the air, into your lungs? I don't know. I don't know if anybody knows. I wish someone did, but until then, here's what I do know:

The scent-ball was over a year old and well used (and I assume off-gassed) when I first tried it, yet it took a few weeks before I could be in the same room with it without inciting symptoms—and that was using a single drop of amber, a scent I'd had no problems using for several months in my nosegay prior to trying the scent-ball. I can use the scent-ball now, over a year later, still with just a single drop of amber, but after about an hour or so, I get a runny nose (an early warning symptom). Is this problem because of the strength of the scent released by the ball, or something about the heated ball itself? I don't know. Maybe you'll have better luck, but I only use this scent-ball thingie in a pinch, when I can't use my clay room diffuser (more on that below).

Why is the scent-ball worth trying? It's light, compact, and the least messy and involved out of all room diffusers I've seen. It can easily slip into a coat pocket, purse, backpack, or briefcase, and it's basically "plug and play." I can keep it in my bag, and then if I go to a friend's house or a doctor's office and there is a triggering odor there that my wee hand-held nosegay can't handle, I can sometimes manage a brief visit if I plug in the scent-ball and sit near it, rather than go all that way, only to immediately flee.

My baked clay room diffuser is my preferred tool for big scent distraction jobs. The diffuser is about five inches tall and hollow and has two pieces. The bottom part looks like a mini wood fire pizza oven. It has an opening in front where I can insert a tea light candle, and a "chimney" hole on top. The second piece, which resembles a palm-sized birdbath, covers the chimney hole. I fill this reservoir with water and however many essential oil droplets. The candle heats the water, which heats the oil, and the scent is released into the air.

Pros and cons: I've tried three of these flame-fueled diffusers—baked clay, marble, and porcelain—with varying results. The baked clay diffuser burned at a lower temperature than the others, which I found to be significant because I could tolerate scents diffused at a lower temperature for a longer period than those diffused at a higher temperature. Baked clay is also lighter weight, so easier to carry around. However, clay is the most fragile. The marble diffuser is more durable but heavy. The porcelain is compact and lightweight yet fragile. Both marble and porcelain get *hot*. The water evaporates at a quicker pace, and I have to monitor it to ensure I'm not just heating a dry reservoir. These two also burn off the oil faster, which results in a big burst of scent and then nothing. So, when I use marble or porcelain, I need to ensure I only put in a drop of oil at a time, and then add more later, with water. A drawback with all flame-fueled diffusers is the potential for fire hazard. It's best not to leave, or sleep with a candle burning. Plug-in diffusers are another option—be wary of the product materials though. All things considered, I react less to the candle diffusers than the scent-ball.

When I go on an excursion and intend to stay for more than an hour in one place, I bring a nosegay (never leave the bubble without it!) and both scent-ball and flame diffuser, along with a few of the most enjoyable scents in my repertoire. When I get where I'm going, I can then decide which scent will work best amidst any triggers inherent in that environment. Sometimes the environment is trigger-free enough that I don't need anything but the nosegay. Sometimes I use a room-size diffuser and it works like a charm. Sometimes I have an immediate reaction to triggers in the new space and have to seek refuge in my car while doing self-talk or meditation, while a diffuser fills the room with a safe scent. Sometimes I can emerge from that car bubble once the diffuser has done its thing, and I find that the new space is manageable from then on. Sometimes the place is simply unmanageable—there could be scentless triggers provoking symptoms, or maybe my intrinsic trigger load is high that day—and I have to turn right back around and go home. Until I find something better, that's the deal, but I can live with that.

A note about steam diffusers: Plug-in essential oil diffusers that send a scented mist into the air have become very popular in recent years. Whether a steam diffuser is made of ceramic, glass or plastic, I find that they usually trigger my Asthma, as well as ILS and MCS, so I can't recommend them at this time. If you decide to try one and find it works for you, great. The more tools you have, the better.

Forgot Your Nosegay?

Every so often I have forgotten my scarf and nosegay and had to find whatever I could in my bag or in the environment that could serve in a pinch. These have worked for me:

- sitting upwind of environmental triggers
- sitting beside an open window or door
- using a piece of peppermint or spearmint gum as a nosegay
- using my peppermint lip balm as a nosegay
- using my ginger tea, hot chocolate, or coffee as a nosegay
- using my snack plate of pineapple as a nosegay
- using my forearm or wrist or hair, sniffing up my sleeve or the inside of my hat (I.E., self as nosegay)
- pulling my turtleneck up over my mouth and nose and breathing through it
- moving a pine cone centerpiece close to me and sniffing it as needed

Get the idea? Try to think of things that make you feel safe or that you find comforting. Hot chocolate never fails for me. Yep, things I think are yummy work great, like maple syrup or pineapple. (By the way, you don't have to chow down on your interim nosegay—you can simply sniff it as needed.)

Some situations and environments are very challenging and can take a lot of concentration—telling my soldiers to back down, telling my brain how much I love pineapple or whatever scent I'm using, breathing deeply, etc. This can make my presence at certain functions exhausting and short-lived. But if I *need* to be somewhere, the above temporary nosegay strategies can give me temporary access and I hope they will, with time and practice, do the same for you.

THE NOSEGAY AS SECURITY BLANKET AND THE WEANING

This is *advanced* advanced information. That is, advanced to the second power. That is, do not even *think* about trying this until you have at least ten to 20 scents solidly in your scent repertoire. That means you can tolerate those scents *any*where and use them as nosegays in triggerful environments, even on high intrinsic trigger days, without inciting a single symptom. If you aren't there yet, DO NOT TRY THIS. I cannot be any clearer. Skipping ahead only causes setbacks and crashes, and neither you nor I want that.

If, however, you have a solid scent repertoire and routinely access triggerful environments as a nosegay ninja (and provoke nary a symptom), then you may be ready to have a look at this level of nosegay technique. (And hey, congrats on getting this far! That took time and patience and a whole lot of dedication to you, yourself, and your health. Let's take a moment to savour the achievement … are you pouring yourself a nice cuppa? I am. *Ahhhhh!*)

The deal is, we don't want to be relying on a nosegay everywhere we go for the rest of our lives, right? We want to teach our brain that most strong smells, synthetic chemical scents, and off-gassing of new products are safe. I've described how to do that. Once we get to the stage where our sensitized brain has re-learned that there *are* some safe scents, we can begin to use the nosegay to teach the brain that there are safe environments that may smell dangerous. Make sense? No? Let me try another way.

Remember Linus, from the Peanuts gang? Linus had a security blanket he took with him everywhere he went. Well, once you get used to using your nosegay for access to all kinds of triggerful places, you may start to feel the same about it—for all intents and purposes, the nosegay *is* a security blanket, right? You use it to comfort yourself in triggerful places, distract your brain from threats, and focus on feelings of safety and enjoyment.

So, what do you think happens when you use the nosegay to gain access to the same triggerful place, time and again, over a period of months or years? Or rather, what do you think *should* happen? The sensitized brain should begin to register that place as less threatening over time. The more you go there and prove to the brain that there is no threat, the more the brain should come to understand that even though the place *smells* toxic—like bleach or new tires or whatever—you are safe there, and the body doesn't need to go into (over)protect mode.

That seems logical, right? Good. Question: if you continue to cling desperately to your nosegay when you enter these well known triggerful places (as you probably did when you first began using your nosegay there) what kind of message does that send to your sensitized brain?

Nothing good. If you clutch your nosegay with a death grip and jam it against your nostrils the entire time you're in that triggerful environment, you are sending a message to your brain that it's *not* a safe place, that it's a scary, threatening place, that you will die without your nosegay to protect you from that place.

I suggest that once you've had ten or 20 successful ventures into whatever triggerful place—a doctor's office, a big box store, or a friend's house—and have left there with no symptoms, you may wish to start the process of weaning yourself off the nosegay in that environment.

What? Stop using the nosegay? But it's my golden ticket!

Yep, I know. Terrifying prospect, but not a cause for panic. Let's put this in perspective, see how far you've come, and determine if you're actually ready to try this next step:

1. You are in crisis phase, you can't breathe anywhere, you are so symptomatic you can barely leave the house.

2. You identify your environmental and intrinsic triggers, you build a bubble and use it to help decrease symptoms and engage your parasympathetic system, you

learn planning and pacing, you determine your functional capacity and respect it, and eventually you become less reactive and enter stability phase.

3. You continue using the bubble, start to notice some desensitization to certain triggers, and work on building a scent repertoire.

4. You start to use a nosegay to gain temporary access to triggerful places while minimizing symptoms.

5. Your confidence in using a nosegay and scents from your repertoire grows and, while there are still countless environments that trigger symptoms even when you employ your nosegay, there are a handful of triggerful places you can routinely enter with your nosegay without triggering any symptoms.

6. You begin weaning yourself off the nosegay in those places where you routinely have no problems.

Feel better? If you have reached Step 5, then you are ready to begin work on Step 6, which I fondly call "The Weaning." (Sounds like a Stephen King novel, eh?) What does the weaning process look like? Good question.

1. Ensure that you are *not* clutching your nosegay with a death grip when you enter one of those "routine" or well-known, triggerful environments. Hold it as loosely as possible without dropping it. You'll probably have to pay attention for a while, and every time you notice your fingers clutching, remind them to let go. Once you can automatically hold your nosegay in a relaxed grip from the time you enter the environment to the time you leave, without having to think about loosening your grip, you are ready to move on to step 2.

2. Engage more specific self-talk each time you enter these routine environments. Instead of the usual "I'm safe here, it's all ok" (a classic in its own right, but not quite appropriate for the weaning) you're going to use something more like this: "Hey, I'm here again! It's been four times this month, eh? Wow, and it still smells like tires. *Quel surprise!* But that smell can't hurt me. I mean, I've been here so many times, and I'm still kicking. I prefer the scent in this nosegay, but I don't really need it because I'm safe here...." So your self-talk needs to go from general to quite specific, reminding your sensitized brain of how many times you've been there, and that although the smell your brain interprets as toxic is still there, it can't harm you. Get the idea?

3. While you're working the self-talk, you're going to start weaning off the nosegay. The tendency, when you walk into a super stinky environment, will probably be to press the nosegay close to the nostrils and block out all other scents. Now you're going to work on doing the opposite. Pull the nosegay away from the nostrils just enough that you can take a gentle whiff of whatever's in the air in that routine environment. If the gentle whiff causes your throat to tighten or nose to run or triggers a migraine or whatever your warning symptoms are, then replace the nosegay and calmly exit the environment. Next time you return, try taking a gentle whiff again. Keep trying until that first whiff triggers no symptoms.

4. Once you can take a gentle whiff without triggering symptoms, you—well, can you guess what's next? Yep, a second whiff. And, if that's tolerated, then a third, and another. The nosegay may be only a few millimeters from your nostrils, just enough to let in some of the environment's odor while you can still smell your

safe scent in the nosegay. Gradually, you want to increase the distance between nosegay and nostrils. This will take many visits, and some days it will go better than others. (Note that while it's important to have confidence in your environmental trigger strategies, your own trigger load fluctuations, combined with the unpredictability of public spaces, require that you remain fluid in your expectations. Just because you've managed in an environment before doesn't mean it will *always* be manageable, so be prepared to enjoy, with the understanding that you may not be able to enjoy, on any given day.)

5. In some environments, I've found it very easy to wean myself off the nosegay, while other places are so challenging that I'm still working on it. Don't be afraid to experiment with this process of decreasing dependency on the nosegay. Sometimes I have better luck with taking one light breath with no nosegay, and then two or three regular breaths with nosegay, and then one light breath without ... alternating like that. If at any time you trigger symptoms, you need to leave *immediately*. Be sure to continue the positive self-talk as you go.

Your ultimate goal, of course, is to be able to smell whatever strong scents are in the air while breathing normally, with no nosegay and no symptoms. And then savor your accomplishment!

Review of Desensitization, the Scent Repertoire and the Nosegay Technique

- Desensitization, or the diminishing of reactivity to a given trigger, may occur after one has passed beyond the ultra-reactive stage. Working with a nosegay and scent repertoire may accelerate the desensitization process, but trying these strategies too soon will most likely elicit greater symptoms, add to the trigger list, and/or cause significant setbacks.
- One should feel safe at all times when building the scent repertoire. One should not try this when intrinsic and/or environmental trigger load is high.
- It may take months to acclimate to one natural scent and become able to tolerate it without triggering symptoms.
- Excursions are stressful, so even when using a nosegay, one must plan for adequate bubble time before and after excursions.
- While the nosegay allows short-term access to places formerly prohibitive, it does not necessarily prevent all symptoms in all places. The nosegay is an access tool only, and a limited one at that.
- While using the nosegay and scent repertoire can help to mask or distract the brain from odorous triggers, the ultimate goal of these strategies is to re-educate the sensitized brain so that it finds enjoyment in most scents, not cause for alarm.

> *The workings of chance are strange. I find it almost embarrassing*
> *that chance can change a mood so drastically, so that it suddenly*
> *seems possible that things will get better. Only now do I realize*
> *I had stopped believing they ever could.*
> —Christa Wolf, *City of Angels or, The Overcoat of Dr. Freud*[15]

5. Coping Emotionally and Psychologically with CS and CSS

Wiffling

The heroine Katniss is climbing the tallest tree, so she can look out across the arena of death. A gladiator in a parallel universe, she strives to make all things right in the world and has only courage and her weapons of choice, bow and arrow, to do so. She's just a character in the movie *Catching Fire*, and a movie is nothing more than a story presented via images, dialogue, and sounds. While watching Katniss' tale unfold, I rely on my brain, as I have for as long as I can remember. I trust it to process the meaning of the images, to translate the sounds into emotion, and to then present the saga to me. My brain is the narrator of the story—of all stories, really—telling me everything in its own words.

I never noticed this brain-as-narrator phenomenon until I got sick.

Now, I witness Katniss standing atop the great tree, boldly assessing the lay of the land, her bow in one hand and a dozen arrows in their ... in their ...

Wiffle.

What the heck is a wiffle? I query my brain, but that's the word it gives me: wiffle. I know what a Wiffle Ball is, and it's not something you hold arrows in. I try prompting with contextual associations, like "Robin Hood has one," which leads to "William Tell split an apple," which leads to "wiffle while you work," to "bells and wiffles," and "not just wiffling Dixie," to a wiffle-stop tour of idiomatic wrongness: "if you want me just wiffle, wolf wiffle, wet my wiffle, wiffle blower—"

The right word is gone. A word I've known for as long as I can remember. A word a kid of eight would know. Nowhere near the tip of my tongue, it's lost, in the fog.

The infamous brain fog of Chronic Fatigue Syndrome wafted into my brain three years ago, following a workplace chemical exposure that also left me with Multiple Chemical Sensitivities, asthma, and an interminable battle with workers compensation. I realized early on that, not only had I lost my health, my job, my home, most of my friends, and my active lifestyle, I was losing touch with my brain.

First I started misspelling things and making basic grammar errors. I'd always been skilled to the point of arrogance with grammar and spelling—friends had long ago nicknamed me a "Grammar Ninja" and relied on me to proofread their résumés and important letters, essays and stories—so when I started having trouble manipulating words and letters, I was shocked, and worried. No, not worried. Deeper than that. I felt betrayed. Without warning, without a goodbye or a chance to let me address its grievances, my brain had run off into the fog somewhere I couldn't follow. It would connect once in a while, but I couldn't trust it to be there when I needed it.

As the cognitive issues increased, my brain trust deteriorated. My vocabulary started disappearing, words and phrases at a time. They often returned later, but I couldn't control when. In the midst of a conversation I would suddenly forget the topic, my argument, my next sentence, my next word, my last word, and/or why I was speaking in the first place. The brain fog would creep in and out, just like natural fog. I never knew when it would show up, when it was safe to have a conversation that mattered.

So, what's it like to lose your language, one comma, one letter, one word at a time? What's it-like having an unreliable narrator telling your stories?

Incredibly unsettling doesn't cover it. For a long time I felt that nothing could or ever would be right with the world again. I was a writer, a song-writer, a good communicator, a quick wit, a smart person, yet the cognitive lapses razed every definition I'd wrought for myself in 40 years of living. My brain was lost, and so I was too.

I wasn't the heroine of some fantasy tale. There would be no two-minute-long montage as I waltzed through the Kübler-Ross stages of grief to a happy Hollywood ending. What I experienced was a terrifying rending of self, followed by a long, arduous crawl through the muck of my own stages of grief. It was—*I* was—ugly and undignified. Unlike Katniss, I plummeted from the top of the world, and my adventure came to a screeching halt. Gravity shifted, or the planet's poles switched places, or maybe I landed on another planet altogether? Up was down was sideways was wrong. It was all wrong.

* * *

Defend.

I've done stupid stuff in my adult life—clinging helplessly to the reins as my rent-a-horse galloped off across the pasture, mistakenly entering the men's bathroom during a Canucks game, taking the Black Diamond ski run instead of the bunny hill—but I'd never believed that I was stupid. Losing that facility with grammar and spelling, losing my vocabulary and ability to carry on a simple conversation, I felt stupid, and vulnerable. Language was my tool and shield. Words were what I did. Words made me. Clothes made the man but words made the writer. And the singer. And they were the key to social interaction. But with increasingly frequency, people were finishing my sentences for me, or talking over me, as I struggled for words. Most gave me odd looks, scoffs, and ultimately, the brush-off.

So I covered my deficiencies up by not speaking, and applied vigorous nodding and shaking of head when applicable. This led to people yammering nonstop about themselves, while I remained mired in silence. Talked out at last, they'd leave me drained and depressed. Desperate for a more balanced dynamic, I tried entering into only short, phatic conversations, but even then there were days when the fog was so thick, I'd get stuck on, "Nice weather we're ... um..."

More like *foggy* weather.

* * *

Rage Against the Me.

When my brain gave me a word like "wiffle," I'd pause the movie and rifle through my thesaurus, looking up *bow* and *arrow* and *holder* and any word that came close to the one I needed, until finally I found it. This stopped working after my comprehension, too, faded. Then, I could read the individual words in the lists but they blurred and danced and meant nothing. Their meanings had become a secret they withheld from me. I'd fling the book at the wall and crumple into a ball on the floor. I think therefore I am. If I can't think, therefore, I am ... what?

I'd yell at my brain, *Why are you doing this to me? What's the matter with you? Get with it! You're young yet! Wait another 40 years; then you can slow down, but not now!*

Self-inflicted anger is not very effective in terms of cures. It is ultimately self-defeating. But sometimes it did feel good just to yell.

* * *

Fear.

I had plunged into the stormy Sea of Uncertainty. Unanswerable Questions sharked at me as I flailed for a handhold or foothold, anything that looked like land, solidity, a place where I could rest and feel safe. *Will my brain kick back into gear? What am I going to do if it is like this the rest of my life? What if workers compensation pays me nothing? How will I survive? What if my condition gets worse?*

Months later, I realized that fear had become my antagonist. I might not be a writer or a Grammar Ninja anymore, or whatever else I had once called myself, but those definitions were not me. The essential *me* hadn't disappeared. I was still the hero of my own story, in the same universe, which contained the same amount of uncertainty as it always had. The difference now was that my health conditions had brought that uncertainty to my attention. My perspective had changed, and the world looked different, but it was the same world.

* * *

Good Grief.

A year passed, and another. There were tears. There was isolation, and silence. I missed the power I had felt when I wielded words. I missed my friends and active life. I longed for the old status quo much the way one longs for the innocence and grandiose dreams of youth. Gradually, though, I came to understand what had happened to me. I'd lost some cognitive ability. Some, but not all. My brain hadn't, in fact, betrayed me. It was busy, working to recover from the workplace incident. I couldn't expect optimal functioning while healing, but I could have faith that my brain was doing all it could.

My narrator's new voice was slower, less precise than before, but it was my narrator all the same. Yes, eventually, grief comes. Like a great wave, it envelops and then ebbs.

* * *

These days I focus on improving my cognitive function and enjoying my life with gratitude for all that I have. I manage my expectations with a "cognitive handicap" I developed using golf handicaps as a model. I scribble scraps of creative ideas in my journal when they emerge from the fog, and over months I piece them together into a story or essay. I ask friends to proofread for me, and I'm comfortable enough with my brain lapses that when I lose track of a conversation I can say something like, "Wait for it..." or, "Slow brain today, one moment please."

These days, I take whatever word comes to mind and I go with it, trusting my brain to give me the real one when it is able. Accepting the wrong word, even temporarily, niggles at me, like putting a jigsaw puzzle together and finding the last piece doesn't fit. But I've learned that going with it—or, *wiffling*, as I call it—can make conversations more interesting and make it difficult for me to take myself, or anyone else, too seriously.

So, Katniss draws an arrow from her wiffle and takes aim ...

My brain continues its narrative, and as the story progresses, I forget that *wiffle* isn't the actual word for Katniss' arrow holder. She is running through the jungle with her wiffle slung across her shoulder, she obtains a new wiffle full of arrows, she tumbles down the hillside amidst an avalanche of rock but her wiffle is miraculously undamaged—

QUIVER!

Flashing neon, bright as a megatron in Times Square, the word bursts from the fog. *Quiver!* Ta-da! I do a little jig in my chair. After 40 minutes of wiffling, my brain delivers. And Katniss survives. And all is again right in the world.[1]

Intro to Coping with CS and CSS

Finding effective ways to deal with physical and cognitive debilitation, manage triggers and rest, and keep oneself fed, clothed and sheltered can be a full-time job for those who have CSS (or CS alone). Unfortunately, living with these conditions also tends to expose core beliefs incompatible with one's new limitations and lifestyle and stir up unruly emotions and challenging psychological and social issues.[2] These challenges, along with everything else, can negatively affect one's mental health and relationships.

In this chapter, I'll discuss some common coping issues and effective strategies for coming to terms with loss, harnessing powerful emotions for your own good, identifying and rethinking core beliefs, and maintaining mental health and authentic relationships. Because coping is an ongoing process, I've designed this chapter to help whether you're currently in crisis phase or stability phase. Once you understand what you're up against and get some new skills and practice time under your belt, you'll discover that you *can* cope—even if you don't feel it now—you can regain hope, meet this challenge head-on, and enjoy a meaningful life. Remember, you're not alone, and I'm right here, talking to you.

Loss

Loss. Life's full of it. Before getting sick, I maintained a hearty resilience to the pit-falls, curve balls and sucker punches of life, but CSS tore the sky open and let loose a deluge that stripped me of everything I'd worked for and believed in. Only a ghost of my former existence remained, haunting me with wispy, hungry memories of all I no longer had: health, active lifestyle, voice, home, savings, job, friends, faith in green architecture and those I'd worked for, future hopes and dreams, sense of safety, and—the greatest loss—my sense of identity.

Loss: of Self
I was a runner.
A singer.
A hard worker.
A social person.
I was a writer,
a gardener.
I was a strong, fit woman.
I was a hiker,
an office manager.
I was a friend.
I was an independent person.
I was a productive person…

And I was *going to be* an extreme marathoner, a globetrotting traveler who had visited every continent, a best-selling novelist. I was *going to be* a singer who made a new cd next year, and several more beyond that. I was *going to be* so many things, I was going to achieve so many dreams, I was … all these things and more.

That is how I saw myself pre–CS, and when I got sick and no longer could do any of those things, I experienced a crisis of identity. Who *was* I without those achievements or labels? What good was I if I couldn't *do things,* or *produce* something? And if I could no longer achieve the dreams and goals I'd had for so long, what did I want? What were my dreams and goals now? Such were my questions.

Somewhere along the way, I'd come to see value in myself only in relation to what I could achieve or produce. I had never learned to value myself for simply *being.* Call me a cynic, but I'd always considered that kind of "you're special just the way you are" messaging as hokey Sesame Street stuff. So when the definitions I'd pinned on myself over the years no longer applied, I could see nothing underneath. I felt like nothing. I felt like a blank, useless slate. Taking up space. (Note, this is how depression can really sink its teeth into people who get CSS. I'll talk more about dealing with that momentarily.)

This is a great example why I believe that chronic illness is a catalyst for transfor-mation, for here I ran into another of those pivotal life-changing decisions people with CSS have to make. I could wallow in the depths of despair and loss for the rest of my lifetime, I could end my life, or I could work at figuring out what my value actually was, who I was, and what I wanted now that these conditions were part of my life.

I decided to try to redefine myself and my goals, reasoning that if I didn't like what I discovered about me, or if I couldn't think of any worthwhile objectives, I could always choose suicide or a lifetime of despair—replete with an auto-renewing subscription to

Netflix, a freezer full of Ben and Jerry's, and a multitude of cats—later. Such was my logic at the time.

How did I do it?

Good question. First, I listed my definitions, like at the beginning of this segment. Then I crossed out all the things I cold no longer do. (With three CSS, and both physical and cognitive debilitation, I had a lot of things to cross out.) Next, I added things I *was,* not things I *did.* This was difficult! It took me weeks to come up with anything. Eventually, my brainstorm resulted in something like this:

TABLE 9. QUALITIES OF ME-NESS

I am …

Musical	Sun-loving	Honest	Loveable
Sensitive	Compassionate	Punny	Curious
Giving	Animal-loving	Intelligent	Dedicated
Beach-loving	Introverted	Emotional	Diligent
Trustworthy	Protective	Creative	Strong

I studied these words and told myself, "This is me, not that previous list of actions and productions." At first the words ran off me like rain off a raccoon's pelt, but in time they soaked in.

Then I asked myself, "What do I want from my life?" Again, I scribbled down any ideas, though they were few at first. How could I envision new goals based on my current limitations when everything I'd dreamed of pre–CSS still dominated my imagination? It took time. Eventually, I decided I would have to live, and dream, with ambiguity. I ended up with a chart that contained two lists, the first of which contained things I wanted to achieve if my functional capacity remained at the same level forever (at the time this was three non-consecutive hours per day); and the second held goals for when I was cured of CSS and CS. (Hey, as long as I'm dreaming, I'm going to dream *big.*) An overlapping section between the two contained things I wanted regardless of my functional capacity. It looked something like Diagram 3.

In addition to helping me accept my current limitations, making this chart gave me dreams to live on. It was a surprisingly revelatory process. It illuminated the fact that I had a lot of Maslow-related needs (food, shelter, and a safe, survivable environment) to satisfy before I could move forward with my life. It allowed me to redefine myself, let go of that old identity, and make way for the "new" me, which was actually the me that had always been there but I'd never recognized. It also taught me that I didn't have to produce much of anything to find meaning, and that there was still much in life that I wanted to discover and experience.

I wonder what you'll find when you explore your identity and desires?

LOSS OF FRIENDS

When I got sick, people I'd known for years acted like strangers. They looked at me like I had leprosy, had slept with their spouse, and was about to steal their silver. I was not prepared for this. I thought my friends would rally around me. I thought I had authentic relationships, the kind that survived everything and kept on growing. And I did have a couple like that; thankfully, I still do. But the majority of people I'd called friend—well, in my opinion, chronic illness works far better than divorce in terms of weeding "false friends" out of one's life and shining a golden light upon the rest. Losing friends on top

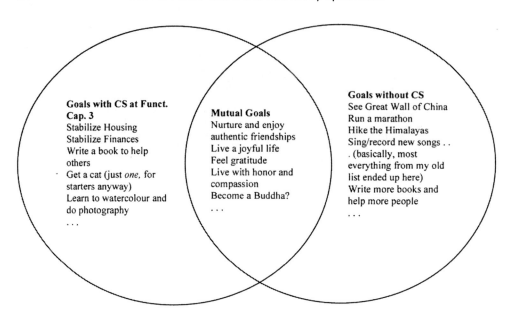

Goals with CS at Funct. Cap. 3
Stabilize Housing
Stabilize Finances
Write a book to help others
Get a cat (just *one,* for starters anyway)
Learn to watercolour and do photography
. . .

Mutual Goals
Nurture and enjoy authentic friendships
Live a joyful life
Feel gratitude
Live with honor and compassion
Become a Buddha?
. . .

Goals without CS
See Great Wall of China
Run a marathon
Hike the Himalayas
Sing/record new songs . . . (basically, most everything from my old list ended up here)
Write more books and help more people
. . .

Diagram 3. My goals

of all the other illness-related loss can deal you a devastating blow, especially if you don't see it coming, but you don't have to operate on the same level of cluelessness I did. Here are my top lessons learned.

Chronic illness is hard for people to face; "invisible" illness, even more so. People's attitudes towards illness and disease run the gamut from acting as if nothing's changed to walking on eggshells around you to disappearing without a word to vast incomprehension, which may result in them saying something like, "I'm sorry you aren't feeling well. Call me when you're better and we'll hang out!" People might make decisions that affect you without consulting you, as if you are no longer an adult, or even a person. Longtime friends might support you for a week or a month or two but then fade away.

Any illness or injury is inconvenient. It's unpredictable, boring, time-consuming, and it's a stark reminder to others of their own mortality. Chronic illness tends to provoke more extreme reactions because it has no clear path to rehabilitation, no expiry date by which time it will disappear and things can return back to "normal," no end in sight. Many people can't or won't acknowledge that such a thing as chronic illness exists, or that it could happen to them. Their fear may cause them to see you as a cautionary tale that they would rather forget.

"Invisible" chronic illnesses like CS and CSS tend to elicit even less compassion than those made "visible" by the presence of a wheelchair, crutches, cane, oxygen tank, or IV stand. I can't tell you how many dirty looks I've received when I sink into a seat reserved for the disabled on transit or in the pharmacy. Or how many times I've heard, "Well, you look fine!" when I'm about to collapse. I've found myself pitted against someone who required the use of a wheelchair in a fight for limited accessibility resources—this was in a *university* setting—and I lost educational opportunities because the administration couldn't *see* my disability. Anyone who remembers several decades ago when people who require wheelchairs were an "unseen entity" and launched campaigns nationwide to fight for ramps and seating space in public places and transit understands that "invisibility" is primarily an education issue. The general public needs to be educated about CS and CSS. We will do that—we *are* doing that now—but it takes time.

Until then, be prepared for these types of reactions and remember, the problem isn't you. It is a problem of people and illness—illness people can see, illness with an ending, illness people have experienced. CS and CSS are none of those.

Friends may blame you. You may blame you. People may tell you, "get over it" or "quit making something out of nothing," as if you've chosen to have this illness and can just as easily choose not to, the way one chooses to get a worm composting bin, take up salsa dancing, or become a vegan. Such interactions can make you feel even worse, especially when you may be having similar doubts, wondering, "Did I cause this illness somehow?" or, "If my doctor doesn't know what's wrong with me, *am* I imagining it?"

I questioned myself a lot at first, especially before getting a proper diagnosis. Pre-CS, I'd had no idea how lucky I was to have such a healthy life. I believed it was because I ate well and exercised. I believed I was in control, but when I got sick, a huge nebulous uncertainty replaced that illusion, and with the uncertainty came people's attacks, mine included. It's normal to question, to deny, or blame, and it's easy to blame yourself, but it's not your fault. You didn't choose CS or CSS and the accompanying discomfort and chaos, and while you can do a lot to manage the effects of your illness, you can't control them. These conditions will ruin enough of your relationships; don't let them ruin the most important one—your relationship with yourself.

Peer relationships may suffer or end. My cognitive issues created a significant disparity between my abilities and those of my writing peers. They could read and write and think faster, they could argue and discuss topics for hours, while Facebooking and changing diapers and cooking meals, whereas I could read for a mere five minutes and had less than half my previous vocabulary at my disposal on a good day, I got woozy at the sight of Facebook, and I lost track of the conversation when talking about the weather.

It took me over two years to accept that I was now one step (or more) behind my peers. First I tried to hide my debilitation, from myself as well as others, but as I came to realize the extent of my functional limitations, I found that I *couldn't* hide them, from anyone. I also discovered that most people can't or won't discuss such things openly. My writing group, for example, began talking around me, making decisions as if I didn't exist. Most of my other writing peers, too, had conversations about my condition behind my back instead of talking *to* me, *with* me. From this present-day vantage point, I suspect their exclusive behavior was primarily due to ignorance, but it felt very hateful and selfish at the time. Only a small percentage of my writing peers showed an interest in discussing ways in which we could continue to work together, or at least relate with one another.

Thus, one more layer peeled away from the onion of my life and left me feeling desperate and terrified. Did I have to lose everything *and everyone* in my life? Were these people even my peers anymore? If they weren't, then who was? Could I only relate to folks with CS and CSS from now on? Don't worry if you have more questions than answers. This happens a lot with these conditions. You don't have to know everything now, and answers will appear in time.

A workers compensation claim will bring out the worst in everyone. I was an office manager at GAS. Unlike most people in the office, who couldn't remember their next-door-cubicle-neighbor's name, I knew all 100 employees. I was good at my job and dedicated, and I went out of my way to make people's lives better there. After the chemical exposure, GAS laid me off, and a total of two co-workers contacted me to see how I was. That's 2 percent.

Because GAS had misinformed workers compensation about the air quality and related issues, I had to seek statements from my co-workers to support my fight for compensation. Only 3 percent of those I asked agreed to help. Some of those who said no weren't merely coworkers, they were friends too, friends with whom I'd shared meals, spent holidays, friends for whom I'd babysat and gone out of my way time and again; yet, when I really needed them, they turned away.

One of my close friends, whom I'd known for over ten years, said she wouldn't write a statement for me because she had just applied for a job at workers compensation, and she didn't want to jeopardize her chances of employment by supporting an injured worker. She could have written a statement for me anonymously, or used only her initials, but she didn't. She knew I had lost my home and savings and would be homeless in weeks. She still said no.

Granted, any workers compensation system that operates with a bias against injured workers and requires them to obtain evidence from people afraid of losing their jobs if they tell the truth has something seriously, inherently wrong with it. Still, what strikes me is that I'd lived over 40 years in such naïve denial of human nature. I'd never expected people to be so selfish.

When I say workers compensation brings out the worst in everyone, I mean me too. Unfair, intimidating, and demoralizing, the system drove me to desperation and I camped there for years. More than once, I found myself *begging* someone to tell the truth about what they saw at GAS, to no avail. More times than not, this ended in me feeling angrier and more rejected than before. I'd lash out and feel ashamed afterwards. I'll talk more about compensation and disability claims later on, but for now, know that the 98 percent who won't support you aren't worth your energy. You don't need to beg them. You can let them go. Focus on yourself and on the 2 percent who bear the torch for humanity.

CS and CSS can shine a light on dysfunction in your closest relationships. Most of the solid friendships I thought I'd built over the years turned out to be one-way relationships in which I gave far more than I received. I like to give, so I was happy to do so, and I assumed that those friends would be there for me if I ever needed them. I thought that was how friendship worked—give when you can and it all balances out in the end. But when I became too sick to continue giving the support and attention those people had grown accustomed to, most of them avoided me, rejected my requests for help, and disappeared. I felt abandoned and betrayed, and also naïve for not having seen the dysfunction in those relationships years prior.

Since then, I've done some work on my personal boundaries (see Appendix F: Recommended Reading and Viewing for my go-to boundaries books). I've also learned that past behavior often indicates future behavior. If friends aren't holding up their end before you get CS, they most likely won't when you become ill. Don't let this get you down. Let it prepare you. The boon here is that you will learn who loves you for *you,* and which relationships to treasure and invest your limited energy in.

How do you know when to speak up? When I got sick and friends began making their exits, I experienced a sudden, desperate regret about losing them, losing everything, losing, losing, *must stop LOSING—!*

Yep, it was intense. I thought that if I could explain a little more clearly what my experience with CS and the syndromes was like, they would understand and come to see this illness as an opportunity to strengthen our friendship, not end it. The thing is, very few people *will* understand. Most will not have a clue. But if you feel inclined to speak up, then do so. Your friend may perceive you as pushy or pedantic or whatever else, but taking care of yourself is your number one job, right? If you need to talk to them, then talk. Afterwards you can ask yourself, *do I feel better knowing that I gave that friendship one last shot by expressing myself as best I could? Or do I feel nothing more than exhausted and deflated from the exertion?* Your answer may help you decide what to say the next time you notice someone drifting away.

I've tried both speaking up and silence, and countless degrees in between, with limited success and satisfaction. Over time I've learned that the best results come when I focus on my needs, not on that idea of "yet another loss." Now, when anxious desperation starts to overtake me, I ask questions like these:

- How does this relationship meet my needs?
- What has this person done for me lately (aka "the Janet Jackson approach")?
- Does interacting with this person drain or feed my spirit?

Tough questions, but once I have the answers, I can see which relationships are authentic and healthy and worth fighting for, and that's the goal.

You may question your judgment, about *every*thing. The hardest part for me was that time of initial discovery. People I trusted were putting distance between us, even lying or offering flimsy excuses instead of being honest. Everything I had thought was solid—writing and singing career, income, apartment, future, retirement—became vapor and, as vapor will, dispersed into nothingness. Even gravity seemed to tug at me from a different direction. I struggled for a handhold, but kept coming up empty. People became one more element in my life that wasn't what I had thought, that I had misjudged, another area where I had misplaced my faith, and this made me question my judgment about everything. Compounding this, after so many people turned their backs, I started to feel worthless. This played into my identity crisis—negative thoughts like, "Now that I have CSS, *do* I have anything to give people, really?" (If you find yourself slipping into negative thinking like this, don't give in. Keep on reading.)

Whenever any illness-related relationship issue gets you down, remember this: These people aren't turning from *you*. They aren't able to deal with the *illness*. It's not fair, I know, but that's the deal. Do your best to focus on the folks who stick around. They're worth more than those who disappear, thousand-fold.

I still do try to convince people to stay sometimes, when fear of losing gets the better of me. I want you to know that there is a handhold for you here, whenever you need one. You aren't alone, though it sure may feel like it, and I'm right here, talking to you.

MATERIAL LOSS

I've had a couple revelations surrounding loss these past few years, one regarding what I call "the Zen progression of loss." First, the furniture, my bookcases, a cherished couch or rug; and then my garden, where I spent so many summer days with hands deep in the soil, or lovingly sculpting jasmine trellis screens; and then my home—the little studio apartment I'd somehow managed to snatch out of the soaring real estate market and call my own (with a mortgage I'd be paying 'til the age of 80 to boot). Everything I'd managed to acquire, and all the money I'd managed to save in my whole life was disappearing at a rapid rate. Those first material losses were the hardest. I clung to each one and fought viciously to hold onto it.

As I began to learn to put my health first, though, I worried less about material losses. It occurred to me that if all my efforts to control the onslaught of loss had failed, then what could I possibly gain by trying to control it? What would happen if I just *let go?* Eventually, I did. I focused more and more on my health and less on the superficial things, and I discovered that there is a wonderful freedom in having nothing material left to lose.

Of course, it wasn't a smooth cruise in the fast lane to get to that point. As I stumbled through the crises of identity, relationships and mega-loss, something nasty got ahold of me. (This is where the other revelation about loss comes in.) I'd been pretty darn lucky for most of my life, able to do most anything I set my mind to. CS and CSS were the first serious issues I'd faced that my will power alone couldn't fix. Feeling so powerless devastated me. I can't tell you exactly when or how it happened, but one day I woke up to find that I'd become what I judged as a "hopeless loser."

In 15 minutes I can run 3k, easy. Then I can run another 3, or 5, or even 10k if I want. Easy. I might have a nap after, but I don't need to rest. I can go dancing that night, or binge on DVDs until dawn.

In 15 minutes I can dance to six pop songs. Then I can sing like Gaga at Karaoke, laugh until my eyes water and belly hurts. Then I can pick up a guy, take him home, have a quickie, go for Chinese at 2 a.m. or stay in bed for more. Wake up at noon, go to brunch, go home and get it up again.

In 15 minutes I can walk across a stage, shake the Dean's hand and collect my Bachelor of Arts Degree. Then I can go to a commencement party, drink champagne, and mingle with well-dressed and sweet-smelling classmates, until the diner on the corner opens for breakfast. The cook serves up my usual when I walk in the door. Then I go for a walk on the seawall around the bay and dream of my future.

In 15 minutes I can get a good job at a reputable company. In the same amount of time, I can sign papers on a little apartment that I will own for the rest of my life. My own home. My heart sings when I think of it.

In 15 minutes I can knead a batch of homemade bread, or prep ingredients for soup and stuff the crockpot full. Then I can do the laundry, clean the bathroom, vacuum the whole apartment. I can go for as long as I want, reading a novel, sweeping the patio, catching up on bills and correspondence. Watching the sun rise and set. Watching whatever I want. Not watching the time.

In 15 minutes I can write 300 words, maybe more. But I don't write for only 15 minutes at a time. Who could? I write for hours. I lose myself in words, in time. I'm working on a novel.

In 15 minutes I can swim in a glacier-fed lake atop a mountain it took me 3 hours to climb. Then I can climb down again, have a beer at the pub, and plan my next adventure.

In 15 minutes I can walk to work along the seawall beside the dawn-painted water of the bay, without breaking a sweat. Then I can start in on a difficult project and keep on working through the morning, through my lunch hour, make my manager smile with my solutions, make my co-workers' day with a funny story.

In 15 minutes I can inhale enough toxic materials at my workplace to develop multiple chemical sensitivities and chronic fatigue.

Then I must rest.

In 15 minutes I can be laid off and told to leave the office where I worked for nearly 4 years, never to return.
Then I must rest.

In 15 minutes I can cough until I fall unconscious to the floor of my apartment building's lobby, at the feet of my neighbor, who wears heavy perfume and won't let me pass until she tells me her issue with another neighbor's dog.
Or I fall unconscious to the floor of the washroom of the grocery store, the restaurant, or the café, each place fragranced by a wall-mounted electric air freshener that smells like Kool-Aid or bubblegum.
Or I fall unconscious to the floor of a brand new transit bus that smells like new car smell and carries sardined people wearing perfume, cologne, and fabric-softened clothing.
Then I rest.

In 15 minutes I can read the official decision letter from the official organization that officially protects workers, the letter that says I will not be compensated because my illness is not an occupational disease, my illness is not real, I'm a faker, get a job.
Then I must rest.

In 15 minutes I can watch three runners and an elderly woman pass from one end of my bedroom window frame to the other, their feet moving through autumn leaves in a wonderful dance I yearn to do again.
Then I must rest.

In 15 minutes, I can watch the clouds dance about the mountaintop—far beyond my window—where I once climbed and swam.
Then I must rest.

In 15 minutes, I can write a line to a poem. Or I can read the first sentence of a story 15 times, not understanding. It depends on the day.
Then I must rest.

In 15 minutes I can try to sing and can make only a croaking, strangled frog noise.
Then I must rest.

In 15 minutes I can open a can of soup, heat it in the microwave, and eat half. Save half for tomorrow.
Then I must rest.

In 15 minutes I can go through my address book and cross out the names of the people who tell me they are too busy to come visit, that I should let them know when I feel better and we'll get together, or that they don't want to be friends anymore because I can't go out to clubs or restaurants or cafés or movies.
Then I must rest.

In 15 minutes I can sign the papers to sell my home at a loss, the real estate market having been inflated when I purchased and the bubble having since burst. I feel cold, but tell myself that at least I have a little money to live on now.
Then I must rest.

In 15 minutes I cannot find a cheap, clean, safe, scent-free room to rent on Craigslist. I must rest, look again, rest, and repeat for many days.

In 15 minutes I can pour hot water from the kettle into a mug of dried ramen and eat some before I must rest.

In 15 minutes I can watch a sliver of sun appear at the edge of the dirty window in the room I rent.

Then I must rest. When I wake, that sliver of warmth has disappeared and it is nighttime again.

In 15 minutes I can move out of the rental room, sell the last of my stuff, and pocket the money.
Then I must rest.

In 15 minutes I can walk one block, feverish and aching, past junkies and dealers, pimps and prostitutes, towards the homeless shelter.
Then I must rest.

In 15 minutes I can buy a gun with my last hundred at the pawnshop next door to the shelter, amble into the back alley and use my only bullet.
Or palm my last hundred to the dealer on the corner, who pops something unnamed into my mouth, then stumble another block to the park bench, where I sit and watch countless runners blur by until I see nothingness.
Or shuffle another block to the seawall I used to strut along every day on my way to work. Then fill my pockets with stones and slip over the wall, into the cold, deep water.
Then I rest.

If you think any of the above thoughts, you aren't alone. I wrote that poem based on my experience, and countless others have had similar experiences because of CS and CSS. If you think the thoughts in the last paragraph of that poem, though, please call someone right now—a therapist, a medical professional, or 911—and ask for help.

Becoming a "Hopeless Loser"

Enough doctors tell you it's in your head,
enough insurance companies tell you you're a liar and a faker and a cheat,
enough people tell you you're crazy or lazy or both, so "just get over it,"
enough time goes by with your world turned upside-down,
enough friends turn away,
enough jobs, money, and stability disperse,
enough time goes by,
enough of all that, years of all that, and your resilience can wear thin.
Loss becomes all you see.
Present and future.
You start to doubt yourself, everyone, every thing
and seek refuge within a quiet, dim pit of despair.
Don't go there—*it's a trap!*

I used to feel so certain about things, but when I got sick, I became what I deemed a "hopeless loser," for years. Is this the fate of everyone with these conditions, you ask? No. It's a trap I fell into, one I'm hoping you can avoid.

Warning signs of becoming a "hopeless loser":

- If you lose your sense of humor.
- If you find yourself using your illness to control others (aka playing the "I'm sick" card to manipulate people who care about you).
- If you see no point in dreaming of the future, or you set out to make a list of future goals and can't come up with anything that you feel is worthwhile.

- If you expect bad news and rejection and it doesn't occur to you that good news or acceptance might come your way.
- If you focus on all the negative things that are happening, and can't see any positive ones.

Some people believe that becoming a "hopeless loser" is part of the grieving process inherent in contending with chronic illness. Some people think of it as "hitting rock bottom," and that you have to go there before you can start climbing out. On the way up, you pass that place where you dropped your faith and hope, and you can dust them off and carefully tuck them into your pocket as you go.

I don't believe that everyone has to hit rock bottom before they can find a joyful life with, and/or despite CSS or CS alone. Some people have more resilience, unfailing support network, and a stronger personal foundation than others. Some people grieve and heal in other ways. I do believe that there is no shame in becoming what I call a "hopeless loser." I believe this is an essential phase in the healing process of some people. And I believe that some people are more prone to becoming a "hopeless loser" than others. I am one of those people.

Part of my problem was the length of time it took to get a diagnosis.

Part of my problem was that I had symptoms that made no sense.

Part of my problem was the lack of support I had.

Part of my problem was the financial pressure I was under.

Part of my problem was the rate at which my stability—income, home, social—eroded.

Part of my problem was that I'd been unprepared for the abusive dynamic inherent in an adversarial workers compensation system.

Part of my problem was that I was contending with unfamiliar health issues while learning to navigate the medical system while learning to navigate the workers compensation system while realizing that my employer and the people I had trusted were dishonest …

Let's just say, I had a city dump of problems.

My greatest problem, of course, the problem that probably would have rendered all the above problems easily manageable if it hadn't been a problem in the first place, was that I had never cultivated my self-worth beyond the confines of what I produced or achieved.

Self-worth. In order to begin climbing out of that pit of despair, I first had to see that I'd become a "hopeless loser." And before I could see that, I had to first increase my self-worth.

Self-Worth

There are entire books about increasing one's sense of self-worth, and this is not one of them, but here are a few ideas to get you going:

- Find that last shred of humor, wherever it may be (mine was in the clothes dryer lint collector, embedded in some pink fluff stuff) and wield it like a weapon against doom and gloom. Make yourself watch a funny TV show or YouTube video every day, and laugh out loud. Laughter is healing. Believe it.
- Take a good honest look at your behavior. If you find yourself playing the "I'm sick" card to control others, stop it. Easier said than done? Sure. Baby steps. First

become aware of your behavior, then start to change your behavior. I'll talk more about this process in the upcoming CBT segment.

- Be sure that your words and actions match your values. If you aren't sure how to go about that, try making a list of the things most important you—like health, happiness, or family, or keeping the cat's claws trimmed, or a month's supply of clean undies, or whatever—and then commit to ensuring that whatever you say and do supports those values.

- Tack your blank or fledgling list of future dreams someplace where you will see it several times each day. Cruise the web, TV or magazines (if their off-gassing doesn't trigger you) and notice what interests you. Maybe a picture of a sunset over a beach, or a story about raccoons taking over Toronto transit or the grand opening of Elon Musk's *Space-ventureland* amusement park. Whatever piques your interest, write it on your list. Don't despair if at first you find nothing. If at first everything seems stupid or meaningless, try, try again. My list was empty for months. I hated it and needed it at the same time.

   Gradually a list of things that excite and interest you will take shape. Don't stop there. Focus on that list every day and consider what it is about those things that makes you smile. Do they remind you of fond memories? Or things you've never done or seen, but want to? What do you want? Keep asking. The answers will come.

- If you find yourself expecting or recognizing only bad news and rejection, start a Güd Book (details in the segment below on more strategies) or make a nightly gratitude list. Before going to sleep, list three things that went well that day, for which you feel grateful.

After over a year of doing the above, I began to regain my old sense of humor and optimism and build up some resilience to the challenges of daily life with CSS. And this time, I didn't feel confident because of something I'd done at work or produced or achieved *outside* of myself, I felt confident because I'd been putting *me* first, caring for and listening to myself, and learning what was important to me. I'd started with nothing and created a solid foundation of self-worth within.

While undergoing that transformation, I also experienced a major shift in my perception of loss. I stopped seeing myself as a victim of loss, as someone who loses. In fact, I started seeing loss as something altogether different. I began to replace the word *loss* with the word *change*.

Emotions

Emotion is defined as "the affective aspect of consciousness, feeling; a state of feeling; a conscious mental reaction (as anger or fear) subjectively experienced as strong feeling usually directed toward a specific object and typically accompanied by physiological and behavioral changes in the body."[3] Constantly alerting and informing, emotions can serve as helpful signals—giving you a warm fuzzy when things go well, a shock when things surpass your expectations, or a warning when you are in danger. It's in your best interest to learn to harness the power of emotions for your own good. This can be tricky because your emotions can, often invisibly, affect your thoughts and behaviors.

How do you tell the difference between an emotion and a thought? Good question. I used to think we had infinite kinds of emotions and had no idea how to discern them from thoughts, but recent research based on "early facial expression signaling" suggests that there are only four categories of "basic emotion communication: … happy, sad, fear/surprise … and disgust/anger."[4] If you perceive a strong "feeling" other than those four—such as guilt, shame, boredom, or excitement—you are most likely experiencing a thought fueled by an emotion. I'll talk more about what that means in a moment.

Strong emotions come with the CS territory. The day you get diagnosed, you may feel elated one minute and grief-stricken the next. Or you might feel overcome by an uncontrollable rage one day when, instead of getting much-needed groceries, you have to stay in bed due to severe symptoms. Or when a friend pops by unannounced, you might experience both surprise at their thoughtfulness and disgust with yourself because your place is a mess. Intrinsic trigger load can also contribute to emotion and mood swings.

Generally speaking, when your conditions stir up unruly emotions it's helpful to let them out. Let yourself smile and laugh if you feel happy—heck, dance gleefully if you are able. Let the tears come if sadness or grief hits you. If someone surprises you, let them know. If you feel disgusted with the state of your home, say so, but don't dwell on it. Simply let it out (and then maybe ask your friend to help clean up!) We'll talk about ways to identify, honor, and release emotions throughout this chapter.

Sometimes it's not in your best interest to release emotions the instant they hit. Some tips:

- When you're in the middle of a meeting with a lawyer or doctor or someone with whom you need to share specific info within an appointment time slot. At these times, if a strong emotion makes itself known, it may be helpful to tell yourself that now is not a good time and that when this appointment is over (or when you get home), you can cry (or dance for joy, or punch pillows and yell) as much as you need to.

- If you have ILS, allowing yourself to freely express strong emotions can trigger an ILS episode, so you may need to temper your releases. Let the emotions out, but in moderate fashion. Instead of full-on laughing, allow a wide grin and chuckle. Instead of uncontrolled yelling or sobbing, punch pillows or jump up and down. Or sit and write down all your angst. Find releases that work for you without triggering symptoms. If symptoms can't be avoided, you know what to do: bubble time.

- When you're at a special event or surrounded by people with whom you don't feel safe letting your feelings show, it may be best to tell yourself that now is not a good time. Assure yourself that when you are in a safe place, your emotions will have free rein.

Note that those who have trouble identifying and/or managing their emotions in a healthy way are susceptible "to whatever will keep [their] feelings contained—alcohol, drugs, food, excessive work, stress, compulsive acquiring, compulsive hobbying."[5] What can they do? According to Anne Katherine, internationally known author and mental health counselor, the best action is to "[get] expert help to learn the skills not learned as children. Therapists, classes, and anonymous programs all offer ways to discover one's hidden self … [and] get back in contact with feelings," safely.[6]

You will develop your own style of dealing with strong emotions when they arise. The important thing is realizing that emotions are assets, and that you need them for your own good.

ANGER—DETRIMENT OR TOOL?

I want to talk about anger specifically because many people with CS and CSS experience a heavy dose of this emotion.

After the workplace incident, I had a lot to be angry about. I'd gone to work and done my job, and in return I'd gotten unemployment, an interminable battle for compensation, debt, chronic health issues, loss of voice, major lifestyle degredation…. My list went on and on. And everything on that list had someone's name on it, someone to blame. I blamed others for their greed, dishonesty and negligence, and I blamed myself, for trusting people, for believing in green architecture, for choosing to work at GAS, for going to work and doing my job, for every single choice I'd made in my 40-something years of life that had lead me to getting poisoned by GAS and developing CS and CSS. Every conversation ended in a rant. Words burst from me faster than the speed of thought. I couldn't control the anger. It had become me, or I had become it. I feared that it would continue to grow until I transformed irreversibly into a violent monster, and I would never again feel curious or excited about life, see goodness in others, or feel peace within.

At that time, I forgot rule number one about emotions, that they act as signals for us. My anger was signaling that something was very wrong in my life. There wasn't something wrong with *me*—I had reason to be angry. I'd been injured and betrayed by people I'd trusted. They had gone so far as to misinform insurers, making it harder for me to survive. No one had apologized to me. No one had compensated me. Instead I had to live with a mysterious debilitating disease, while fighting an interminable bureaucratic battle while somehow managing to keep a roof over my head and food on the table. Even without a compensation battle, CS and CSS cause a whole load of unwarranted crap, and the natural reaction to a load of unwarranted crap is anger.

The second thing I noticed was that my anger was keeping me alive. During the first few years with CSS, not a day went by that I didn't feel tempted to give up, go camp on the front lawn of city hall and drown my sorrows in cheap gin. Some days that temptation prodded and poked at me every minute. Some days I even got drunk and went to bed before noon. But I woke up angry, and that anger helped me to keep on fighting, for a diagnosis and cure to my illness, for compensation, for my own happiness and peace.

And now? I'm still angry about what happened to me. Every time I experience a relapse after walking more than five minutes on a beautiful day, or I laugh out loud and my throat muscles tighten, I feel a twinge of anger. Every time I have to flee a public place because of environmental triggers, I feel it, although the intensity of that anger has diminished as the years passed—less supernova and more glowing embers. Perhaps one day it will fade away completely.

Resentment, though, is another story. Deep-seated anger—the stuff that has distilled down to intense resentment—will consume your energy and joy and leave a hopeless, lifeless void in its wake. One way to oust resentment is to let go of blame. Ask yourself, *who do I blame?* Make a list if it helps. Include everyone, and then forgive them. Easier said than done, I know. This can take years, but if you can bring yourself to forgive everyone—including yourself—you'll be all the better for it.

Not at the forgiving place yet? Then try to burn excess anger off rather than steep in it. I always used to run to rid myself of excess emotion. When I got sick and couldn't run, I did some pillow punching for a while, and eventually I gravitated towards therapy and meditation. I also tried to distract myself from feeling stuck in a mire of injustice.

I'd focus on things that were going well, or things that made me happy, like sitting in a pile of sunshine, or napping near the ocean. Relishing the simple pleasures is way more healthy and enjoyable than steeping in bad feeling about the injustices of life that are beyond my control.

Finally, take it from a hothead, anger can unground you, but it doesn't have to, no matter what insurance companies or fate or people throw at you. I try always to stick to my daily plan. If I am on my way out for walk when I receive a letter from workers compensation that says I won't get paid a cent until I disprove 20 lies GAS concocted, I go for my walk, savor the fresh air and sunshine and natural beauty. I go about my day. Then, during my next planning and pacing session, I schedule time to focus on the letter and respond.

Review of Loss and Emotions

- CS and CSS often cause loss. These conditions also may reveal existing problems in your relationships or cause people to blame or turn away from you. None of this is fair or easy to deal with and can be upsetting and discouraging. Know that the issue is *illness* and how people relate to it.

- CSS or CS alone may cause you to experience an identity crisis, but you can rediscover yourself, redefine your goals, bolster your sense of self-worth, and emerge from crisis with strength and direction.

- If significant losses are getting you down, you may find it helpful to think of loss as *change*. Change is an inherent, uncontrollable element of life and doesn't carry the negative connotation that *loss* does.

- Living with these chronic conditions can stir up strong emotions: happiness, sadness/grief, fear/surprise, or anger/disgust. Generally speaking, it's better to *feel* or experience your emotions than to try to repress them. Better out than in. Seek a professional's help if you need to.

- Emotions can act as helpful signals to us. Anger, especially, can cause harm but also can serve as an important tool for survival and source of strength in times of crisis.

- Grief is welcome. Let it wash over and through you until it ebbs away.

Be kind to yourself, dear—to our innocent follies.
Forget any sounds or touch you knew that did not help you dance.
You will come to see that all evolves us.
—Rumi[7]

Hunkering

Hunkering. I'm hunkering down like a soldier too loyal to go AWOL though she questions the judgment of her shell-shocked commander. I hunker like a soldier at a bunker. Yes, I bunker. I'm bunkering in the front bedroom of a little bungalow owned by a woman whose only son moved out last week to go to junior college across town. Within moments of moving my stuff in this afternoon, I thought I smelled cigarette smoke, and I said to Lucy, my new housemate and landlady, "Do you smell that?" I say that a lot, and most of the time, the person to whom I address the question gets a confused look on their face and shakes their head. No, it's only me. Me and my over-sensitive sense of smell. Lucy assured me there was no smoke in the house. "The downstairs tenant," she said, "has lived here for years, but he smokes only outside."

Outside not in. No smoke inside.

But I detect it. Stale cigarette smoke. Inside my closet. Inside my walls. For hours the pungent odor has been scratching at this point high inside my right nostril.

Inside, not out.

I didn't unpack. But I didn't cut and run either. I can't keep running. This is not the first time, and I need a home.

So I made my bed, with my soft flannel sheet and my fluffy white comforter, and the buckwheat pillow my dear friend gave me when I left her apartment this morning. She said, "Trust yourself," and saw me off. She knows me better than most but even she cannot understand that trusting myself has become the hardest thing for me to do. I climbed into my new bed, pulled the clean unscented comforter over my head, pressed my cheek against the pillow, and hunkered down. That was hours ago.

I'm still hunkering now.

The walls are paper-thin in this little house, the house that I found charming when I first came to view it, with its real oak floors and old-style central heating. The house I wanted to make my home for several months or years, until my brain reset itself, I regained my energy and could rebuild my life. I can hear Lucy in the front room. She's on the phone, speaking Mandarin or Cantonese, I'm not sure. When I viewed the house, I asked her if she'd teach me her native language and she said yes. I was looking forward to that. I thought we would become friends. I was looking forward—

No past tense. I mustn't think in past tense like that. No giving up. I pull the comforter tighter around my nose and try to distract my mind from the smoke. The smoke I smell that Lucy doesn't. The smoke that cannot be here, that my mind believes is. The smoke that I sense weaving its way, cobwebby fog-finger-like, through the folds of the comforter, into the pocket of air around my head. It fills that space with its bitter, sharp tang and stings my eyes until they produce water—

I'm bunkering.

"No smoke," I whisper to my brain, "You smell nothing, *absolutely nothing*." I say it like I'm Sargent Shultz from that old television show *Hogan's Heroes*, rejecting what I perceive so that I can survive.

Every fight or flight molecule in my body has been urging me to run out the door, for hours now, since I first smelled the smoke, but I deny them all. This isn't going to be like last time. There's no threat here. That place had mildew. Only I could smell it. I lasted three days, then returned to the doorstep of my friend, buckwheat pillow in hand, with swollen lungs and throat, full of tears and unbelonging. The place before that had fresh paint. The one before that started a balcony restoration with no notice. Prior places had contained laundry room exhaust that bled into the building's main ventilation system, melamine shelving or laminate flooring off-gassing formaldehyde, PVC in-floor heating pipes, or damp parking garages. Today's was my eighth move in three years. It couldn't happen again. I would fight for my place in the world, even if it meant betraying my brain.

"You won't smell anything when you wake up," I whisper. "You just need rest." It's 2 a.m. Only five hours to go until sunrise. I smoosh my nose into the buckwheat pillow and repeat the words again and again. The smoke smells so real that to deny it feels like lying to my brain. But my brain's been lying to me for three years now, so can't I lie to it? Fair is fair, right?

No, none of this is fair.

Three years ago I was a professional singer, emerging writer, and marathon runner in training. Then I was exposed to unsafe levels of toxic chemicals and particulates at my day job, an incident that took my income and savings, my home, my health, and my voice, and left me with asthma, multiple chemical sensitivities, chronic fatigue, and irritable larynx syndrome—Central Sensitivity syndromes. Some say brain disorders differ from mental illness, but I don't see how. Any condition in which the brain becomes unreliable and out of balance, anytime the brain trust between self and the mind is breached, that's mental illness. And, although I dislike the label, because it is like a bad tattoo that can never be removed, I have come to accept that it accurately labels me, me and my mind.

Not only did I acquire hyper-finicky lungs and a sense of smell that can outsniff a bloodhound, but my brain overreacts to every odor it perceives with its new souped-up olfactory system, and takes action by tightening the muscles around the larynx to protect my lungs, effectively choking me. For the first year and a half, there were countless coughing fits, unconscious spells, puking sessions, you name it. I had to avoid public places, new materials, and chemical fumes well into the second year before I could manage the larynx issue, so that my airway no longer went from open to closed faster than a Lamborghini goes from zero to 60 mph. My sensitivity to some trigger scents has decreased somewhat the past few months, and I have fewer severe larynxial episodes now. But I still can't do mildew, and I can't do cigarette smoke, fabric softeners, paints, formaldehyde, or perfumes.

I checked this house out before committing. It smelled like boiled cabbage when I viewed it, a strong aroma but not offensive. I went through the list of things my lungs and mind couldn't tolerate and Lucy nodded and smiled and said she understood, no problem, welcome. So why hadn't she told me about the smoker downstairs? Did she really *not* smell it?

The worst part about mental illness is feeling like I can't trust myself, my instincts, or my experience. Everything is seen through a veil of survivalism, reptile brain, and desperation. Do I trust a brain that resists rational thought and perceives mortal dangers where there are in fact very few? Or do I trust my sane-looking new landlady? Siding with her feels like the worst kind of betrayal of self, but where do you go when you have a "Maslow-nian deficit," when you can't find a safe or secure shelter anywhere, because you have no money left, because a giant corporation screwed you and workers compensation turned out to be an insurance company with no legislative imperative to compensate workers? What do you do when you simply cannot breathe in a chemically-saturated world?

You hunker. In your bunker. And you lie to your brain all night. You wait until the landlady leaves for work in the morning and you get up. You have a steaming shower and tell yourself the water is a purification ritual. It will cleanse your sense of smell, it will reset your brain's alarm system, and wash this whole terrible night away. And you will begin again, in this sweet little house with the nice landlady and the primroses along the front walk. You will set up your desk by the window that looks out on the quiet street with cherry trees already budding in February. You will hang your clothes in the closet, and you will remember what Lucy said when you first asked her about the smoke and she swore there was none.

"This is your home now," she said. "If there are any problems, you tell me, and we will fix them."

You repeat this to yourself as you step out of the shower and dry your skin. You love the sound of the words and say them again out loud as you enter your little room and unzip your big blue suitcase in search of clean clothes. And you start to cry as you dress, because you want more than anything to believe that someone could make it all better the way Lucy thinks she can. But you see, beyond your blue suitcase on the floor, you *see* cigarette smoke puffing out of the heating vent like malicious grey clouds. And you know she can't fix that. Even if she kicked out the downstairs dweller, even if she scrubbed the walls with bleach and then repainted her home to cover the odor stuck in the walls—the odor you detected all night, the odor you lied to yourself about all those hours while you hunkered and bunkered—you still couldn't stay because of the bleach, and then because of the paint fumes and then, the outgassing. For months, maybe a year, the paint would trigger your brain, which would trigger your lungs and larynx.

Now you have visual proof. This mission is officially a bust. As you tug on the same clothes you wore yesterday, sobs lurch out of you. They form in your core like bald baby gerbils and grow into ferocious rats that can chew their way out of anything. They run up your centre, claws in your belly and throat, and thrust their way out of you, heaving like throw-up, wracking your entire form. Suddenly the stress you've carried during three years of losing feels unbearably heavy—

And you don't think.

Not at all.

You haul box after box at a half-run out the front door of the little house and dump each one into your car. Breathless, snotting, crying, coughing, shuddering, you carry it all, every last bit that you lugged in the day before. Your throat constricts each time you enter the increasingly smoky house, and then loosens a smidge with each emergence into the fresh air outside. And when everything is in the car, you stand in Lucy's yard, teeth chattering, limbs quaking, breath huffing in and out as if you've run farther and faster than a body could be expected to. Any body. Anyone.

With shaking fingers, you hit the speed dial on your phone and when your dear friend answers, you sputter and slur as though speaking a tiny language with a mouth made for bigger words, "It's starting to feel like there is no place for me in the world.... I don't know what to do."

"Come back and sleep on my couch," she says, though her apartment is so small it seems like it will burst with another's presence. "You will find a better place."

Like a good soldier, you march to the car without thinking. You pour into the seat, and your little Toyota Echo feels like a tank around you, solid and powerful. You sit with your hands on wheel, feet on pedals, until the tremors cease and your breath deepens again. This takes several minutes. Moisture from your breath creeps up the side windows. You turn on the engine and crank up the defogger.

In the rear-view mirror, you glimpse "traitor" stamped on your forehead. You want to apologize for the overnight deception session, for your illness, for not being stronger emotionally, physically, mentally—but it would change nothing. The part of you that betrayed another part of you last night served as a whip-cracking, drill sergeant hero during this morning's evacuation. It's as if your mental regime hit a minefield three years ago and you've been patching up the survivors and winging it since then. Every part of you knows this, yet you still yearn for resolution, coherence, and certainty.

Who doesn't? You laugh, knowing you will be eating uncertainty again for dinner tonight, and for many nights to come. You should develop a taste for it, you tell yourself. Then your brain could rest. Then you could rest.

Then rest.

Then breath.

"Hunker down," you say, wiping your face with your sleeve. "Retreat is not defeat." You speak the words to yourself, and to your mind, and in this moment you detect no breach, and no resistance.[8]

Maintaining Mental Health with CS and CSS

If you are reticent to discuss mental illness, you aren't the only one. Most folks would rather not. The topic carries a stigma heavier than a concrete albatross the size of the Statue of Liberty. When my GP told me I had developed a mental illness secondary to the CSS, my brain immediately envisioned a helpless me, strapped to a gurney in a grungy asylum full of screams and despair, reeking of bleach and urine, like in an old horror movie. I was terrified my GP could sign away my life to evil Frankenstein-ian doctors who would experiment on me there forever.

See? Intense fear surrounds mental illness. No one wants to experience it, but the truth is that many people do at some point in their lives, and the sooner one recognizes and treats it, the better. CS and CSS are challenging enough without the added element of mental illness, so you need to know what to look for.

Let's start with a definition: "Mental illnesses are health problems that affect the way we think about ourselves, relate to others, and interact with the world around us. They affect our thoughts, feelings, and behaviours. Mental illnesses can disrupt a person's life or create challenges, but with the right supports, a person can get back on a path to recovery and wellness."[9] CS and CSS are not mental illnesses, nor do they cause mental illness. However, many people with these conditions develop mental illness. To give you an idea, up to 75 percent of those with Fibromyalgia develop depression and/or anxiety.[10] Why? A major reason is that CS and CSS affect so many aspects of people's lives that they become "at-risk" for developing a mental illness.

I'll use a garden-variety analogy to illustrate: If your tomato plants are strong and healthy, a couple caterpillars won't be able to inflict much damage. They'll eat a few leaves, and your healthy plants will easily generate plenty more. But if your tomato plants are underwatered, stressed, and don't get enough sunshine, those caterpillars will likely eat faster than the plants can produce. Like the tomato plants, your brain, while occupied with all the challenges inherent in CS and CSS, may become prone to mental illness. That's a problem, but it's not the big problem.

The big problem is, many of those with CSS or CS alone who develop a mental illness don't seek treatment. Despite the incredible work that UK Royals Kate, William and Harry are doing to obliterate stigma, those of us who've had the taboo of mental illness ingrained from toddler-dom have a lot of fear and cultural programming to overcome. Who wants to think of themselves as "crazy" or "mental" or any of the numerous derogatory terms our culture has created to marginalize and dismiss people with mental illness? Who wants to entertain the thought that they might need psychiatric help? Who wants to worry that their friends or neighbors might ostracize or think less of them because they have a mental illness? Who wants to think less of themselves for having a mental illness?

In addition to fear and programmed prejudice, there's denial. When my CFS specialist asked me to take a test to determine if I had become depressed from the impact of CS and CSS on my life, I agreed, but I didn't take him seriously. *Duh, anyone could see I'm not depressed. I'm not "mental."* (Such was my thinking.) The test was frustrating, clearly meant for someone without CS or CSS. I mean, of course I had lost interest in things I once enjoyed—I could no longer *do* the things I once enjoyed because I had CFS, ILS, and MCS! And naturally, I had stopped being social—I couldn't breathe in social situations! Of course I felt tired all the time, I saw little hope for my future, and I wasn't eating right.... But those things were all because of my conditions. People with severe fatigue, pain, and cognitive issues don't have the ability to cook properly for themselves, and they can't do many of the things they'd hoped to do in future, and feeling tired is one of the symptoms of CS and CSS! What a stupid, useless test, I thought. It didn't mean that I was *depressed*. It just meant that it didn't accurately assess someone who had my conditions.

Then my doctor explained that it didn't matter *why* I'd lost hope in my future. If I was feeling hopeless, that was a symptom of depression. It didn't matter *why* I was not social, or *why* I had lost interest in things I enjoyed. What mattered was the current mental state of me. Somehow, when I was busy dealing with CS and my syndromes and workers compensation and wasn't paying attention, mental illness had snuck up and sunk its teeth into me. And I did everything I could *not* to see it.

My subconscious had its reasons. I had extreme terror fueling that denial. I had my Frankenstein-ian nightmare. And I'd seen Claire Dane's bipolar breakdown in *Homeland*. I didn't want my few remaining friends to dismiss me as "crazy." If word got out, people could lock me up in an institution, I would no longer be seen as an actual person, with actual rights, more as an "irrational freak" who couldn't make decisions for herself. I didn't want to be labeled—and discredited because of that label—for the rest of my life. As if intense denial and fear weren't enough to dissuade me from accepting and seeking treatment for my mental illness, my recent loss of autonomy due to CS and CSS intensified my defiance. I was desperately clinging to the minute amount of control over my life that I still had. Unfortunately, this type and degree of resistance is as common as it is unhelpful, and it means that many folks who develop mental illness after getting CSS, or CS alone, suffer needlessly.

When depression's twin brother anxiety came to visit and wanted to stay, I decided to see a psychiatrist who specializes in working with folks who have CSS. I'd probably get nothing out of it, I figured, (yep, that's depression talking) but at the very least I could learn my rights as a citizen with a mental illness and avoid becoming a lab rat in some institution.

Seeking treatment in this way turned out to be one of the best decisions I've ever made. If you suspect you're becoming depressed or anxious, or should you find a mental illness diagnosis staring you in the face, I encourage you to confront your fear and denial and whatever else impedes you from seeking appropriate treatment. You deserve to be as healthy—physically, emotionally, *and* mentally—as you possibly can be. There is no shame in having a mental illness. There is no shame in taking steps to treat your mental illness. There is only a desire and quest for health. Remember, you aren't alone, and I'm right here, talking to you.

Keeping Emotions, Thoughts and Behaviors in Balance

As I mentioned earlier, your emotions often influence your thoughts and behaviors, and this can be a helpful thing. That said, your emotions, thoughts, and behaviors must work in a state of equilibrium in order for you to have a healthy cognitive-behavioral process. If one of the three dominates the rest, problems can occur that endanger you or wreak havoc on your life. For example, if your emotions influence your thoughts and behaviors overmuch, you can make unhealthy decisions and take unhealthy actions. This imbalance is not uncommon for many of those dealing with the chaos of CSS, or CS alone, especially when in crisis phase and/or during prolonged isolation and longer-term challenges. Some examples:

- After yelling into the phone and hanging up without listening for a response, Suzy punches the wall and breaks several bones in her hand.
- Tears blur Pat's vision as she kneels on the floor and sets the huge pile of creditors' collection notices aflame. She watches in shock as the entire room catches fire.
- Joe decides not to call friends anymore since friends aren't calling him.

Can you tell if a thought, emotion, and/or behavior has taken control in each scenario?

Suzy is clearly driven by anger. She isn't thinking about the consequences of what she's saying or doing. Emotion is dominating both her thoughts and behaviors. Emotion fuels Pat's behaviors and thoughts too, but this time the driving emotion is probably sadness, not anger. What about the third example? Joe makes a decision and bases his actions on that decision, so does that mean his thoughts are dominating both emotions and behaviors? Not entirely. His decision not to call anyone is based on negative emotions, probably sadness or fear. If you don't see that, don't worry, I'll break this concept down further in a moment.

Emotions are tricky things. We can make up our rational minds in a moment, but emotions don't change just because we tell them to. They remain, and manifest in all kinds of ways. They can transform healthy actions into self-defeating ones and twist helpful thoughts into unhelpful ones. They can paint a new reality over the old one, and make that new reality seem *REAL*, so real that it taints our view of ourselves and everything around us. Who can live a sensible, joyful life with a warped, emotion-driven reality in the way?

I sure can't, so I use the meditation, self-talk, and visualization techniques discussed earlier in the book to help keep emotions working for and not against me. I also employ Cognitive Behavioral Therapy, the most powerful tool I've found for defeating unhelpful thoughts and behaviors and restoring balance to my cognitive-behavioral process.

COGNITIVE BEHAVIORAL THERAPY AND HOW IT CAN HELP YOU COPE

Some people get turned off by the name "Cognitive Behavioral Therapy." It sounds like electrodes may be involved, doesn't it? Or intensive sessions with a psychiatrist who charges $400 an hour and wears sloth-skin shoes? Truth be told, Cognitive Behavioral Therapy, aka CBT, is simple, and you can do it all by yourself, electrode- and sloth-free. (By the way, don't let the names of strategies or therapies deter you in your quest for healing. Often times, people with no imagination make up these names, and you can always rename it something that suits your taste. I've adopted a "take what I can from wherever it makes sense" attitude with strategies and treatments. After researching and discussing risks versus potential benefits with my doctor, I try a strategy, and if it works, great. If not, I try something else. Perhaps a similar philosophy will benefit you.)

CBT is "a form of psychotherapy that emphasizes the important role of thinking in how we feel and what we do."[11] There are several types of CBT, some dependent upon a therapist's involvement and others purely independent. Even with a therapist, the bulk of the work falls to the patient, who should practice CBT daily to affect positive and lasting cognitive-behavioral change. "The goal is for you to become your own CBT therapist," says Jason M. Satterfield, Professor of Clinical Medicine, at University of California, San Francisco, "but there aren't any shortcuts or magic. The CBT process can be quite difficult, it takes practice and commitment."[12] CBT is based on the premise that one's thoughts, behaviors/actions and emotions all influence each other in a kind of feedback cycle that looks something like Diagram 4.

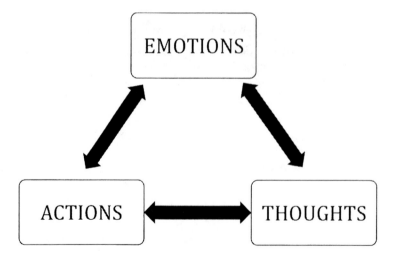

Diagram 4. Cognitive-behavioral cycle

Remember the example in the previous segment in which Joe's negative emotions generated unhelpful thoughts?

Here's a more detailed example of the same phenomenon.

Say Betty passes her coworker Rina on the street, and Betty says "Hey, Rina" as she passes (action). Rina looks at Betty, says nothing, and keeps on walking. Betty walks away feeling sad and angry (negative emotion). Why would Rina snub her? Betty wonders. She decides Rina must be mad at her (negative assumption), or that Rina is a jerk for not saying hi (negative thought), or that maybe aliens came and took Rina away and what Betty just saw was merely a shell of the person Rina once had been (catastrophization). Betty decides to avoid Rina unless Rina approaches Betty first and says something un-alien-like (negative action). See how Betty's emotions influenced her thoughts, which in turn influenced her actions? This may seem like an extreme example, but lots of people behave this way when negative emotions dominate their cognitive-behavioral process.

If this imbalance operates long enough, then people can develop *situational* or *automatic thoughts* based on those emotions and get stuck in a harmful cognitive-behavioral rut without even realizing it. According to Amy Wenzel of the Department of Psychiatry at the University of Pennsylvania, "a great deal of work in cognitive therapy is geared toward the identification, evaluation, and modification of situational thoughts (i.e., automatic thoughts) that patients experience on particular occasions and that are associated with an increase in an aversive mood state."[13] That is, much of CBT involves noticing, considering, and then changing unhelpful thoughts. In order to do so, we have to first understand that "we all view the world through a subjective lens."[14] Once the patient gains an awareness of her/his subjectivity, s/he can perceive emotions, thoughts and actions with greater objectivity and choose how to respond to any given situation, rather than merely react.

CBT operates on the assumption that if we change one of the components in that feedback cycle, the other two will automatically change in response. Therefore, if I change my thoughts, my actions will automatically change, and in turn my emotions too will change. Let's see how Betty does it.

Say Betty passes her coworker Rina on the street, and Betty says "Hey, Rina" as she passes (action). Rina looks at Betty, says nothing, and keeps on walking. Betty walks away feeling sad and wonders why Rina would snub her. It's not like Rina to be snooty, she thinks (non-emotional thought). Maybe Rina has a lot on her mind (non-emotional thought). Or maybe she got abducted by aliens (off the map, possibly fear-fuelled thought, or maybe just a geeky thought). Betty decides to check in with Rina next time they meet and make sure Rina's ok (positive action). She feels happy (positive emotion) and starts humming (positive action) as she continues on her way.

What a different, and much healthier result! Of course, it's not easy to identify negative thoughts or unhelpful behaviors in the moment, but with practice, self-awareness and time, you will improve, learn to control your responses, and generate a happier, healthier, more connected and open life.

As you work with CBT, you may find that certain unhelpful thoughts are more difficult to change than others. Often this is because those thoughts are based upon *core beliefs*, "fundamental, inflexible, absolute, and generalized beliefs that people hold about themselves, others, the world, and/or the future…."[15] Core beliefs that are "inaccurate, unhelpful, and/or judgmental (e.g., 'I am worthless')" can cause serious detriment to one's "self-concept, sense of self-efficacy, and continued vulnerability to mood disturbance."[16]

If we don't practice CBT or other therapy, it can be very difficult to recognize core beliefs because they influence us at a subconscious level. As well, "core beliefs are much more difficult to elicit and modify … relative to situational automatic thoughts. They usually develop from messages received, over time, during a person's formative years, oftentimes during childhood but sometimes during times of substantial stress during adulthood."[17]

When we must make drastic changes to our lifestyle, expectations, and goals because of CS or CSS we often run into core beliefs such as these:

- If I can't make it perfect, it's not worth doing
- All or nothing
- No pain, no gain
- You have to work to earn a living
- People on welfare or disability are just lazy
- I'm unworthy of love

Do you see how such beliefs can cause deep-seated internal conflict for people who become debilitated by CS or CSS? How would you feel about being unable to do anything "perfectly"? What if you could no longer do all your laundry and cleaning in one go, but had to chip away at it in ten-minute intervals over a span of days or weeks? What if you believed "no pain, no gain," but had to stop yourself from pushing through in order to avoid relapse or crash? What if you couldn't work anymore and had to apply for welfare or disability insurance to survive? What if you believe you are unworthy of love—a common core belief—and you need to ask others for help because you can no longer do everything for yourself?

Though tenacious and able to undermine your intentions to be happy and make choices in your best interest, unhelpful core beliefs can be debunked. With time and practice, CBT helps you identify them and choose healthy, accepting, empowering core beliefs instead.

Examining myself through the CBT lens and studying my developmental missteps has been both uncomfortable and challenging. Who wants to do that? I sure didn't, especially considering all the other stuff I had to manage in my life with CS and CSS. But I did want to be happy, and I was miserable enough to try anything. CBT made a big difference. I hope it can help you too. Ask your doctor or therapist if you'd like to learn more.[18]

More Coping Strategies

In the first couple years, I wanted my life back exactly the way it had been pre–CS. That was my singular goal, and it caused me no end of misery. I resisted my new reality and wound up feeling more beaten and displaced than ever. It finally dawned on me that my resistance was *causing* most of my suffering. I couldn't have my life back the way it was, no matter what. Even if I were to be completely cured today, right now, my life would remain changed. Because *I* am changed. Sure, I'd go running and hiking and sing until the cows came home, but everything would be different because of my experience with this illness. I would know the meaning and magic of gratitude, my favorite things would seem novel, my relationships would be far more authentic, my boundaries more defined, and I would have different expectations, of people, of myself, of life.

That suffering was optional, and when I eventually opted out, by surrendering rather than resisting, things got a whole lot better for me. I became able to accept my current level of debilitation while maintaining hope that my health would improve in future. And with acceptance and hope came joy. This didn't happen overnight, nor did it simply come to me. I had to work for it.

But there are different kinds of suffering, right? In addition to resisting things we can't control, there's suffering from physical pain, and suffering from what I call "Maslownian deficit," such as lack of adequate food, clothing, shelter, love, or safety. Yes, of course. Remember what I said about symptom control way back in the crisis phase discussion? It will never be perfect. We seek to control the symptoms we can, as much as we can, starting with the ones that most affect our quality of life. Decreasing the severity and longevity of symptoms is one aspect you can control (primarily with bubble time), as is planning and pacing to develop a manageable lifestyle (primarily by limiting triggerful excursions and affording your central nervous system sufficient rest—again, bubble time), and engaging the parasympathetic response.

After reading this far, you know that I am no paragon of the peaceful warrior. I have been angry, and bitter, and a "hopeless loser." I have been bitten by both depression and anxiety, and I still feel those illnesses at the fringes of my mind once in a while, scratching for a way in. Along with CBT, the strategies that follow have enabled me to pull through the worst of my experience with CS and CSS, and continue to help me contend with the challenges of living with my conditions. I hope they may help you too, on your own path to healing and happiness.

MINDFULNESS

I've talked about meditation, but what about mindfulness? Are they one and the same? I've found that the lines can get blurry here. Some say mindfulness is a type of meditation, while others say meditation is part of a "mindfulness practice." For me, meditation tends to be more of a situational thing, while mindfulness is more of an "anywhere, anytime, all the time" way of looking at life and being. "The founding father of the mindfulness movement is Jon Kabat-Zinn, PhD, a molecular biologist who ... established the Stress Reduction Clinic [at University of Massachusetts Medical School] and developed the now-famous Mindfulness-based Stress Reduction program."[19] Zinn's program provides intensive mindfulness training to help patients cope with chronic pain. The source of this mindfulness training is Buddhist meditation practices. See? Blurry.

This definition, by Dr. Kristin Neff, Associate Professor at the Department of Educational Psychology, University of Texas at Austin, is my favorite: Mindfulness is holding "our experience in balanced awareness rather than ignoring our pain or exaggerating it."[20] Mindfulness "means we don't have to believe every passing thought or emotion as *real* and *true*. Rather, we can see that different thoughts and emotions arise and pass away, and we can decide which are worth paying attention to and which are not.... Mindfulness provides us with the opportunity to *respond* rather than simply *react*."[21]

When do we "hold our experience in balanced awareness"? When do we watch "different thoughts and emotions arise and pass away," and "decide which are worth paying attention to and which are not"? While meditating, or while doing CBT. It seems to me that meditation and CBT directly engender and nurture mindfulness because while we practice these techniques, we are focused on noticing and naming our thoughts and emotions. And that, in turn, gives us the power to keep our emotions, thoughts, and behaviors in a healthy balance. Over time, the process strengthens our resilience so we can contend with any challenge that arises, and that, my friends, leads to healthier, happier living.

Mindfulness doesn't mean walking through life with a fake smile and Pollyanna attitude, blind to everything that isn't working for me. It's more a perspective of intention. My intention is to enjoy my life as much as I possibly can, given the current limitations of CS and CSS. So I focus on ways to make that happen. My intention is to live free of dictatorial emotions, and to choose helpful thoughts and behaviors. So I focus on that. My intention is to solve the problems I have while maintaining emotional equilibrium, and to handle whatever life throws my way with grace and confidence rather than fear or resistance. Mindfulness, as defined above, helps me to fulfill all those intentions.

What about when we aren't "officially" practicing CBT or meditation at a specific moment? Can we do mindfulness then, and if so, what does it look like? Some examples:

- Since managing CS and CSS requires that I stay home much of the time, I don't tend to think of myself as particularly lucky. I acknowledge that it's not a great situation, and sometimes I cry or feel anger about it and have a good release. But I don't get let grief and anger rule me. I choose not to. Instead, I consider how much worse my health could be, or how awful it was being homeless last year, and then I feel an extraordinary amount of gratitude for my current hovel, for the small amount of energy I have, and for the view outside my window. My health problems are still here, and I continue to work on finding a cure and increasing my functional capacity, but me choosing to focus on the good rather than the bad, that's mindfulness. Me choosing not to react to intense grief or anger, but merely to acknowledge the emotions and let them pass, that's mindfulness.

- How about a day when I wake up with major inflammation and pain? I don't want to focus on the pain, or on the fact that I'll have to stay in bed until it subsides, or on the fear and dread that maybe it never will subside, and what will I do if that happens…?

  I focus instead on an image of me on the beach, with warm sun cascading over my body. Or I focus on how glad I am that the pain isn't half as bad as it was at this time last year. Or I put some classical music on and focus on that. These are all mindful choices.

- How about a day when I have minor symptoms and really want to go running or take a long walk in the sun, but I have to pace myself, so I won't over-exert. Pacing like this makes me feel sad and angry, at me and the world. I don't want to live in grief and anger, so I acknowledge that it sucks, I may even shed a tear or two, and then I use mindfulness. I go on a five-minute walk outside, and I drink in as much of the sights and sounds as I can, and I relish that walk. Maybe I take photos while out there, or simply commit all to memory, so I can enjoy them later. If I'd stayed in a bad mood, I wouldn't have enjoyed the small amount of freedom I had, and I might have inadvertently increased symptoms, but mindfulness saved me from that negative mire.

Recent research has shown that the brain has a "default setting" that causes it to automatically focus on certain mental activities when you are not paying attention to the present moment, and when in this default mode, the brain works on "finding fault with yourself, finding fault with others, imagining better alternative realities, thinking about the past, all the stuff that we think of as really creating a lot of suffering of the mind...."[22] Fortunately, it is possible to create a new default state for the brain, through mindfulness training: "You can actually see a shift in the brain from this fault-finding and evaluating state into a direct experience.... The brain pays more attention to sensations and less to the stories."[23] How do we make that happen? Practice.

Practicing mindfulness involves an element of *conscious* gratitude or *conscious* distraction at first. What I mean is, you will probably have to *tell* yourself to pay attention to something else, or *remind* yourself not to get stuck focusing on the negatives. Be careful not to criticize, just acknowledge and redirect. Gradually, the need for you to issue such directives will decrease, and your brain will no longer automatically go to places of intense dread or anger or negativity and want to stay there. Your brain will learn to let go of past regrets and future worries and focus on the present moment or activity, on the beauty and wonder or whatever it is that you have or enjoy, and on things farthest away from thoughts and feelings that can ensnare you in suffering.

Using Mindfulness to Disrupt Ruminations. Some folks with CSS or CS alone have some especially persistent negative thoughts, aka ruminations, chewing up a good portion of their time and energy. According to Dr. Neff, to ruminate is to "repeatedly or continually think about something.... Rumination on negative thoughts and emotions stems from the underlying desire to be *safe*."[24] Remember when I said safety is key? Rumination may be signaling that you need more bubble time, need to engage your parasympathetic system more, and/or need more stability or support. You may be doing all you can in those areas but still finding it hard to disrupt ruminations. Unfortunately the longer one ruminates, the more challenging it can be to stop.

Mindfulness can help with this. For example, when an anxious thought interrupts my sleep in the middle of the night, churns into a rumination, and does all it can to convince me that what it says is real and true, I use mindfulness to ground myself in place and time. This means I take my focus off the rumination and place my attention on my environment and the present moment.

To do this, I say to myself, "Hey, there, nice and easy now...." (Yep, when I wake up ruminating at 2 a.m., I talk to myself the way I would talk to a spooked horse.) I say, "Hey there, it's ok. Look, you're in bed, under your snuggly white comforter with the little grey flowers on it. You just washed it the other day and it still smells like clean cotton. And this is your wee hovel, and look, everything is fine in here. Nothing is wrong, you've done nothing wrong. You've tried hard, and things haven't all gone your way. But you're still here, and everything's ok."

First of all, notice how I pointed out specific details to myself, like the color of the comforter and the design on the fabric? Details help bring my attention out of my head and into the environment. Now, at this point, I'm probably pretty calm, but if I'm feeling extra upset or fearful, I will delve into detail of the room even more, something like this: "There's your closet, and the door that squeaks when you open it, and here are your clothes bins, and the book you've been working your way through for the past month...."

If even that fails to disperse the dervish of negative thoughts, then I add an element of what I call "distracting the two-year-old brain." (Yep, the same strategy I use when having an ILS episode.) This involves absolutely anything I can think of to refocus my brain on something other than the current topic of rumination: "The building sure is quiet this time of night. Even the ever-barking dogs. There goes the air conditioner next door.

Must be hot in their place. This comforter rocks. It was only $15. Remember when you got it from Ikea? It was pre–CS, when Ikea smelled *normal*! You got these pillows then too. For $5 each. This one is *still* hard as a rock…." I reminisce on funny stuff that's happened to me, or I recite the names of all the books in my bookshelf, or the names of my favorite bands or composers. I talk to myself as if I'm a wee child and just dropped my ice cream cone on the ground and all of life went from ecstatic to horribly horrible in a split second. That'll do it.

Mantra Making

I mentioned earlier that I sometimes use mantras during meditation. I also use them when I'm outside the bubble and catch myself thinking unhelpful thoughts. I make up affirmations, song lyrics, poems, and mantras and then recite them aloud or silently, over and over, to disrupt negative notions before they become ruminations. You may worry that you aren't a guru or mystic poet, so how could you possibly write a mantra? Nonsense. The only requirement here is that you debunk the negative thoughts. Usually my DIY mantras end up sickeningly punny, because that's my sense of humor. Make yours to suit your own serious or funny bone. They can be as simple or complex as you like.

These first three are of a more visionary and dignified nature. Each verse can be used separately, or combined into one long mantra:

> The human body and mind can achieve most anything.
> Both can heal, given proper time and attention.
>
> My body is strong, my mind resilient and resourceful.
> My mind is strong, my body resilient and resourceful.
>
> Each day I am stronger
> Each day I breathe easier
> Each day I am more grounded
> Each day I recover some energy

Remember that whatever you affirm, you need to believe it is true. (You can't lie to your brain. It always knows.) According to Dr. McGonigal, reciting affirmations you don't believe can "backfire" on you and decrease your confidence and/or self-esteem, so it's far more helpful to focus on something true instead, such as the opposite of the untrue affirmation.[25] For example, if you fear that you aren't recovering energy every day, it won't be helpful to say, "Each day I recover some energy." But maybe you believe that you can work to make healthy choices each day, in which case it would be helpful to say something like this: "I have the courage to face this illness and do what I can to improve my health every day." Then, instead of reinforcing fear or doubt, you are affirming your courage and strength; and that mantra will yield far better results.[26]

I find sing-song poetry to be exceptionally effective in debunking negative thoughts. These might annoy anyone around you, but I find they stick in my head better than commercial jingles. Here's *Climbing the Walls*:

> This is my life
> It's not so bad
> Got four walls to climb
> More walls than some have

And I've got the sun
It's warm and it's bright
Keeping me company
Until it's night.

Silly stuff, right? Try creating your own next time you catch unhelpful thoughts marauding around your mind. As with most things CS-related, you need to tailor your mantras to you. If they banish the negative thoughts, then they're doing their job. And if they make you laugh and fill your mind with happy thoughts, bonus.

> *The outside world is the vital*
> *component of my inner life.*
> —Eudora Welty, *One Writer's Beginnings*[27]

Photo Dwelling

I started taking photos when I was too sick to do much else than recline in bed and watch most of my day go by. When I ventured outside for a minute or two at a time, I took photographs and would later toy with them on the computer. This enabled me to do something creative without struggling with language or taxing my energy overmuch.

I've discovered that looking at and playing with images is soothing, expansive, and incredible. They remind me that there is a big wide world out there and that anything can happen. These reminders help me to refocus my thoughts from pain or resistance to thoughts of serenity, healing, and strength.

You don't have to take photos in order to benefit from photo dwelling. You can find images on the web and purchase and download them. You can flip through magazines, tear inspiring images out and pin them to your bubble's wall. If triggered by printed publications, you may find old and pre-out-gassed magazines at a thrift store or ask friends if they have some at home.

Walkabout/Sitabout

Traditionally, a walkabout is a walking journey undertaken by an Australian Aboriginal adolescent male as a rite of passage. Crocodile Dundee fans will recall that one may go on walkabout any time for spiritual cleansing and/or transformation. A walkabout doesn't have to last for months and span three continents. A few minutes' walk can effectively overrule unruly emotions, negative thoughts or looming depression or anxiety.

Some days the hardest thing is to get out the door, but once I do I immediately feel better. Sunshine or rain—the energy invigorates me. The thudding of my boot heels on the pavement and the rhythm of my steps ground me. The earth seems to absorb all my tension and negativity and leaves me feeling lighter, buoyant, and free. The negative chatter within loses its hold over me, and I can marvel in nature (even urban "nature") and enjoy myself. On walkabout, I feel more connected, more like part of the world, than I do when indoors.

When my symptoms reached a certain severity that prohibited walkabouts, I developed the "sitabout" technique. This involves sitting outside my apartment with feet firmly planted on the ground. This is usually done in sun, but I've been known to sitabout in the rain with an umbrella. If it's warm and dry enough, sitabout works best with bare feet. I sit and rest with eyes closed. If my mind turns to ruminating or negative thoughts,

I focus on noticing as many details about the outside world as I can: sounds, smells, the movement of the breeze, etc. Soon my mind fills with wonders of the world, my spirit feels lighter, and instead of feeling trapped in sickness, I feel expansive and full of potential.

You may wish to combine the walkabout and sitabout techniques by using a wheeled walker that has a seat, or by using a chair cane (which goes by many names, such as "walking chair stool" or "portable chair cane thingie"). These tools allow you to walk a while and sit when you need to. After a seated rest, you can choose to walk further (if your GET program allows) or turn around and head home. I find this particularly useful if I head out for a five-minute walk but symptoms arise mid-way through. Without a walker seat or chair cane, I'd have to sit on the ground to rest (and risk not being able to get back up) or walk back to the bubble without resting, which might trigger a relapse or crash. Bringing a seat along allows me to rest immediately before returning to the bubble. Chair canes and wheeled walkers with seats also serve me well when I have to park a distance from my destination. If the only parking is a seven-minute walk from my doctor's appointment, I break that walk up into manageable segments and rest in between. This minimizes the severity of the inevitable post-exertional malaise.

Finally, a walker or chair cane can help steady you while you walk, if needed.

Fear Posting

CSS and CS alone tend to inspire a large amount of fear, and you may find that some of your most persistent ruminations revolve around that emotion. If so, you are not alone. Fear is a normal reaction to illness or trauma—fear of loss, illness, unbelonging, an uncertain future … the list goes on. (Please note that in this segment I'm referring to the above kind of fear that comes at us in reaction to serious and chronic illness, not the kind of fear that helps keep us from physical harm, like when you stand atop a tall cliff and fear jumping, for example.)

Fear posting is not about wallowing in fear—quite the opposite. It's a way to identify your fear, acknowledge it, and let it go.

Step 1: When you catch yourself ruminating on something that frightens you, write down your fear(s) in sentence form, using one of these prompts: *Right now I feel afraid that …* or *Right now I fear that….* A couple common fears for folks with CSS would look like this:

> *Right now I feel afraid that no one will ever love me again.*
> *Right now I fear that I'll never be able to support myself again.*

What do you notice about these fears?

They are not real or proven facts. Fears develop from our own negative assumptions about people and situations and about what might happen five minutes, an hour, a year, or ten years from now.

Step 2: After you post your fear, read it while taking slow, relaxed breaths. Acknowledge that it is a fear, it is *not* reality. This may be enough for that fear to lose its power over you, at least for a little while.

Step 2.5: Often you may need to dig to get to the powerful center of a persistent fear. For example, with that first fear, I can ask myself why I feel afraid no one will ever love me again.

- Answer: Because I can't go to restaurants or bars and be social and do lots of fun things.

- Question: So are you only loveable if you can go out socially?
- Answer: No … well, yes … well …

I find that when I start stammering or vacillating, I've hit the chewy center of the fear, which is often an unhelpful core belief. In the case of the above example, the core belief is something like, I'm only loveable if I can *do* lots of things, or *go* lots of places with people. Realizing that I have this unhelpful core belief may be enough to debunk it. If not I will do some CBT around it and rationally disprove it.

Step 3: If the same fear returns, post it again. You may also find it helpful to perform a ritual with greater finality, like burning the paper upon which the fear is posted as you tell yourself that it is nothing but fear and has no power over you. Repeat these steps as necessary until the fear no longer dominates your thoughts or makes you anxious.

Step 4: Keeping a running list of my fear postings has helped me to reinforce the idea that fears have no power over me. As time passed, I would scan the list and notice my progress. Fears that had terrorized me in weeks or months prior no longer frightened me. That's the goal.

Da Güd Book

I started my güd book in crisis phase, when my symptoms were still increasing and I had no idea what was wrong with me. Depression had a good grip on me, I think, like a mean dog gnawing a postal delivery person's leg. I felt beaten in every aspect of my life, and my efforts made nothing better. Powerless. Afraid. Lost. Hopeless. Depression. Yep, that's how it happened. My acupuncturist told me to try writing a gratitude list. Have you ever tried to do this when you're REALLY down? For me, it involved staring at an empty page, scouring my brain for a tidbit of gladness, and coming up empty. This made me feel even worse.

Some people use The Bible, the AA Big Book, or the texts of another established religion or organization to help them through challenges that threaten to steal their hope and faith. None called to me at that time, so I decided to make my own good book. This is not as hard as it sounds. You don't have to be a brilliant writer or even a good writer. You just need to dedicate yourself to helping yourself, every day, a little at a time.

I wrote "Da Güd Book" on a notebook small enough to fit in my back pocket, and I kept it with me at all times. *Why did I call it* Da Güd Book, *you ask?* Good question. I wanted a book with good things in it, so "good book" seemed a natural title. And I tend to find comfort in languages other than my native tongue, some of which use umlauts. I also believed my good book would seem more legit and, well, old, if embossed with a pseudo–European title. Such was my line of thinking at that time. Thus, *"Da Güd Book"* seemed good to me (pun intended).

Anytime I noticed something, *any*thing going right in my life, I wrote it down, one event per page. My life was a shambles, remember, so I had to start small. Some sample entries:

- *My oatmeal was delicious this morning.* (Ok, I had to start *really* small, but hey, get excited about the little things. Like the Springsteen song, "From Small Things [Big Things One Day Come]." Believe it.)
- *Today I got an old bus to town instead of one of the brand-new ones, and no one was on it! No off-gassing, no perfumes, minor diesel fumes. Victory!*

- *My fave choco bar was on sale today—50% off—so I bought two!*
- *The sun was out today—in January—for a* whole hour! (If you lived in my region, you'd celebrate this too, believe me.)

Painstakingly, the little pages in my book filled with wee "me victories" and brief moments of beauty or magic that I experienced. I read *Da Güd Book* every day. I studied its palm-sized pages endlessly on a bad day. And I told myself while reading, *good things do happen to me, good things do happen to me. There is good out there for me, there is good* … like a mantra. I could see the proof in my book, so I had to believe it.

Over time, I found it easier to identify good stuff. I also noticed that positive events seemed to be occurring with greater frequency, and they seemed to be getting *bigger*. No longer was I scribbling about the weather and chocolate. I was writing about someone who rented an apartment to me even though they knew I had no job, or how I got to see a world-famous healer even though I had no money, or how my GET had brought me up to five-minute walks, three times a day …

Over a year later, my optimism returned. *Da Güd Book* saved me. I hope it does the same for you.

Therapy

As I mentioned, I've done some therapy with a psychiatrist, Dr. H, who specializes in patients with CSS. Working with Dr. H enabled me to gain perspective on CSS-related issues—the loss, the emotions and cognitive-behavioral imbalance, the mental illness, the ruminations and revelations … you get the idea. Dr. H also served as my "sanity barometer." I discussed earlier how I began to question my own judgment and how I feared becoming an angry monster, or becoming so depressed that I couldn't help myself. So I asked Dr. H to tell me when/if I went too far; after all, who better than a psychiatrist would know what a "crazy" person looked like? Dr. H had my back, which made me feel safer and more free to explore my experience and my feelings about it, while developing strategies for living a happier, more meaningful life with my conditions.

Note, sometimes you may not "click" right away with a therapist. This may be due to conflicts between personalities or communication styles, or you may not like the way that particular therapist works. I didn't like working with Dr. H for the first several sessions and almost stopped going altogether, but then I started seeing progress and was hooked. I suggest you give it at least three to five sessions. If you don't feel it's helping, you can try working with someone else, or try another strategy or treatment altogether for the time being.

A note about therapists' offices for those with environmental triggers: before making an appointment, ask if their office is scent-free. (More on visiting medical offices in Appendix B.) Some actually do have scent-free policies. While the building may still be triggerful, and while some patients won't respect a scent-free policy, every little bit helps. I tend to think that any doctor willing to implement a scent-free policy potentially knows more about CSS and CS than the doctors who don't ban fragrances.

Group Therapy

Going someplace unknown and talking about your "stuff" with people you don't know can seem intimidating, but there are lots of good reasons to participate in group therapy. Maybe you want to try therapy and can't afford a private session. Maybe you have been doing lots of bubble time and need to get out for a little semi-social time in a relatively safe place. Maybe you are having trouble relating to your friends since getting sick and want to meet others with similar conditions. Whatever your reason, once you decide you want group therapy enough to attempt to attend a meeting, then the next step is to look at how to manage the environmental triggers you may find there.

I find it incredibly challenging to be in a closed room with a bunch of people who don't have CS or CSS, even in a "scent-free" environment. Most don't really know how to be scent-free and think that not wearing perfume or cologne is all it takes. So they come to group therapy after having used scented soap and shampoo, hand lotion, and/or laundry products; wearing hours-old nail polish; drinking strong-smelling fruit drinks; flipping through PVC binders and glossy brochures and new books. They use Sharpies to write nametags, and dry-erase pens to outline things on the whiteboard. I've tried using my nosegay and scarf techniques in such situations, sitting back from the table away from others, sitting by an open window. But sessions tend to last an hour or more, and with all the environmental triggers inherent in the building itself, I don't last long.

I have managed successfully, however, in a group of people with CSS, most of whom had some environmental triggers and better understood "scent-free." By planning extra pre- and post-session bubble time and relying heavily on my nosegay and scarf techniques during sessions, I could attend and participate without decreasing my average functional capacity. This was *wonderful*. Once a week, I got out of my bubble, socialized, and participated in discussions focused around CS- and CSS-related experiences and issues. My group-mates were *brave*, and *strong*, and I loved the camaraderie and the inspiration I gained from those sessions.

A counselor facilitated the sessions and actively enforced the scent-free policy. I believe it's crucial to have a counselor present at group sessions in order to moderate discussions and prevent strong personalities from dominating and creating an unhealthy and/or unsafe dynamic. Also, unruly emotional and cognitive stuff can arise unexpectedly during group sessions, and it helps to be able to talk with a counselor when that happens.

Overall, big thumbs up, as long as the sessions are manageable enough that they don't significantly worsen your symptoms or decrease your functionality afterwards.

Writing/Journaling

When I first began working on coping strategies, I found it near impossible to identify my emotions. I'd never excelled at knowing what I was feeling, and the years of distance running, during which I learned to dismiss pain and "just get on with things," hadn't helped. But writing was another story (couldn't resist a little pun!) and when I got CSS, writing called to me more than ever before. I believe writing saved my life many times in crisis phase. It gave me a place to vent, sift through overwhelm, and break problems down into manageable bits. I began using writing then as a tool for illuminating what was going on inside me when I felt troubled yet clueless. I'd write whatever came to mind and soon enough, fears, worries, anger, grief, or whatever scurried out on to the page. *Ah*, and then *relief*! Why is that?

Writing allows us to notice and name what's at the root of strong emotions or beliefs. Similar to the concept of fear posting, *naming* the troubling emotion or thought is like pulling the curtain back and revealing the mystique of the wizard. Naming helps us to take away the power of that strong emotion or thought and remove its hold over us. In addition, once we put the emotion or thought on paper, we can step back from it instead of automatically engaging or reacting to it. We can then take time to decide how we want to act; thus, the emotion or thought no longer controls our actions. (Meditation can do this too, and so can CBT and therapy. That's why these strategies are healing for so many people—they all involve digging to the root of cognitive-behavioral problems and revealing what's there. Once exposed, the roots lose their hold and the problems begin to wither away.)

Writing provides a safe place to examine and/or simply record one's experience, thoughts, and feelings. Maybe you'll read it later. Maybe you'll never read it. Maybe you'll burn it in a transmutation ritual and toss the ashes into your garden. The important thing is to let the strong emotions and beliefs out, identify them, acknowledge them, and then benefit as their power over you diminishes and disappears.

Writing is also a great way to clear your head of stuff you have to remember to get on the next grocery store run, or stuff you mustn't forget to do in the next couple days, weeks, or months. Once you write something down, your brain can let go of it. You'll stop worrying about forgetting something and have more energy for enjoyable things.

Prescription Medication

As I mentioned earlier, prescription drugs often prove effective for treating debilitating symptoms. They also might provide a solution for someone experiencing severe emotional issues, sleep issues, anxiety or depression, brain chemistry imbalance, and/or other problems related to coping. I encourage you to consider prescription medication for coping-related issues if your doctor recommends them. **Always research any treatment your doctor recommends before trying it.** Review how to do this in the section discussing prescription medication for pain and other symptoms. Whether or not you decide to try prescription treatments for coping issues, doing bubble time and using the strategies discussed thus far will provide long-term support and bolster your health throughout your lifetime.

Review of Mental Health, CBT and Coping Strategies

- A mental illness interferes with a person's thoughts, feelings, and behaviours and can cause one to develop unhealthy perceptions and beliefs about oneself, others, and one's life.
- People with CSS may develop a secondary mental illness due to the far-reaching impact these conditions can have on one's life.
- Anxiety is neither fear nor an emotion. Anxiety is a mental illness and should be treated as such. Depression is neither sadness nor grief. Depression is a mental illness and should be treated as such.
- Like physical illness, mental illness is nothing to be ashamed of.
- Unfortunately, many people with mental illness suffer needlessly because fear and/or denial get in the way of timely diagnosis and treatment.
- Cognitive Behavioral Therapy helps people transform cognitive-behavior imbalances and live happier, healthier lives by teaching them to notice and identify unhelpful thoughts and respond to them in a positive way.

- Mindfulness involves becoming aware of our experience and choosing how we want to respond or engage with issues that arise, and ultimately choosing how we want to live.
- Core beliefs and ruminations can cause unnecessary suffering, but the coping strategies in this chapter work to debunk them and teach the brain to focus on positive, healthy topics.

> *O wondrous creatures,*
> *by what strange miracle do you*
> *so often not*
> *smile?*
> —Hafiz[28]

6. Longer-Term Symptom Management, Living Skills and Healing

Demystifying the Healer

My symptoms sounded unbelievable, even to me. I was used to running at least 5k every other day, and doing hour-long workouts three times a week. Now, if I went to the gym or for a run, or even took a walk around the block, my joints and muscles became severely inflamed and my limbs felt heavy, like lead, for days or weeks afterwards. When my GP ran some tests and came up empty, I began to suspect what any normal, fit, 40-something in Vancouver would: that I was dying of some rare temperate rainforest disease.

My GP referred me to a specialist but I'd have to wait to get an appointment. In the meantime, I endured a terrifying year of increasing symptoms, decreasing energy, and diminishing hope. Cognitive problems joined the physical ones. I couldn't move or think clearly after exerting the smallest amount of energy, like washing dishes or doing laundry. Even watching television wore me out. The proud multi-tasker within devolved into a bumbling one-thing-at-a-timer, and my short-term memory dwindled to nothing.

My olfactory system, though, developed a dog-like sensitivity. My nose could detect synthetic chemicals everywhere—emanating from new materials and buildings, cleaning products, people's skin and hair and clothing, even plastic shopping bags—and they triggered sneezing and coughing fits, nausea, migraines, fluey aches and sweats and more. Breathing in public, taking the bus or train, stopping by the post office or drug store—it all transformed into an extreme sport, and I was crashing and burning daily. I didn't even know what arena I was in.

I stayed home as much as possible to conserve energy and avoid odors that made me sick. This isolation proved detrimental to my social life and, along with my active lifestyle, my job, and my health, I lost most of my friends. Forced to quit taking transit, I spent a chunk of my precious savings to buy a car—an expense and hassle I didn't want—so I could manage necessary errands once or twice a week.

The only things that helped to relieve symptoms and keep me sane during that period I have since deemed the "time of great loss, isolation, and unknowing" were journaling and acupuncture.

On a particularly sluggish day, my Acupuncturist suggested I try Chee Gong.

A raised eyebrow was all I could muster.

"Chee—spelled Qi—Gong, an ancient Chinese healing practice," she was writing it down, knowing I had little hope of remembering it. "It cultivates and builds your life-force, your energy."

"Sounds like just the thing." With a spark of hope, I dragged myself over to the library, checked out a DVD called *Qi Gong for Healthy Joints and Bones*, and tried it out at home.

* * *

Healer Myth #1: Qi Gong masters are all ancient Chinese men with moth-eaten robes and unkempt beards that trail along the packed dirt floor of a dim, smoky cave in the hills of some little known East-Asian province.

* * *

The Healer on the library's DVD was a clean-shaven white guy from California, 30-ish, who used to be a soccer star. The program consisted of the Healer demonstrating movements similar to tai chi—but slower, gentler—while talking about Qi, life-force, energy. "Energy is life," he'd say, "breath is life." Move the Qi between your hands, shift it into your belly.

I didn't feel any life-force, except once in a while, when my arms would tingle after doing a particular movement, but that was probably just poor circulation. My blood pressure tended towards the low side. I thought it quite possible that the Healer was nothing more than a charlatan cashing in on his empirically good looks, Star Wars fanatics' desire to feel the Force, and the desperation of the chronically ill to get well. The guy wasn't my type, and my jury was still out regarding the Force, but I *was* one of those desperately ill people, so I followed his lead as often as I could.

After three months, however, something changed. During my daily DVD session, the energy outside of me suddenly seemed almost tangible. I could feel it surrounding me like a blanket made of something nebulous—like layers of cotton candy, without the sticky factor. I could push it up or down or gather and compress it into a ball and move it from side to side, like a kitten with a yarn ball—no, this was Qi Gong after all—like a dragon with a Qi ball. I looked at the space between my splayed fingers and palms and saw nothing, but I *felt* it—mass, heat, power—Qi. When I brought my Qi ball up over my head and let it go, a sensation of warmth cascaded down, over and within me, like a sunlit waterfall. When I pressed Qi into my belly, it was like feeding a furnace. Heat shot up and down my limbs. Every part of me tingled and hummed. I gathered and poured Qi over me, and pressed it into my core again and again, reveling in a euphoria, like a child who has just discovered the wonder of swimming or being propelled into the sky by a trampoline, finding a way into another universe.

I suppose that's when I became a believer. One *could* manipulate life-force energy. *I* could manipulate life-force energy. Qi Gong was real.

Could it make me better? The Healer seemed to think so. He sold a CD and DVD set entitled "Self-Healing with Qi Gong" on his website. While purchasing mine, I saw that he taught classes in Santa Cruz and New York.

Someday he would come close enough that I would be able to meet him, I told myself, and work with him in person, one-on-one. Maybe I'd become his apprentice and embark upon a Healer's life myself. At the very least, I'd get my health back.

But as time passed, my illness progressed and I had to reduce the amount of Qi Gong I did with my DVDs. I could no longer summon a Qi Ball, or stand for 45 minutes and do the movements without suffering for days afterward. Soon 30 minutes was too much, then 15, and then five. Ultimately, I could manage only a few minutes of gently shaking my wrist and elbow joints, thumping with half-closed fists on my chest, or pressing on key acupressure points.

I turned my focus to the CDs, on which the Healer taught the history and philosophy behind Qi Gong and led the listener through meditations. I had so much brain fog by then that the Healer's voice drifted in and out. I couldn't focus, and I remembered very little, but I listened as well as I could, I kept breathing deeply and imagining my belly full of a limitless supply of energy.

Over a year after my symptoms began, I got to see a specialist who could pin the names on my ailments: Chronic Fatigue Syndrome (CFS) and Multiple Chemical Sensitivities (MCS). At last, in all the vast space of unknowing, I knew something. Though apparently incurable, my conditions were known entities, and there were tools I could use to manage symptoms. After a year of scrabbling blindly in the brush, I had reached the head of my healing trail. There I found little respite, but solace aplenty.

My specialist introduced me to the "energy envelope," a conceptual tool used to help folks with CFS objectively assess and visualize the limitations on their energy. People without CFS have a seemingly bottomless energy envelope—they can do whatever they want, whenever and for as long as they want, and their bodies can keep on going. But those with CFS have a much smaller envelope, one that regenerates energy at a fraction of the pace of a healthy person. And if they expend energy beyond their limits, they wind up back in bed with a smaller envelope than before, and they gotta start all over again, slowly building up energy. It's like a brutal instant karma game with no known exit.

I spent the next year learning the limits of my envelope, which was basically a process of try—crash—recover—try a little less—crash—recover—try still less.... Each crash forced me back into bed for weeks, blurry-minded and in pain. I practiced very little Qi Gong during that time, but I played the Healer's CDs, and I listened as well as I could, breathing deeply, sometimes wishing for the misery of life to end, sometimes dreaming of getting well.

My envelope turned out to be about three non-consecutive hours a day. When I managed to stay within it, the pace of my health's downward spiral slowed, as did the frequency of my crashes. Managing all my daily living activities—cleaning, cooking, eating, laundry, bills, shopping, seeing doctors, and fighting for disability payments—within that three-hour limit required me to prioritize ruthlessly. I found it difficult to justify using my already insufficient energy stores on Qi Gong or meditation before attempting a household chore or attending to my ongoing disability claim. The doctors told me I would be debilitated like this forever; there was no hope.

And yet I had some. CFS was new, a stubborn voice within me argued, and Qi Gong was ancient. The practice would not have endured if it had no efficacy. I suckled hope from its tradition and ruminated on a morsel of wisdom I retained from my bed-ridden CD sessions: "First ecstasy, then the laundry." The proverb tickled my mind like a *koan*.

* * *

Healer Myth #2: Healers speak in metaphors and riddles. Only a life-long disciple can make sense of such things.

* * *

What *was* ecstasy? All that came immediately to mind was sex—and James Spader, naturally—but the Healer hadn't spoken about either of them. His teachings focused on Qi Gong, so there had to be a connection. Life-long disciple or not, I could work a *koan*—I had studied the *Upanishads* in university, after all.

Eventually the answer came: ecstasy was the bliss I had experienced when practicing Qi Gong. Thus, cultivating energy had to be a priority, or else I would lose myself in the daily drudgery, isolation, and uncertainty of chronic illness. And so I started again. At first I could manage only ten seconds of Qi Gong movements, but I worked up to two minutes once or twice a week.

Over the next year, I lived primarily within my envelope, and my conditions stabilized. I still crashed when I over-exerted or endured significant stress, and I still had pain and cognitive symptoms, but three non-consecutive hours a day remained my general functional rule. This relative stability was good, I told myself, far preferable to decline. All the same, I was stuck in a rut. My attempts to sneak beyond the three-hour limit, via infinitesimally small increases in exercise, only resulted in crash. I believed Qi Gong could help me, yet how could I generate more energy when I couldn't practice for more than two minutes a day, a couple times a week? When I couldn't even gather a Qi ball?

I needed to break the Healer's lessons down, to find kernels of Qi Gong I could do at my current level of debilitation and upon which I could build. But I didn't know enough. What aspects of Qi Gong would be most beneficial to someone with my conditions?

It was time to see the Healer.

* * *

Healer Myth #3: One must travel to the Healer by burro, or camel, or on the back of a rice wagon pulled by wasted, ribby oxen, or by walking a pilgrim trail across three continents and through seven ecosystems with only the clothes on one's back and a ten-pound sack of cane sugar, with which one will pay the Healer.

* * *

Three years after I first heard about Qi Gong, I got to meet the Healer in person. (I paid online by credit card and then was driven in a car from Vancouver to Seattle—a mere 143 miles—drinking coconut milk tea and listening to Todd Rundgren's song "The Healer" the whole way. So much for Myth #3.) By that time, I had concocted and bought into no small bit of a mystique surrounding this Healer. Not in an obsessive or stalkerish way, more a subconscious way.

Images and portrayals of various healers on television and in media had certainly influenced my perceptions throughout my lifetime. This particular Healer's self-presentation had also made its mark. Divine gongs and new-agey background music pervaded his instruction materials, which depicted him practicing Qi Gong on a broad, flat stone in the middle of a serene pond, or a sheltered cove in Lake Tahoe—yes, like walking on water—or in a giant Zen garden with symmetrically placed rocks and raked sand. And symbols graced each location, like koi fish, lily pads, or cranes and herons—maybe cranes *are* herons? I can't remember. And the Healer glowed, always, bright with health and energy.

When you are ill, and you don't know what's wrong with you, or even if you do and you have been told there is no cure, you want badly to believe that there is someone out there who *can* make you all better, or at the very least, improve your health. If 21st century medicine can't help, you think, then maybe ancient practices can. What do you have to lose? So you watch the Healer on DVDs and listen to his voice on CDs, for years, and if you are a creative person like I am, you start to develop a mythology about your energy Yoda. I wasn't aware that I had done so, of course, but it became apparent to me the moment I met him.

* * *

Healer Myth #4: Healers don't joke around or laugh aloud. They live in a constant state of composure and balance. (In extremely humorous circumstances, they may crack a smile.)

* * *

I promised myself that I wouldn't allow my health conditions to force me to live the rest of my life in a bubble, and so far I've managed to maintain much of my autonomy, but I am required to spend a significant amount of time in seclusion. Venturing out of my safe zone into unfamiliar territory is always a shock. Going anywhere tires me, and with MCS, I have to be cautious about unfamiliar environments. Any synthetic chemical trigger can cause a coughing fit, nausea, migraines, or worse. When I can't avoid unknown places or people, I prepare for the worst, but being acutely aware of the risks can take the fun out of things. When adopting caution and preparedness, I sometimes lose track of delight and fall prey to a gnawing sense of dread.

My friend Suz picks up on that when she drops me off. "Are you nervous?" she asks.

"A little dread-full," I say, "about breathing. It's a new space for me, and filled with people. Lots can go wrong."

"Pray for the willingness to let it be wonderful," she advises. I've never been much for prayer in any orthodox sense, but her words lift my spirit like glitter in the air.

"Oh, I'm willing," I say, "I'm willing and open to wonder...." I repeat the phrase like a mantra as I enter the yoga studio and take shallow breaths. The room has serene paper lantern lighting and hardwood floors. The air is thick with the smell of warm bodies and the faintest tinge of sweat. It's a safe place, I tell myself. You can breathe here.

When I approach the Healer, he smiles, shakes my hand and says, "I'll be ready in a few minutes, once I say good bye to these people. The owners gave me the keys to the place, so we have plenty of time."

"You have the keys?" I say, still taking shallow breaths, "If I'd known, I'd have invited some friends and—"

"We could have a party!" we say in unison.

The Healer laughs out loud—a full, unrestrained laugh. (Looks like Myth #4 is toast.)—then grins like an innocent, and leaves me. Holding my breath, I weave through the blissful crowd and sit on the floor near the far wall. I close my eyes and take deep breaths, willing the shock of the new place and the exhaustion from the long drive to dissipate, coaxing my sense of wonder to come out and play.

* * *

Healer Myth #5: Healers never get sick.

* * *

While waiting for our session to begin, I hear the Healer blowing his nose like a Snuffleupagus in the bathroom down the hall. When he sits in front of me, his eyes look feverish and his lids, heavy, like he's struggling to keep them open. My conclusion: The Healer has a cold.

"Tell me what's happening with you," he says, sniffling softly.

I'd expected I might feel a little star struck when I at last sat face to face with the actual Healer, but when I see that he is *ill*, I feel only doubt. Insatiable, it gnaws at my faith. I remember Dorothy discovering the Wizard of Oz behind the curtain. Maybe The Healer *is* a charlatan after all and I've come here for nothing, I think. But only for a moment. Then I remember the feel of energy between my palms, the need that drove me to come all this way. It's real enough. The man sitting before me may have a cold, but he radiates vitality like a small sun. I look down at my list of health issues and goals for our session. So tired, my brain feels sloshy, and I must wait until the words stop dancing on the page. The Healer sniffles and attends with patience.

At last I read to him. He listens.

* * *

Healer Myth #6: All Healers are steeped in patchouli oil, or myrrh, or frankincense, or garlic. Something like that.

* * *

The Healer wields energy the way a western doctor employs prescription pad and pen. The Healer utilizes tools like acupuncture needles and tea. He moves with the grace of an eagle, the power of a bull, and a step as silent as midnight. He has me sit on a chair with palms pressed together, hands in lap and eyes closed, while he practices medical Qi Gong on me. I feel him move around my body, close but not touching. I feel heat and see flashes of light behind my eyelids. I don't know what he's doing, exactly, but he's doing something.

One of the gifts/curses of having MCS is a nose like a bloodhound. I can smell a donut shop from a mile away. (Gift.) However, I can also detect perfume, cologne, and fabric-softened clothing from 50 yards, I can smell someone's deodorant fragrance or lip balm at two yards, and hair products and hand lotion—well, you get the idea. (Yep, curse.) But as the Healer moves around me, I can't sniff a scent on him. No menthol or licorice cough drops, even. I note something though—not a scent so much as a texture—something almost waxen, but more enduring. Something that would burn hot. A resin? The Healer is wearing a resin? Or is made of resin? Like a great tree. Or, perhaps he is no longer human, I muse, merely a conductor of energy. But that would make him a god. Do gods get colds? (You see? This is how myths are born.)

* * *

Healer Myth #7: Healers work in mysterious ways. The Healer's gift to you may not be what you wanted, but it will be what you need. (For more detail, check out the Rolling Stones' song.)

* * *

I return my focus to what's happening with my body, which is nothing less than incredible. It never occurred to me that the Healer would do something like this, give me such a gift. I thought he would provide me with a list of basic exercises to do at home. That's what I had asked him for, after all, a plan of baby steps that would help me to gradually get stronger. It occurs to me now that what I asked for was very western—like a prescription—and he complied in the first part of our session. But this, what he's doing now, is so much more, so much better.

At home, when I practiced my two minutes of movements, I felt a weak tingle of life-force trickle down my arms or into my belly, but soon after I finished, the Qi drained away and left me feeling weak and tired, empty and cold. Like a dead car battery, I couldn't store energy anymore like a normal person could.

But when the Healer concludes his work and steps away, the Qi stays put. I can see it inside me, gleaming white and gold—my core is full to bursting. What do you know? The Healer gave me a jumpstart!

My mind grapples for comprehension while my body sings, and zings and hums. I bask, I steep, I pulse and throb. I am electric—

This is how it felt, I fathom, to have an unlimited reserve of energy, the way I did before I got ill. I couldn't perceive my life-force then—I took it for granted—but I behold it now. Oh, wonder, and rapture—and yes, *ecstasy!*

"How do you feel?" The Healer smiles down at me.

"Like you stuffed my belly full of Qi," I say, laughing, and gleaning that he did more than that. Faith had brought me here, but I had carried no hope for this, the greatest possible outcome. At some point I had resolved myself to believing that while I might succeed in increasing my energy somewhat, I'd never feel this, this vital, ever again. Or perhaps, since I'd had no clear sense memory of this feeling, I couldn't envision or hope for its return.

How did the Healer know what I lacked, besides the obvious? How did he know I needed invigoration of spirit as well as body? (I suppose some myths are based in truth, after all.) I rub my belly, expecting sparks to fly from it. "Thank you." My whisper sounds like a prayer.

He puts his hands together at his chest and makes a small bow in farewell.

* * *

I'm supposed to wait for Suz to pick me up outside the yoga studio. Or was it across the street? I can't remember. I bounce down the hill in the rain, reveling in the abundance of energy crackling in my belly, before I think to call and tell her where she can find me.

"I forgot the plan," I say, tasting raindrops and grinning like a five-year-old, "I didn't think—I just started walking—it feels so good, like I could walk forever!"

Intro to Longer-Term Brain Health and Healing

"Long term" sounds so permanent, doesn't it? I prefer "long*er* term." It has a more open-ended feel and better reflects my belief that I won't be dealing with CSS and CS for the rest of my life. Maybe I read too many Nancy Drew books when I was young, but I want to leave the fate of my conditions wide open, let the possibility of cure hang in the air like a mystery about to be solved, you know?

This chapter discusses what comes after you've spent some time in *stability phase* and have developed a solid base for longer-term living and healing. Are you ready? Let's see if you meet the criteria. By this point …

- you've built your bubble and become a planning and pacing ninja
- you have learned how much bubble time you need to reduce environmental and intrinsic trigger load, minimize symptom severity and duration
- you have used the bubble to reduce a significant percentage of symptoms, on average
- you have identified your warning symptoms and decreased relapse and crash frequency, and the majority of crashes you now experience are planned.
- you have sought treatment for mental illness if necessary
- you practice coping strategies to minimize suffering and maintain mental health and authentic relationships (with others as well as yourself) *daily*, not just on bad days
- you practice techniques to engage the parasympathetic system *daily*, not just on bad days.

If you found yourself answering no to any of the above, I suggest you go back and review and practice in those areas before reading on. If you said yes to all of the above, CONGRATULATIONS! It took a lot of courage and love to get here. Take a moment to savor your accomplishments and your devotion to yourself and your health. *Ahhhh!*

Once I reached this point, I found I could at last investigate and address areas I'd back-burnered during the chaos and desperation of my 24/7 survival-driven *crisis phase* and the fairly steep learning curve of early *stability phase*. Questions such as these took center stage: How could I *increase* functionality? Could I find a way to *heal*? How could I establish longer-term financial security? How could I manage the other intrinsic triggers? What did longer-term life with CSS and CS look like, and how much joy and satisfaction could that life bear? Nothing to do but start digging.

Sleep

Like many people, I slept great until CS and CSS came along. Then, I stopped sleeping deeply, I tossed and turned for hours most nights, and in the mornings, I felt groggier than I had the night before. Dr. Norman Doidge, an M.D., psychiatrist, and psychoanalyst on the faculty of the University of Toronto's Department of Psychiatry, reports that it's not uncommon for patients with brain issues to sleep poorly and experience fatigue.[1] The brain flushes most of its waste products during sleep, which means lack of sleep can lead to oxidant build up, and prolonged sleep problems can cause the brain to become toxic and less functional.[2] Nutshell, we need sleep.

First, my GP prescribed sleeping pills. I'd had minimal experience with doctors and prescription drugs at that time and believed that the patient had to do whatever the doctor said (unhelpful core belief). So I took the drugs, without research, without question. Then I slept, sort of. I didn't toss and turn anymore, but I awoke feeling strangely non-rested, and I wandered through my days in a dopey haze. That was the end of the sleep drugs trial for me.

Next, my GP taught me about sleep hygiene. (Yep, like dental hygiene but for sleep. Who knew? I've often thought that they should teach stuff like this in school, and that school should be taught well into adulthood. I forgot so many things from 11th grade that I need to know now. Like the role of the amygdala, for instance—what a revelation!) Practicing good sleep hygiene involves steps such as these:

- Install thick blinds so bedroom is as dark as possible.
- Wear a sleeping mask if you require more darkness.
- Wear earplugs if ambient noise in your bedroom disturbs sleep.
- Limit naps to one a day, one hour long, max.
- Do slow, relaxed breathing or meditate before bed (and if you awaken in the middle of the night in a panic) to engage the parasympathetic nervous system.
- Use your bed only for sleeping or for sex, so your brain understands that when you go to bed, it's for one of those two things (and not for staying up all night).
- If you can't sleep, get up and do something until you can. Don't toss and turn for hours.
- Establish a sleep routine: Go to bed and rise each morning about the same time. Don't sleep in if you were up for a few hours the night before. You may not sleep well the first few nights and then stumble drowsily through your first few days, but if you stick to the routine your body will work to adjust.
- Ask your doctor for guidance with sleep hygiene.

After I established a sleep routine and installed blackout curtains, I slept better—not great, but better. That was in crisis phase. When I reached stability phase, I saw a marked decrease in sleep interruptions, and now, after over a year of stability and practicing CBT, mindfulness, Qi Gong, and meditation daily, I have the rare morning when I wake up feeling fairly rested.

Some folks have had success using non-prescription supplements such as Cortisol Manager, 5-HTP, or Melatonin to promote better sleep. With the support of my naturopath and psychiatrist, I tried all three, with mixed results.

I began with Cortisol Manager, an Ayurvedic sleep aid containing Ashwagandha

Root, Magnolia Bark, L-Theanine, and Phosphatidylserine. The Cortisol Manager didn't improve my sleep but I did feel calmer and more grounded in the mornings. My naturopath posited that I had acceptable nighttime cortisol levels but elevated cortisol in the morning. (Months later, testing revealed my cortisol levels were within normal range. Unfortunately, my testing didn't take place until I'd reached stability phase. Ideally, one is tested in crisis phase and prior to trying supplements.) Since mornings were manageable and my goal was to improve sleep, I discontinued this supplement.

Next I tried 5-HTP, aka 5-hydroxytryptophan, which is thought to help raise levels of serotonin and thus improve mood, but research to date is inconclusive.[3] Note that 5-HTP is also suspected of causing "a severe neurological condition, but the link is not clear."[4] I tried 50mg of 5-HTP before bedtime and within a week I was sleeping like a baby and feeling rested upon awakening. "I'm cured," I cried, "I'm *cured!*" Not so fast. After about ten days, I noticed depression slowly sinking in. I consulted with Dr. H, who theorized that my brain might not be able to tolerate the boost in serotonin (as I understand it, it's a chemical balance thing). She suggested I stop the 5-HTP and try melatonin instead.

The brain's production and secretion of the hormone melatonin is triggered by onset of darkness and slowed by the return of light; thus it is theorized "that melatonin is involved in circadian rhythm (the internal body clock) and regulation of diverse body functions…. The most common use of melatonin is to aid in sleep."[5] I took 10mg of Melatonin before bed for three weeks and saw no improvement in my sleep. Perhaps you'll have better luck. Remember, never try supplements without thoroughly researching and consulting your doctor.

FOOD

Preparing food, cooking, and cleaning up can be a challenge when you have CSS. In crisis phase, I didn't have enough energy to cook and clean up. I also couldn't tolerate anything with a strong smell, and for a while *everything* had a strong smell—not just onions and garlic—even butter and sugar did. For over a year, I survived on smoothies, protein bars, and pre-roasted chickens. I don't recommend that diet, but when you're single, living alone, and in crisis phase, that may be all you can manage. Maybe you live with someone who can cook and clean. Maybe you can afford healthy pre-cooked or packaged meals. However you get food into you, *get food into you*.

Eat well, even if you don't feel hungry, even if you feel hungry all the time. Pay attention to what you are eating, and how much. Some people add different foods to their diet, or overeat, when they get sick. Others drastically cut calories in an attempt to compensate for reduced activity. Be careful with such changes. Sure, physical activity may decrease, but the sensitized central nervous system is working overtime and therefore consuming more fuel than that of a sedentary person without CS. If you don't know how many calories you need per day, find out. Work with a dietician who understands CS and CSS. If you can't see one right away, calculate your Basal Metabolic Rate (BMR) and estimate your energy needs from there.

Your BMR indicates the number of calories your body uses in a 24-hour period to carry out its basic functions—breathing, circulating blood, adjusting hormone levels, and growing and repairing cells—when at rest, that is, if you did nothing but lie still in one place all day and night. BMR is determined by several factors, including body size and composition (larger bodies, and bodies with more muscle burn more calories), gender (men generally have less body fat and more muscle than women of same age and weight and thus burn more calories), and age (amount of muscle tends to decrease and fat tends to increase with age).[6] You can estimate your BMR by visiting one of the many BMR calculation sites online that do the math for you, or by using one of these formulas:

> Women: BMR = (10 × weight in kilos) + (6.25 × height in cm)–(5 × age in years) -161
> Men: BMR = (10 × weight in kilos) + (6.25 × height in cm)–(5 × age in years) + 5[7]

Once you know your BMR, you can estimate your daily caloric needs on a BMR-calculating website, or by multiplying your BMR by the appropriate activity factor, as follows:

- Little or no exercise: BMR × 1.2 = Approximate Daily Calories Needed
- Light exercise (1–3 days/week): BMR × 1.375 = Approximate Daily Calories Needed
- Moderate exercise (3–5 days/week): BMR × 1.55 = Approximate Daily Calories Needed
- Heavy exercise (6–7 days a week): BMR × 1.725 = Approximate Daily Calories Needed
- Very heavy exercise (twice per day, extra heavy workouts): BMR × 1.9 = Approximate Daily Calories Needed.[8]

Note, the above is a general approximation and does not take *you* or the energy requirements of CS or CSS into consideration. I offer it as a guideline to help you to estimate how much to consume should your activity suddenly and significantly decrease due to your illness. I encourage you to consult with a dietician experienced with CS and CSS in order to attain a daily caloric intake guide tailored specifically for you.

What kind of food should you eat?

Here lies controversy. You will need to do some research and decide what's best for you. And I mean, put in the time and do *real* research. Going online and searching for "best diet for [insert CS or a specific CSS here]" isn't going to do the job. Your brain and your body are much too important to throw away on free internet advice from people touting an all-in-one cure. I recommend that you get advice from a CS-knowledgeable dietitian on what you should and should not be eating. Lots of folks with CS have Irritable Bowel Syndrome (IBS), cranky guts, and/or food sensitivities and intolerances. If your dietician understands CS, s/he will most likely recommend a diet that avoids foods known to irritate the gut or cause bloating and/or allergic reactions—usually gluten, dairy, processed sugar, high-glycemic or high–FODMAP foods, stuff like that. (FODMAP stands for Fermentable Oligosaccharides, Disaccharides, Monosaccharides and Polyols. FODMAPs are molecules (in foods) that tend to be poorly absorbed by the small intestine and thus can cause or exacerbate gut issues.) Remember what I said early on about CS and the gut? Whether or not you have IBS, or even minor bloating after eating certain foods, if your dietitian doesn't mention IBS or gut issues when you say you have CS, find another dietitian. When you find one who knows and understands CS, and they recommend a special diet, research it before trying it.

You say you don't have IBS, and you tested negative for food sensitives so you can eat *any*thing—test results don't lie, right? Well, here's the deal: With CS the nervous system is highly reactive, right? This means that, even if you don't have any known food allergies or intolerances, your body may react to some of the more allergenic or irritating foods because of your sensitized system; thus, certain foods may be intrinsic triggers for you. And triggers are cumulative, remember, so the more you are exposed to on a given day, the more likely, and more severely, your sensitized nervous system will react. Avoiding known food allergens and irritating foods is another way of reducing your trigger load, giving your central nervous system a break, and working to decrease symptoms. According to Dr. Doidge, patients with ADD or depression experienced significant improvements after removing particular foods—sugar, wheat, or other grains, for instance—from their diets.[9] Do you have to remove "trigger foods" from your diet forever? Probably not. Many people eventually can phase them back in.

If you can't find a qualified dietitian in your area, you might be able to find an M.D. or Naturopath who knows CS and/or who is certified in Functional Medicine. Medical professionals who practice Functional Medicine examine factors such as your past and present health concerns, lifestyle, and genetic predisposition, and then generate a healing plan based on that information. They use a patient-centered approach (necessary for treating CS and CSS) and tend to consider lifestyle and diet changes before reaching for their prescription pads.

Whatever you end up doing, remember, there is no perfect solution for reducing symptoms and decreasing exposure to/impact of all triggers. We can only do the best we can with the resources we have at hand, and then see how they work for us. If there is absolutely no one qualified in your area to work with you on diet, perhaps you can crowd-fund some money to pay for a visit to the nearest specialist. Or maybe a friend would be interested in driving you on a low-budget road trip? Remember, there is no single avenue for getting help, and if you hit a roadblock, there is always another way.

Remember also that people with CS and CSS tend to present symptoms in different ways and respond to treatments with varying results. It follows that a dietitian's recommendation will work for some and not for others. This can be discouraging, but just because figuring out your diet may be complex and complicated, that doesn't mean you can't do it. Give yourself time, usually from 3 to 12 months, to figure it out. When I hit on the right diet, some of my symptoms disappeared. (Yep, disappeared. Soldier on …)

What if you try the dietitian's recommendations and don't get the results you want? This could happen. For example, my CS-savvy dietitian advised me to eat small meals with protein every two to three hours, on a low–FODMAP diet (i.e., avoiding foods that are high in FODMAPs) that totaled about 53 grams fat, 70–100 grams protein, 253 grams of carbs, and 1600–1800 calories per day. The frequent consumption of protein helped even out my blood sugar and the diet helped decrease bloating, both good things; but the diet also caused my body to store fat, primarily around my waist, and did nothing to decrease brain fog or increase energy. I found this unsatisfactory, so I did what I'm going to recommend that you do should you find yourself in a similar position: more research. I'll share more of my findings with you momentarily.

THOUGHT AS FOOD

Some people will tell you to "just think positive" because they don't understand CS or CSS at all and don't know how to be supportive or what to say. This can feel dismissive and, after the hundredth person says this, it can get downright annoying, I know. But I'm telling you to think positive because I *do* understand certain things about CS and

CSS. Being mindful about how you think about what you put into your body can make a difference in your thought patterns and your health.

Remember our CBT discussion? If you believe a negative thought to be true and think that thought enough times, it can become an automatic thought. Fortunately for us, positive, helpful thoughts have that same potential to become automatic. So, when you consume, try thinking of your food as fuel that will help your central nervous system heal and decrease symptoms.

Neuroplasticity—Your Most Important Tool for Healing?

After reading two books by Dr. Doidge, I became convinced that neuroplasticity is a major key to decreasing CS and CSS symptoms and longer-term healing. *If neuroplasticity is so important,* you ask, *then why aren't you talking about it until now?* Good question. The truth is, I have been talking about neuroplasticity throughout the book, albeit unofficially, but there was no point in throwing a bunch of the science at you until you were safely out of crisis phase and able to focus on it. When people are in fight-or-flight-mode, feeling anxious and/or desperate, they aren't able to learn or heal well.[10] This is why we build a safe bubble and move from crisis to stability first. Now we can work on healing.

Healing the sensitized nervous system is complex and complicated, and researchers have a long way to go to crack this egg. They know enough, however, that we have a few places to start. For simplicity's sake, I'll organize this information into two realms: creating positive neuroplastic change, and promoting brain health. Neuroplasticity first.

Neuroplasticity Primer

Back in the late 1960s or so, scientists learned some amazing things about our brain: when the brain performs an activity its structure *changes*, and the brain streamlines its processes for repetitive activities, *and* it can even "re-purpose" certain parts of itself to do tasks that a damaged part of the brain used to do.[11] Sometimes the brain can replace dead brain cells, sometimes the way we think or behave can cause genes to switch off or on, and sometimes efficient brain "circuits" we believe to be permanent can be changed.[12] The scientists called these adaptive abilities of the brain neuroplasticity—*plastic* indicates something that can change or modify itself, and *neuro* stands for *neuron,* the type of nerve cell found in the brain and nervous systems.[13]

Remember when I described how CS develops? Technically, CS "is a form of maladaptive [inappropriate/detrimental] neuroplasticity,"[14] (as is chronic pain and other CSS issues, which I'll get into in a moment). Upon learning this, I hypothesized that if the brain's plasticity enabled it to develop CS and CSS in the first place, then that same malleability can make the brain *un-develop* these conditions—that is, re-learn proper sensory perception, signaling, and responses—by creating positive neuroplastic change. (Go with me on this for now; I'll discuss plastic potential momentarily.) How can we facilitate positive plastic change? Good question. First we need to understand some basic laws of neuroplasticity:

1. **Neurons may fire together or fire apart:** When you acquire a new skill or learn a new idea, the clusters of neurons processing that skill/idea simultaneously send

out an electrical impulse (aka "fire together") and connect to each other (aka "wire together") into "circuits."[15] When that new activity is repeated, the brain streamlines those circuits, and the neurons fire stronger, faster signals.[16] The more streamlined the circuits, the harder they can be to break, but if you stop doing an activity, over time, the related circuits will weaken and even break, or "fire apart."[17] For example, consider how you toiled to learn French in high school, but since graduation you haven't used it; and now, years later, you can't remember more than "Bonjour." This loss of neuronal connection and thus, knowledge, means that the neurons that had once fired and wired together to learn and use French have since fired apart because of disuse. Those neurons then can fire together and form circuits with other neurons to process new activities and information. Neurons that fire apart and then form new circuits are commonly said to be *rewiring*.[18]

2. **Plasticity is competitive:** There is limited brain real estate and a lifetime of learning to store there, so if you stop using a skill, the related neurons will rewire to replace it with a skill you use frequently.[19] Basically, if you don't use knowledge, you will lose it.[20]

3. **Attention is necessary for long-term plastic change:** Studies have shown that long-term plastic change requires focused attention.[21] When we pay close attention, the brain secretes two neurotransmitters—acetylcholine and dopamine—to strengthen the new neuronal connections involved in what we're learning or doing.[22] We need acetylcholine for learning, as it assists us in concentrating and forming sharp memories.[23] Strong memories create strong neuronal connections.[24] Dopamine, a "reward" neurotransmitter that makes us feel good and increases energy, plays a role in strengthening the new neuronal circuits, which is necessary for long-term plastic change.[25]

4. **Repetition can limit plasticity:** Everything we do or experience alters our brains, for better or worse, but plastic potential is affected by some factors, one of which is repetition.[26] For example, have you ever noticed how quickly ruts form on freshly groomed ice as skaters pass over it time and again? Each time they circle the rink, the easier it becomes to get caught in those ruts. This is similar to the brain's way of wiring. At first, the brain is a "blank slate," but as we go through life and learning occurs, neural connections, or mental "tracks" are made upon it; and with enough time and repetition, those tracks can become *rigid*.[27] Rigid neural tracks or circuits have become so efficient, fast, and strong that changing them can pose quite a challenge.[28] Think about breaking a stubborn habit, like biting your nails or procrastinating. Habits, automatic thoughts and core beliefs, and some of our disorders are all products of plasticity and repetition and are, to some extent, rigid.[29]

Now that you understand the basics of neuroplasticity, aren't you *excited*? Aren't you wondering if you can rewire your brain and cure your CSS and CS? Aren't you wondering if anyone can change *any* unhelpful automatic thought or behavior, even if it's become rigid? Don't you feel like dancing in the streets, or at least doing a quick jig in your bubble? Perhaps you prefer to temper your excitement for now. Perhaps you aren't yet convinced. I understand. Using neuroplasticity to cure CS and related syndromes sounds idealistic and impossible, and most of us have never noticed neuroplastic change happening, so it's easy to underestimate what the brain can do.[30] Let's look more closely at the brain's capacity for healing.

Everyone is born with "plastic potential," and some people retain a high level of plasticity throughout their lives, but others develop rigidity, primarily due to repetition from things such as work, lifestyle, or neuroses.[31] Over time, with repeated activity, rigid circuits can become "self-sustaining."[32] Are the circuits involved in CS and CSS self-sustaining, and if so, can self-sustaining circuits be broken? Good questions. At time of writing, researchers aren't yet sure.

Some studies propose that a type of neuroplastic change called *kindling* may be involved in causing CFS[33] and MCS.[34] The kindling theory posits that "repeated exposure to an initially subthreshold stimulus can eventually exceed threshold limits" and cause a long-lasting "hypersensitivity to the stimulus" which eventually causes automatic and problematic physiological issues.[35] Many believe the effects of kindling to be permanent. One study states that if kindling is involved in CS and certain "structural changes in the neurons have occurred ... then it might be extremely difficult to recover from such an illness [as CFS]."[36] Sound discouraging? Well, nothing is conclusive yet. Until you know for sure what kind of structural changes, and the degree of rigidity your brain has developed, there's only one way to discover the extent of your healing potential: by ensuring that your brain's neuroplasticity works *for* you as much as possible, and not against.

When I got sick, my brain wired some unhelpful connections that cause it to treat all strong scents and other environmental triggers as life-threatening. Even intrinsic triggers like an emotional stressor or hormone fluctuation cause my central nervous system to go into red alert and overprotect. Over time, these neuronal connections have become strong, efficient, and to whatever degree, rigid. So how do I get my brain to unwire the CS- and CSS-related connections and rewire healthy ones? First step: I use neuroplasticity for healing every day.

When wet paint fumes trigger an ILS episode and I fix my attention on the smell and strength of the fumes and believe they can hurt me, what will my brain focus on? *Strong, nasty smell! Danger, danger! Wet paint! Red Alert! Soldiers, defend! Close down that airway on the double!* That is what my brain will learn, and the connections will become faster and stronger and more rigid with repetition and time. But if wet paint fumes trigger an ILS episode and I fix my attention on other things—like the safe, comforting, and pleasurable smell of the hot chocolate in my cup, or an image of Sergeant Shultz putting my soldiers to bed, or telling myself I am safe regardless of the smell of paint fumes— what will my brain learn? *No danger. Ooo—do I smell hot chocolate?! Soldiers not needed. No threat. I am safe.* If I don't use the neurons that formed the red alert circuits, then eventually, they should fire apart and wire themselves differently. Given enough time, they could rewire and become rigid circuits that respond normally to the smell of paint fumes.

All it takes is a distraction, you ask? Not exactly. Long-term plastic change requires fixed attention and genuine belief or interest, so dopamine and acetylcholine will be involved in the process, right? I can't just say, *I'm safe here* and expect change. I have to *believe* I'm safe, or else the brain will use the same over-reactive, fear-driven neural circuits. If I tell myself I'm safe—or whatever I tell myself—I have to believe it in order for it to work. If I imagine my soldiers going to bed, I have to really believe I don't need them. If I decide to use my hot chocolate, then perhaps I become engrossed in wondering how the hot chocolate was made, or what its ingredients are. I don't have to do math problems, although math could work. So could solving a puzzle, working on brain games like *Posit Science* or online geography quizzes, learning a language or how to play a musical instrument, meditation, CBT, teaching myself to use my recessive hand to do things… With fixed attention and genuine interest or belief these can all incite positive plastic change.

In addition to working some of the above strategies into your daily life, you may wish to try treatments that have had some success in causing positive plastic change. I'll introduce options momentarily, but there's no point in trying them without first ensuring you have optimal brain health on a cellular level. Untreated cellular problems will only impede the brain's attempts to heal.

Promoting Brain Health on a Cellular Level

With some brain issues, "miswiring" occurs because a mineral deficiency, infection, chemical exposure, or a triggering food disrupts the neurons and glia [cells that protect the brain from invading organisms], but we can support neural function by treating infections promptly, decreasing chemical exposure and detoxing if necessary, and addressing any mineral or nutritional issues.[37] As I've already discussed detox, this segment will focus on the latter only.

When digging deeper into diet and nutrition, I wanted to work with a medical professional certified in Functional Medicine, but those in my area charged a fee that in my case was cost-prohibitive, so I did the next best thing: I signed up for the Institute of Functional Medicine's free introductory online courses and learned the basics of Functional Medicine. I discovered many things there, chief among them that food could be used as medicine. This led to more research, which led me to two game-changing revelations regarding mitochondria and the brain's favorite food.

The mitochondria are the "powerhouses" of the body's cells. Basically, they generate energy for the body to do all it does. According to Dr. Dominic D'Agostino from the University of South Florida College of Medicine, "The healthier your mitochondria are, the greater capacity you have to deal with stress, the more efficient you can convert food into energy."[38] But over time, and with chronic stress and/or trauma, the mitochondria can degrade, and their ability to generate energy decreases. Mitochondrial dysfunction has been found in CFS and Fibromyalgia.[39,40] I'll delve deeper into these findings soon. First, feeding the mitochondria.

You may recall that I've sung the praises of sitting in sunshine for its invigorating properties. That's not just a "me thing." Sunlight actually affects our brains.[41] Our mitochondria use sunlight to incite the generation of a molecule called ATP (adenosine triphosphate), which is like a battery that stores energy in each cell, energy essential for the cell to do its job.[42] Everyone needs to support their mitochondrial function and ATP production, especially those with CS and CSS who have fatigue, low exertion tolerance, and brain fog—and sunshine is *free*.

There are supplements said to boost mitochondrial function, to help them repair themselves and increase energy production. One such is N-Acetyl-L-Carnitine, an amino acid that the body produces naturally. When I started taking this supplement (under my Naturopath's supervision) my brain fog all but went away within two months. I also experienced a lovely side effect that decreased my minor depression symptoms. Is N-Acetyl-L-Carnitine guaranteed to eliminate your brain fog or depression? Nope. There are no guarantees with CS, remember. My Naturopath said some patients see improvement with that supplement and others don't.

Next, I tried Coenzyme Q_{10}, also known as CoQ10 or Ubiquinone. This substance is naturally produced by the body, can be found in every one of our cells, and is reputed to increase brain function. CoQ10 has also been shown to reduce CFS symptoms.[43] To understand why, you need to know more about *oxidative stress*.

Nutshell, oxidative stress is an imbalance between the body's antioxidant defenses and its production of free radicals (chemically reactive by-products of normal cellular functions). Normally the body produces antioxidants that help eliminate free radicals before they can do harm, but an over-abundance of free radicals and/or a deficiency in the body's production of antioxidants can lead to cellular damage by free radicals. Several studies connect oxidative stress to CFS, including work by Dr. Martin Pall, who has proposed that oxidative stress plays an important role in the pathophysiology of CFS.[44] According to Dr. Pall, when the channels that control ion (electron or signal) flow through neuron membranes are stimulated by allergies, toxins, microbes, bacteria, or viruses, these channels (aka NMDA receptors) produce nitric oxide (a free radical).[45] Nitric oxide can combine with the free radical superoxide (a mitochondrial by-product of energy/ATP production) to make peroxynitrate, an oxidant.[46] Peroxynitrate can lead to genetic damage and to elevated levels of both nitric oxide and superoxide, thus creating its own "self-sustaining cycle."[47]

CoQ10 binds to superoxide and, in so doing, prevents nitric oxide from combining with superoxide to make peroxynitrate; this ultimately results in decreased oxidative stress.[48] Klonopin and Neurontin, two prescription medications that down regulate NMDA (and thus decrease nitric oxide), have also been shown to reduce CFS symptoms.[49] Women generate more nitric oxide than men,[50] and more women have CFS. The above discoveries support Dr. Pall's theory and suggest that oxidative stress is an important piece of the CFS puzzle.[51] Researchers have taken their suppositions one step further, theorizing that kindling could be the catalyst of the neurotoxicity and help create the perfect environment in which oxidative stress can flourish.[52] While much of this is still to be proven, I want you to be aware of possible correlations between oxidative stress and CS and CSS, should you wish to investigate potential treatments such as CoQ10, Klonopin, and Neurontin. Although I have not tried the latter two, I am still taking CoQ10 today.

While researching this chapter, I learned that depletion of *glutathione* (an important antioxidant) has been found in CFS patients.[53] Although I haven't yet investigated further for my own health, I want to include it here for you. Glutathione, a neurotransmitter "composed of the amino acids glutamate, cysteine, and glycine," plays an important role in the body's antioxidant defense, learning, memory, and numerous other physiological processes.[54] Studies have shown that glutathione protects cells from oxidative stress, and that depletion of glutathione can "promote"[55] or "enhance"[56] oxidative stress. Does this mean folks with CS and CSS should seek to increase glutathione levels? It may not be as simple as that. A 2015 review by Dr. Yunus noted that glutamate, a component of glutathione, "is increased in the brain in several CSS."[57] (Higher levels of glutamate, yet lower levels of glutathione, which is one-third glutamate? Yep, it's complicated.) Another report found that "deterioration of biosynthesis of glutamate in the anterior cingulum [a part of the brain dealing with autonomic function, emotions, and more] might cause autonomic imbalance and prolonged fatigue,"[58] two conditions common in CS. Much is still unknown, so until scientists can clarify connections between elevated glutamate, decreased glutathione, and CS, I recommend you keep this on your radar for future research.

My naturopath and I also added a Vitamin B50 complex, Vitamin D3, Zinc, and Iron to my regimen, along with supplements I mentioned in the detoxification segment. We added one at a time and tested for efficacy before adding the next. If it remedied deficiencies found through testing (such as zinc and iron), or helped decrease symptoms or improve functionality, we kept it in the regimen. If no effect, we dropped it. Thus I began learning how to promote brain health at a cellular level, with supplements in pill form, anyway, but supplements are expensive and can be unreliable, and I would far rather use *food* as medicine.

My research led me to Dr. Terry Wahls, an M.D. who has progressive Multiple Sclerosis (M.S.). Previously athletic and active, Dr. Wahls became wheelchair-bound by her disease over a period of several years and, determined to reverse the effects of M.S., she began experimenting with food as medicine. Using functional medicine and paleo principles, she developed a successful protocol and a year later, was back to working full time and riding her bike! Sound too good to be true? Read her book[59] and see what you think.

Here's the thing that caught my eye: Dr. Wahls has M.S., a disease that affects the brain, and she based her protocol on two key facts about the brain and healing:

1. The brain, like any other part of the body, needs nutrients to heal, and
2. because at least 60% of the brain is made up of fat, the brain runs best when consuming fats as fuel instead of carbohydrates. (This process is called *ketosis* and involves the liver transforming fatty acids into molecules called *ketones*, which the body converts into energy.)

A growing body of research supports the idea that ketosis can promote brain health at a cellular level. According to Dr. D'Agostino, "[Fats] function as a very high, dense source of alternative energy for the brain…. Ketones increase brain blood flow; they also increase blood flow to the periphery."[60] The body must oxidize ketones to produce ATP. This process occurs in the mitochondria. A ketogenic diet forces mitochondria to increase their efficiency and "probably stimulat[es] mitochondrial biogenesis [reproduction]," says D'Agostino.[61] So, to optimize brain performance and healing, Dr. Wahls developed a three-tiered, nutrient-dense diet protocol (the top level of which is *ketogenic*). Are you making the same connection I did? My thought process was this: I have CS, a condition that affects my brain and mitochondrial function. I know that my brain needs desensitizing, but what else does it need? What else do my mitochondria need? And what level of healing could my brain achieve if I fed it its favourite food: fats? I couldn't wait to find out.

I needed to know more about the mechanics of ketosis so, more research. Kristen Mancinelli's book, *The Ketogenic Diet: The Scientifically Proven Approach to Fast, Healthy Weight Loss,*[62] delivered the comprehensive information I needed. (Note, despite the title, this book is not just for weight loss. It was the clearest and easiest-to-understand out of countless other books on ketogenic diets that I read. If you want to work with ketosis, first read Mancinelli or another reputable book on ketosis mechanics.) Once my Naturopath agreed to supervise, the trial began.

Three months in, I was recovering faster from symptoms, including relapses and crashes, and I had enough energy to cook most meals. My functional capacity remained at three hours per day, but quicker recovery and better meals significantly improved my quality of life. My naturopath and I decided to try the diet for another three months and re-evaluate then.

This is where the aforementioned food controversy comes in. My dietician was very much against a ketogenic diet for me, to the point that she would not agree to supervise it. I had to go to my naturopath. This was not a big deal, but it serves to illustrate that the effectiveness and safety of ketogenic diets in treating CSS and CS needs official research. It also should drive home the idea that experimenting with your diet can have serious repercussions and must not be done without a medical professional's supervision. I am emphatically NOT suggesting that you try any diet you can find, willy nilly. I am stating that I have had some success with a nutrient-dense, ketogenic diet that I adopted from Dr. Wahls' book and had supervised by a medical professional. Always thoroughly research diets, take your findings to a professional, discuss them, and then follow a plan your medical professional agrees to supervise.

Oxygen as Food (aka "Take Ten")

This is my final point related to promoting brain health at a cellular level. Think for a moment about how crucial oxygen is to our bodies. Our brain and all our cells rely on oxygen to function properly. During a stroke in which the brain is deprived of oxygen for a few seconds, what can happen? Paralysis, loss of speech function, loss of other cognitive functions …

So what happens to our brains when we have trouble breathing due to an Asthma, ILS, or MCS episode? What happens when chronic pain or anxiety causes our breath to get shallow and stay that way for minutes, or hours, weeks, or more? Do we end up with an oxygen deficit for that hour or that day or for however long it takes us to breathe normally again? Do brain cells suffer from such oxygen deprivation and never recover? I don't know, and I don't see a need to research this in depth.

I know enough about the importance of oxygen for brain and body function to believe that proper oxygenation is an important key to healing CS. Thus, I view and use oxygen as a medicinal food. Whenever I catch myself breathing shallowly due to symptoms, anxiety, or negative rumination, or whenever I wake up feeling worried or dreadful, or like I haven't slept deeply, I tell myself to "take ten," and then and there I take at least ten deep, slow breaths. While I take ten, I imagine oxygen flowing throughout my body and brain and clearing out any illness, negative thoughts or emotions, or negative perceptions of stress. I imagine the oxygen feeding and rejuvenating every cell. I picture my brain absorbing the oxygen and glowing a bright white or golden light of health and balance. *Yep, mine is a happy, well-fed brain!*

On any given day, after implementing the "take ten" method, I find that I breathe deeper than usual throughout that day, and over time I've noticed a deepening in my breathing in general. This means my oxygenation strategy is serving a dual purpose: not only am I getting more oxygen than before because of periodically taking ten, but the deeper breathing is also helping to engage my parasympathetic system and override my fight or flight mode. All that, from a little breath. That's some powerful food!

Neuroplastic Treatment Options for CS and CSS

By now, you're using simple strategies to create positive neuroplastic change on a daily basis and doing all you can to support your cellular health and optimize brain function, right? Good work. This segment is for those who wish to augment their established brain health regime with a treatment. Caution: There are a lot of purported neuro-health-related treatments available and much experimentation happening these days. Always conduct research based upon your condition, circumstances, and healing goals—and discuss with your doctor *before* trying any treatments.

One way to help the brain rewire, decrease symptoms, and/or support healing is by a process called *neurostimulation*. Because thought activates certain neural circuits, it can revive or activate (aka *neurostimulate*) brain cells, and so can vibration, physical movement (walking, for example), sound (as I mentioned in Chapter 2 regarding music), light, or electricity.[63] I could write an entire book about each of these, but that's not this book. Just know that they are possible avenues for you to investigate if you wish.

Low level laser therapy (LLLT), also known as light therapy, NIR, or cold laser therapy (nope, this doesn't involve light sabers, sorry) is a neurostimulation treatment that I feel has great potential to help those with CS and CSS because of its many health benefits. It releases serotonin and acetylcholine and triggers ATP production, which is essential for cell function, growth and repair, and different laser wavelengths can support healing by improving circulation and oxygen usage, and activating new blood vessel growth.[64] There's more. Got inflammation?

Laser light applied to chronically inflamed areas can decrease swelling, inflammation and pain.[65] Laser light also fights inflammation by causing the immune system to secrete more cytokines, proteins that fight inflammation by increasing the amount of "macrophage" (cells that evict harmful and unrepairable cells), and decreasing the amount of "neutrophil" (cells that can add to chronic inflammation).[66] There's more. Got oxidative stress?

Recent studies suggest that LLLT can reduce oxidative stress.[67,68] Another study reported that LLLT had increased ATP and caused "normalization of the overloaded sympathetic nerve system."[69] If you'd like to research this type of therapy, check Appendix F: Recommended Reading and Viewing for some good places to start.

In addition to helping on a cellular level, neurostimulation can trigger the brain's self-regulating process called *neuromodulation*, which helps the brain restore homeostasis (the body's natural balance of healthy functioning).[70] Basically, neuromodulation re-establishes a normal sleep cycle and restores balance to the autonomic nervous system by engaging the parasympathetic nervous system. The brain can do this successfully with a variety of brain problems,[71] but not with CS. Nevertheless, we can do things to support the brain's efforts towards neuromodulation, such as practicing good sleep hygiene and treating severe sleep issues appropriately, and practicing the strategies I introduced earlier in the book that help engage the parasympathetic nervous system, such as meditation, Qi Gong, and yoga.

Recent research suggests that neurofeedback (aka neurobiofeedback) can support neuromodulation and improve cognitive functions.[72] In this method of brain retraining, a computer shows the patient what the brain is doing in real time. Neurofeedback is commonly used to treat several conditions, such as sleep issues, chronic pain and fatigue, some learning, brain, and mood disorders, fear, epilepsy, and more.

Whichever techniques or treatments you decide to try (or not), remember that there are variables—including genetics, neuroplasticity, your condition and circumstances— that may impede or contribute to your success. As I've said time and again with CS and CSS, symptoms, triggers, treatment success—all vary with the individual. The important thing is to focus on your healing goals, take daily steps, and see how far your brain's cellular health and inherent healing powers can take you.

Neuroplasticity and Chronic Pain

Chronic pain is another great example of neuroplasticity gone wrong. Many times, chronic pain develops after an acute injury. When injury occurs, the nerves do their job, sending pain signals to the brain, but the central nervous system may not interpret or respond correctly.[73] Constant "false alarm" signals are sent, signals amplify.[74] Even long after the acute injury has healed, the patient continues to experience real pain.[75] The patient with chronic pain feels far more pain than s/he should because as the pain signals amplify, more and more neurons are involved.[76] A specific area of the brain processing acute pain should use only about five percent of its neurons, but the incessant firing and wiring that occurs in chronic pain takes up more neurons—about 15 to 25 percent—in that brain area.[77] Basically, chronic pain recruits an extra 10 to 20 percent of the patient's neurons, sometimes from adjacent areas of the brain that process pain for other parts of the body.[78] The patient may then develop "referred pain," which means the patient feels pain in a part of the body other than where the injury occurred.[79] As more and more neurons responsible for processing pain are recruited, and as those neurons fire with increasing frequency, they begin to fire so readily—even when triggered by a tiny stimulus—that the patient eventually experiences severe, constant pain over a great portion of the body.[80]

The above can occur because our brains are plastic. So, does that mean neuroplasticity can make it "un-occur?" As with much of CS science, research involving the use of neuroplasticity to treat chronic CS- and CSS-related pain is in rather infantile stages. The best-known options now include neurofeedback, visualization, and neurostimulation (such as magnetic, electric, or low level laser therapy). More are being researched as I type, some of which I'll introduce when I discuss the future of CS and CSS. For now, let's look at a neuroplastic success story.

Dr. Michael Moskowitz, a psychology and pain specialist and former chronic pain patient, discovered that the parts of the brain that fire during chronic pain process things other than pain in their "downtime"; that is, they process emotions, memories, ideas, sensations (other than pain), physical movement, etc., when their circuits aren't busy processing the chronic pain.[81] His findings explain why we may experience diminished cognitive or motor function, tolerance of light or sound, or emotional control when we are in pain—because the areas of the brain that normally regulate such things have been commandeered by the chronic pain signal.[82] Moskowitz supposed that, in order to rewire those commandeered neurons and get them to serve their original purpose (which was something other than pain processing), one would have to first weaken the circuits made strong by chronic pain.[83] (Remember, circuits can be weakened by disuse.) Moskowitz theorized that by doing other activities—moving, remembering, thinking intellectual thoughts, etc.—when in pain, he could weaken those recruited chronic pain circuits and eventually rewire them.[84] Moskowitz used visualization in his process: every time he felt a twinge of pain, he pictured the areas of the brain that were involved in processing that pain, and he imagined them *shrinking*.[85] After six weeks of practicing this neuroplastic therapy, he saw marked improvement in his level of pain, and within 12 months, he became almost entirely pain-free—after 13 years of chronic pain.[86] That's the power of neuroplasticity, and visualization.

VISUALIZATION

Throughout the book, I've encouraged you to use visualization as a tool for dealing with various CS- and CSS-related issues. Now that you have an understanding of neuroplasticity and how it relates to CS and CSS, we can dig deeper. Officially, visualization, or mental imagery, "is the process of envisioning specific physical or cognitive activities or perceptual experiences with the intention of altering the facilitation of neuronal networks."[87] It can improve cognitive performance, memory, and motor skills, and is also commonly used to treat certain psychological disorders.[88] Visualization is a powerful healing tool because a significant portion of the brain is dedicated to visual processing.[89] Visualization can take many forms, such as structured therapeutic work guided by a medical professional, or simply imagining yourself sunning—relaxed and healthy—on a tropical beach, or picturing your soldiers standing down, your successful drug store excursion before it happens, or the shrinkage of brain areas commandeered by chronic pain. Musicians and actors use it in preparation for a performance; athletes, for a competition.[90]

Neuroscientists have proven that when we visualize with intention and attention, we can actually cause neuroplastic change.[91] Turns out, imagining doing something and actually doing that thing aren't all that different from our brain's point of view.[92] The act of visualizing requires both memory and imagination.[93] When you visualize an activity, you use the same neurons as when you *do* that activity.[94] If you visualize or remember something bad that happened to you, the neurons that processed the negative emotions you initially had in response to that bad experience can fire again and strengthen their circuits; conversely, if you imagine or recall a happy experience, the circuits that fired when that experience first occurred can activate and strengthen.[95] This is why it can be helpful to imagine yourself relaxing on a tropical island when you feel anxious, why mentally practicing your drug store or grocery run before you go can improve your in-store performance, and why the soldiers visualization can work wonders.[96]

Visualization enables us to wield neuroplasticity for our own benefit. So does positive and believable self-talk, CBT, the scent repertoire and, well, most of the strategies I've recommended in this book. I encourage you to review them now, to deepen your comprehension, your practice, and ultimately, your ability to heal.

Review of Neuroplasticity and Chronic Pain

- Neuroplasticity refers to the way in which the nerve cells (neurons) in our brains and nervous systems are malleable or changeable throughout our lifetimes.
- Neurons make connections amongst themselves by using electrical impulses. This is commonly referred to as neurons "firing." When neurons connect, this is commonly referred to as the brain "wiring" itself and creating "circuits."
- As we refine our abilities or understanding, the brain "rewires" and reinforces those connections to make them as efficient as possible. Over time, enduring or

persistent thoughts, beliefs, behaviors, and/or sensory signals can form "rigid" circuits in the brain.

- Neuroplasticity can work *against* us, as in the sensitization of the central nervous system or the development of chronic pain.
- Neuroplasticity can work *for* us—if we apply focused attention and intention—to reduce CS and CSS symptoms, to support a healthy cognitive-behavior process, and to live happier, healthier lives.

> *They can be like a sun, words.*
> *They can do for the heart*
> *what light can*
> *for a field.*
> —St. John of the Cross[97]

Self-Care

Some people have amazing self-care skills. They learned when young that putting oneself first was their number one job. I don't mean in an unkind or sociopathic way, nor do I mean they possess the skills necessary to survive on the streets should they become homeless. I mean that some people learned a way of prioritizing themselves that provided them with a healthy foundation for self-worth and well-being. Self-care is about intentional, self-initiated care of oneself. Good personal hygiene, eating right, sleeping enough, keeping one's living space, possessions, and clothing clean and well-maintained, removing oneself from unhealthy relationships—these are all aspects of self-care.

Different people do self-care in different ways. Some make the bed first thing after getting up in the morning, so it's exactly as they like it when they retire that night. Some roll out of bed and meditate for an hour before doing anything else. Some go for a walk, some hop in the shower, some make the perfect cup of coffee—you get the idea. What small self-care step do you do for yourself that makes you feel good, that makes you feel like everything's ok, that you're putting your best step forward, or that makes you feel well taken care of? (As you might guess, I couldn't answer these questions easily and had to brainstorm a list over time. If you have the same problem, you know what to do.)

With CS and CSS, self-care takes on an added dynamic that encompasses daily decisions about managing the illness. You can't go to the doctor for help or advice every time you have an ILS or MCS episode, IBS or Fibromyalgia flare-up, or fatigue-related crash, can you? Nope, you have to learn how to manage your condition(s) on your own, and how minimize the illness' impact on your life. Bubble time, pacing and planning, meditation, mindfulness, medications, special diet, sleep hygiene, therapy, CBT, and any other treatments or strategies you use—anything you do to manage and improve your health and well-being—now belong in your self-care portfolio. (Anything safe and legal, that is. If you rob a bank because your chronic illness prevents you from working and you need money, that doesn't exactly fall under self-care.)

When my conditions forced me to be more attentive, I realized that I'd never mastered basic self-care when I was young. I wasn't a swine rolling in mud and refuse, but I lacked skills in certain aspects of basic self-care, such as setting healthy boundaries or having balanced relationships, for example. Poor self-care, turns out, is closely linked to low self-worth. Lucky for me, and for all of us with CSS or CS alone, self-care can be learned at any age, and one can keep on improving it over time, like any other skill. It just takes practice.

BACK TO BASICS

Putting self-care first meant focusing on the basics. Once I had adequate food, clothing, safety, and shelter, I focused on taking time to prepare good food; ensuring my clothing fit, was clean, and pleased me; finding ways to feel safe despite crumbling finances and mysterious health issues; and keeping my shelter clean and homey. I'll explain.

Remember when I said that I felt this compulsion to *do something* in my early days with CSS, to fix everything? It stayed with me for a couple years or so. My doctors told me to meditate, to be mindful, and I tried, but I was fighting to keep my home, to find a safe place to live, to get compensation—*everything* was a battle, and a lot of basic skills got shoved onto the back burner, or into a crevice, forgotten, while I contended with the pressing things. It wasn't until much later, when I got back to basics, that I could see the true import of self-care and move it higher on my priorities list. How did I see it, finally?

I had this epiphany one day, while cooking myself some lunch. (I know, the word "epiphany" is so disused these days it sounds hokey, right? But it's a perfectly good word.) As I've said, for the first few CSS years, I survived mostly on smoothies, juices, and protein bars. I ate enough. I ate pretty well for someone who didn't cook much at all—far better than folks who eat frozen fried chicken dinners or fast food. At first, I believed there was no time to cook. I had too much life stuff to contend with and not enough hours in the day. And then, once my fatigue and cognitive issues became severe, I simply couldn't cook. Once I started practicing self-care, though, I made a concerted effort to prepare and cook at least one quality meal per day. (Incidentally, this began as an onerous chore but eventually became enjoyable.)

So, one day I was cooking lunch—and I'm not a great cook so it was probably something like bratwurst, Brussels sprouts, garlic and mushrooms fried in ghee. *Mmmm, yummy!* I turned the stove dial to level four and set my cast iron pan onto the burner. After scooping some ghee from the jar, I thudded it into the pan. The blob of ghee was bright yellow against the midnight black background, like a miniature sun, I thought.

My stove sits on an angle, so the ghee slid across the pan, making a greasy rivulet, and pooled at the edge nearest me. I was watching the ghee burble, preparing to add the meat and veg, when I realized, all I was thinking about was making lunch. All I was thinking about was ghee, and how it looked like a bright sun, and how black the pan was. I wasn't thinking about the upcoming deadline for the umpteenth workers compensation review, or researching various therapies for my conditions, or loan applications or real estate woes, like always. I wasn't feeling irritated that I had to spend time cooking instead of doing things that "really mattered." All I was feeling was safe, and happy, and *satisfied*.

After years of survival mode and intense dissatisfaction and chaos caused by my illness, safety, joy and satisfaction had returned to me. While I was cooking. For myself. (Do you hear the heavenly chorus of *Ahhhhh!* when I say that? I do.)

Such was the epiphany. When I took the time to cook for myself, to clean up afterwards, to put things in order around the apartment, to meditate, to work on CBT, to brush my hair instead of ignoring it—or on bad days when all I could do was put on a clean pair of undies or socks—this all mattered in an invisible yet magnificent way.

Practice everyday. Baby steps, like practicing scales on the piano. Think of how you learned things when you were young. Short walks. Then rest. Controlled movements. Controlled environment. Controlled expectations. Food, cleaning, self care. It's ok not to focus on what lies beyond these basic things for a while. You don't have to try to control how it's all going to turn out. You can let go, and focus on the basics.

When we take the time to do the basics of self-care, we invest in ourselves, our self-worth increases, our sense of well-being improves, and we are actually then better prepared to deal with the big issues. We develop more resilience to the crises. And eventually, even the crises don't seem so huge and insurmountable. It sounds unlikely, doesn't it? How can self-care connect to overcoming our hugest fears and problems? It does. I'm living proof. Believe it.

SELF-COMPASSION

Self-Compassion is part of self-care, and—you can probably guess—it's something I didn't learn very well until I got sick. Even now, I'm no self-compassion ninja, so this will be brief.

During my early CSS years, I got pretty depressed and often woke up to the same self-debate, something along the lines of this:

> "Well, looks like I'm still breathing. I better carry on."
> "Yep, *barely* breathing. And no one knows what's wrong with you. What's the use?"
> "Hang in there, things will get better."
> "Yeah, right. Life is nothing but suffering. I just want it to stop."

You get the idea …

I noticed that when someone called or wrote me and said, "hang in there," I felt far better than when I said the same words to myself. Why was it I could not comfort myself? Why did I seem to want and need someone else to do that instead? Why was it that I blew off any compassion I tried to give myself? Shouldn't I value what I say over what anyone else says? Shouldn't I be my own best mate, through thick and thin, no matter what? Yep, so then why did I discredit my own attempts to comfort myself?

The major reason was resentment: I still blamed myself for what had happened to me. I held myself responsible for things I could not have controlled: I took that job with GAS, I went to work that day, I trusted them to be ethical and competent, *I let this happen to me!* The problem with self-criticism is that "it activates areas of the brain that are associated with punishment, threat, and inhibition, as if you're trying to prevent yourself from making another mistake. And so literally, the brain starts to shut you down."[98] Self-compassion, however, activates other parts of the brain that allow you to feel safe and connect—with yourself and with others—and enable you to be self-aware.[99] As I've discussed, self-awareness plays a big role in helping us change our thoughts and behaviors. Thus, by learning self-compassion, I would be able to stop self-criticizing and, finally, forgive myself.

Unfortunately, self-compassion was not a tool I carried in my skills toolkit. But I wanted it. I wanted it bad. I wanted to be there for myself, no matter what. I wanted to value my own opinion and stop discrediting myself, and I wanted to be able to make myself feel better no matter what life threw at me. This prompted a deep exploration into self-compassion. I started by reading Dr. Neff's book on the subject.[100] This gave me a good idea what I was going for. Then I made a list of all the things friends said that I found comforting, I said them to myself every day, and I told myself to believe them.

"It's going to be alright."
"You're so strong to deal with this."
"Things will get better."
"You are so brave to face this."
"Your life is going to turn around."
"You are smart and creative and resourceful. You will find a way to survive."

At first it felt hokey to be offering myself compliments and affirmation—I mean, really, *Who talked like that to themselves?*—but I wanted to learn self-compassion, so I persevered.

I found it helpful to consider the ease with which I could express compassion for others. *How did I know what to say to friends? Why was it ok to comfort them but hokey to comfort myself? Boy, was I messed up!* (No, scratch that. I wanted to stop negative self-criticism.) *I'm not messed up. I simply am not skilled at self-compassion yet.* I decided to imagine that I was talking to a friend when I talked to myself, a friend I really cared about, who was hurting and needed comfort. Then I outlined my plan for mastering self-compassion:

- Be there for myself, acknowledge painful things, and offer compassion daily.
- Forgive myself for mistakes I make and don't blame myself for things that are out of my control.
- No more talking disparagingly to or about myself.
- Treat myself as my best friend, always.

Remember, it's important that you use affirmations you *believe*. You can't lie to your brain. Maybe you need to take baby steps towards using affirmations—that's ok. Even affirming your *willingness* to show compassion to yourself or be supportive of yourself can help you toward your goal of improving your self-compassion skills. A willingness would sound something like this: "I want to have the thought that … or I want to have the belief or emotion that … so I'm going to try it on now as a way of planting the seed."[101] Affirming your honest desire in such a way will lead you to honest and real demonstrations of self-compassion. It just takes practice and time.

I hope this may help you find an appropriate starting point for your own explorations into self-compassion. As I said, I'm no ninja at it now, but I've developed some skill, and now there's always someone there for me.

FAITH

"Since developing all these breathing issues, anxiety has become my constant companion," I said. "I fear everyone I come into contact with, I fear every environment I enter, every vehicle that goes by, weather shifts, season changes, getting too tired, laughing too much … this level of hyper-vigilance is exhausting. And on top of all that, I am constantly visualizing and self-talking my soldiers to 'settle down, throat closing not needed today, thanks,' so the energy drain is double."

Dr. H nods. She can convey a lot with a nod, sometimes an acknowledgment that she's heard me, sometimes a sign that she's understood what I said, sometimes encouragement to continue.

"I used to fear not achieving all I wanted to in my career before I died. I used to fear never being a successful artist, I feared an abusive boss, an asshole ex-boyfriend. I feared road-ragers when I was a bike commuter. Bad pizza. Bad dates. *Hm-hm!*" I try to clear my throat against the wad of mucus residing there. "I think now I fear finding no solutions. *Hm-hm!* … Every time things get a bit easier, like I have a good day with only one major breathing episode, or a day with loose throat muscles and less coughing, I start to believe I'm getting better. *Hm-hm!*" I take a slow breath. "Or every time I figure out a way to do something, go someplace that before was smell-prohibitive and now is somewhat survivable, I then believe that strategy will *always* work for me. I cling to that belief like it's a certainty. Like there's a checklist in my mind and I can check that one off forever. As if I could develop and collect enough strategies that my life would become normal again." I feel like I might start to cry. I know lots of people do it—heck Dr. H has tissue boxes strategically located around her little office—but I hate crying in front of Dr. H. "Then, the next day, things don't go well, and I get even more anxious. I feel like I'm not getting better when that happens." Phlegm floods my throat. I try to clear it every few seconds to keep talking. "*Hm-hm!* I feel like I will never again have that denial that most people have as their daily default—*hm-hm!*—the denial that allows them to walk into a room, any room, any where, and feel safe."

Dr. H nodded. She has this way of listening without showing any emotion on her face. I guess that's her job, but I've always been a person who cannot hide the slightest emotion—everything lights up my face like a neon sign whether I want it to or not—so I marvel at her skill.

"Is this a sign of immaturity or mother abandonment or something Freudian, that I want so desperately to cling to a *certainty*?" My throat gets tight like it always does in this office. It's partially the dying lily smell and partially the fact that I can't talk about emotional stuff anymore without my throat closing up. I can't even *feel* emotional. No laughing, and no crying. What's an artist to do? "Why can't I just accept that there is no certainty in the world, and function like that? *Hm-hm!*" The mucus remains, like a gelatinous glottal shield. I imagine my soldiers standing down, Schultz yelling at them in German.

Dr. H says, "That denial allows people to feel calm and secure, to find some peace. It's normal to want that, and to feel you need it. Everyone needs some degree of that kind of denial in order to function in our culture, don't you think?"

"*Hm-hm!*" I nod. "Will I ever get it back?" I smile and wipe my eyes. "That invisible opiate for the masses?"

"Perhaps, to some degree," she says. "But once a bubble bursts…"

"It's gone?" I imagine my existence up until now as a miniature me floating in a bulbous bubble like the ones I used to blow on the lawn at my childhood home. How vast and sunny the sky appeared—full of promise and wonder—as I rose into it, cushy and safe in my soapy rainbow-tinted bubble. Then, for no perceivable reason, my bubble met the demise that all soap bubbles do—*pop!*—and suddenly miniature me tumbled into the lawn that needed mowing, an endless, treacherous jungle, no safety in sight. "You once told me that *shoulds* are the language of the depressed, but *shouldn't* I have expected this?" I say. "*Shouldn't* I have known what would happen? Don't most people know how messed up life can be? I mean, everyone says *shit happens* but I guess, when it gets dumped on you by the tractorload…"

I'm not sure where I'm going with that. Probably venting. Wishing I were different.

Being disgruntled. "I still feel angry at myself, I guess, that I let this happen to me, that I trusted GAS not to poison me, that I trusted they were an *ethical* corporation."

"It isn't fair of you to expect yourself to have known what would happen. You didn't know then what you know now, two years later," she says, kindly, even though this is an old discussion for us.

"I know. I accept that. But I don't know how to reconcile the fact that the people at GAS did this to me, yet they remain unaccountable. Their lives have gone on, unchanged, whereas my life has been altered, it's at a standstill, and I've lost a huge part of me. *Hm-hm!* I have to deal with all the repercussions of what GAS did, yet I can't blame them."

"You don't think so?"

"Well, yes, they are to blame for the exposure, but I can't blame anyone for my problems. So I have to blame myself."

"What difference does blame make? Why is blame important?" She's got that gleam in her eyes again, as if I'm becoming a more intriguing case study.

"Good question." I take a moment. Clear my throat. Wipe my runny nose. "I think it's important because if GAS had been penalized, fined and forced to undergo safety inspections, then maybe all these people who act like I'm not sick, who turned away from me, maybe all those people would see that I'm not making it up. They'd see that GAS really did make me sick, that workers compensation really is a demoralizing shit show that's wearing me down, bit by bit, dollar by dollar, and they'd … I don't know, treat me better. Or at least believe in me again."

"You feel like they don't believe in you anymore." As soon as she says it, I realize she's right.

"Yeah, they just believe GAS's story. The easy lie. The comfortable one. The one that allows them to go on with their lives, guilt-free." I blow my nose. Clear my throat. I suspect that what we're really talking about is how I'm losing faith in myself, amidst this long, horrible haul. What was it like in my soap bubble, looking at the open sky with awe? It was easy to have faith then, I bet. What we're really talking about is that I'm yearning for easy now. I'm always yearning for easy. What we're really talking about is that I am feeling empty and looking outside of myself for a sign of faith.

> Some people have to see something to believe it.
> Some believe only what they hear.
> Some believe without such proof. They just know. And they move through life with a certainty—somewhere on the spectrum between righteous and humble—an unshakeable certainty that grounds them in times of trouble, grief, confusion, and enables them to carry on.
>
> I am not one of those people. I do not trust what I see, for sight is limited. I do not trust what I hear, for the tales others tell cannot be trusted.
>
> I place my faith in my nose.
> You will laugh—most do—but *Oh, the things I have smelled!*

Recovery

Prior to getting sick, I associated the term *recovery* primarily with 12-step programs that help people recover from drug addiction. Since then I've learned that recovery is an integral part of healing and self-care. One may recover from crisis phase and reach stability.

One may recover from CS- and CSS-caused financial devastation and live again with financial security. One may recover from a functional capacity of three to a functional capacity of five. One may recover from a crash or relapse. Get the idea? I've experienced a great many setbacks and recoveries since getting CSS and have come to see *recovery* as the process of regaining or rediscovering what I need after a time of great change—not necessarily what I *want,* but definitely what I need, for sustenance and to bring me closer to my goals of living a healthy, happy, and meaningful life.

You *can* recover from CSS or CS alone. Do I mean there is a guaranteed 100 percent cure? Nope, I don't know that to be true, yet. What I mean is, these conditions take a toll outside of the physical and cognitive—a psychological, emotional, financial, social, and spiritual toll. I've already discussed ideas for recovering from the psychological, social, and emotional issues, and I will talk about finances momentarily; right now, I'm going to discuss recovering from spiritual losses. To be clear, by "spiritual" I don't mean religious; I mean spirit, inherent driving force, or *joie de vivre.*

I've spent a lot of time thinking about spirituality since getting sick. I find this interesting because pre–CSS, I had little interest in "religion" and in fact wasn't sure how it differed from the idea of spirituality, and once I got sick, I didn't realize I'd lost something spiritual until I was living without. Things were bad then, during that time when I couldn't sing, could barely talk, had discovered that the compensation process was a long, demoralizing battle, and had no idea why my health was diminishing. My sense of humor went on hiatus and, like I said, things were bad then. I came to believe that all of life was suffering, that we were simply meant to suffer and that I must learn to endure it with grace. I came to believe that all the dreams I'd had of having a happy, satisfied life in a safe place, with good people around, good food, a little hard cider and chocolate, were things only a child believes, childish things, things of child. Things I should be glad were gone. I should be glad that I was at last seeing the world with an adult's eyes, mature, knowing.

Looking back now, I can see that I'd always based my faith on those dreams of a simple life. I'd believed in and valued simple things. But when I got sick, that belief didn't carry me through the hard times, the way people say faith does. That belief didn't serve as a steadfast handhold, an anchor in the storm. My faith seemed to vanish, and for over two years anger sustained me—anger and some intrepid, fierce instinct to survive. I acted out of desperation and fear. Most days I felt like my feet were dangling in mid-air while I scrabbled at the eroding edge of a cliff. I tried again and again to find a quiet, deep pool of grace and douse the flame of anger in it, but I failed. Anger trumps grace, I decided. Anger rules all. I finally gave in and let it drive me where it would.

Then a miracle occurred—and I use the word in its truest sense, as something inexplicable—my voice began to come back. As the chronic congestion waned, my speaking voice started changing from a high, raspy thing to its pre–CSS low register. I felt a frisson of hope then, that I would sing again, that things could get better again, and I suddenly felt wholly certain that suffering did not comprise all of life. There was more to life and living—lots more—and I wanted to experience it.

At that moment, anger relinquished its control and faded to the background of my consciousness (where my emotions hang out when "off-duty." I picture a set of four bunks in a room with an automatic espresso maker, water cooler, microwave, cases of Ramen, Kleenex, beer, and chocolate bars, a punching bag, maybe a Jacuzzi, and a card table.) At that moment, my dreams of a better life returned to the forefront of my vision and served again as my sustenance.

Sometimes I think this means that my faith stayed with me all along. How else would it have abruptly appeared in full force—after being MIA for over two years—at that exact moment I noticed my voice was returning? Maybe my spirit had buckled down when things got real difficult. Some part of me knew that only anger could successfully propel me through that horrible time. Only anger could save me, and it did.

Alternatively, sometimes I think this means that I skated by in life with no faith other than belief that my sheer will could solve any problem, get me through any hard time. And when I got sick and learned that my will could only do so much, I had a crisis of faith, and nearly two years had to pass before I could develop a more enduring faith, that something or someone outside of me would help and support me when I needed it. Something or someone outside of me—that sounds like a God concept, eh? I tend to think of it more personally than that. I think of all the people who helped me during that dark time, and who continue to help me still, when I can't do something myself. And I include the amazing and inexplicable events, like the return of my voice, that I call miracles and serendipities. My faith lies in people and wonderful occurrences, the fount of which is some divine mystery, and I'm ok with letting the mystery be just that.

Sometimes I think I have no idea what faith really is, and that I am just a tough egg who found what she needed, within and without, to survive a messed up situation and emerge from it with humor intact. Maybe my faith is in humor, maybe we can lose nothing that cannot be recovered, or maybe we never really lose anything—we just let go. Maybe I let go of my anger, rather than it letting go of me …

Am I helping?

Perhaps no one can tell anyone about faith—it is what it is, to *you*—as the poem by Rabia says:

> *Since no one really knows anything about God,*
> *those who think they do are just*
> *troublemakers.*[102]

These days, I carry my humor and my faith with me, and they sustain me when life gets turbulent. I hope you will find what sustains you and gives you solace and shelter in any storm, and I wish you speedy recovery.

Well-Being

Well-being describes a sense or attitude about one's health (mental as well as physical), economic, spiritual and social state. Well-being is generally gauged in terms of positive sense or negative sense. The term is usually used to indicate one's quality of life.

Causing loss of income, detriment to relationships and/or social life, feelings of physical endangerment, loss of housing/displacement, debt, loss of savings/security, mental illness, and/or spiritual apocalypse, CS and CSS can really do a number on one's sense of well-being. With so many aspects of their lives affected, it's no wonder people with these conditions tend to react with catastrophic thoughts at first. Who wouldn't? The important thing to remember is, we don't *have to* see this as catastrophe forever. We can reestablish our sense of well-being by nurturing self-worth and self-compassion, working on mental health, focusing on the basics, recovering and discovering what we need, and mastering self-care.

Maintaining Autonomy

In our modern world, autonomy revolves around two things: your ability to manage and physically carry out your daily living activities, and money. If you can't take care of your household affairs or work for a living, you become dependent, upon your family or friends, the government, an insurance payout, savings, handouts on the street, or other sources of money. CS and CSS can make it challenging to impossible to maintain autonomy. Severe CFS, POTS, Fibromyalgia, and other pain syndromes can prohibit one from doing more than a few minutes of any physical activity each day. In this segment, I discuss what to do when your illness interferes with autonomy.

Finances First

If you become unable to work or have to cut hours way down due to CS or CSS, you may be eligible for various kinds of disability. I recommend that you try for it, even if you have savings. You don't know how long you will be sick, or to which degree, so reserve your savings for as long as you possibly can. Depending where you live, you may have options such as these:

- Medical unemployment insurance (temporary)
- Regular unemployment insurance (longer term)
- Welfare or income assistance
- Short-term disability insurance
- Long-term disability insurance
- Personal health insurance policy
- Federal disability pension
- Low-income housing
- Pro bono legal services for low-income earners
- Workers compensation (see next segment)

I know, that's a lot to investigate. And there's a learning curve. Each organization has rules, eligibility criteria, fine print, and application forms and protocols, and the sad truth is that most of us have no experience with, or knowledge about these things before we get sick, and then have to figure it all out while we're dealing with physical and/or cognitive debilitation and all the chaos inherent in life with CSS or CS alone. Yep, it's a slog. The good news is, there are programs and organizations that can help you stay afloat.

So, prepare yourself: the above will take some time and energy. Plan time each week to research and fill out forms. Don't try to do it all at once. Chip away at it. First figure out what you are eligible for and then prioritize the applications. There is an art to, and a specific language for such applications, I've learned. Ask for help from your doctor and look for a local organization that helps people with disability claims. Social workers and community centres are a good bet.

Each year, conduct research to identify any new programs and organizations you may be eligible for. Also, check in annually with the ones you couldn't apply for in the past, to see if they have changed their eligibility criteria. In many cases, neither CS nor CSS is accepted or seen as valid or truly debilitating—except sometimes when severe pain or cognitive impairment is involved—but I believe this will change soon, as more and more people get diagnoses, move from crisis to stability, and become able to lobby for assistance.

I had no debt when I got sick. I had money in the bank and a healthy start to a retirement fund. I even had six months' worth of income set aside in case of sudden job loss. This led me to believe I was all set financially for whatever came along. If I'd known what was wrong with me sooner, and that I'd be sick longer term, I'd have done things differently, but many of us don't know all the facts right away. We make the best decisions we can with the information we have and carry on.

I was very careful with my money from the start. That's just how I am, financially cautious. I created a strict spending plan and adhered to it, with the exception of accommodations like buying a car or moving to avoid triggers. I didn't buy new clothes. I didn't get my hair cut. I was the embodiment of FRUGAL. By the time I got a diagnosis, I was beginning to understand that I would run out of money long before workers compensation would offer a settlement, *if* they would at all. I adjusted my financial goals so they were more "*chronic*-illness–minded." Minimizing spending and making the money I had in savings last as long as possible were my foremost goals, and I also began looking at which disability income options I was eligible for. I researched different ways to go into debt too: which would allow me the easiest recovery from the financial toll of chronic illness when I did finally get some disability income? I made smart decisions about my money. I never avoided the issue. I did all I could. Nevertheless, two years later, I was out of savings, tens of thousands of dollars in debt, had to sell my home to survive, and I was still fighting workers compensation, with no end in sight.

"If you have a lot of currency, it seems as if anything is possible. If you don't have a lot of currency, you may think that nothing is possible, *including getting a lot of currency.*"[103] If you think nothing is possible, that's fear talking—don't believe it. After creating a conservative spending plan, examine your debts. What is the total amount you owe? What are the various interest rates? Find out if any of your creditors offer deferment on payments for people with chronic illness. Be careful with this: some offer deferment, but at an elevated interest rate, so it might be better to move that debt somewhere with a low rate, or pay it off completely with part of your savings or retirement fund (beware of penalties if you decide to do this). A low-interest loan could help you pay off debts and/or give you money to live on. You generally need a job in order to get a loan—I learned this the hard way when I tried getting a personal loan *after* I had to stop working—so, consider this option *before* you quit your day job.

Lines of credit tend to charge lower interest rates than credit cards, so you might wish to get credit lines on your bank account(s), for emergency use (that is, in case you can't access disability income right away, deplete your savings, and don't want to run up your high-interest credit cards. You don't have to *use* the credit lines, and you aren't penalized if you don't use them, but if you anticipate a long wait before you can get disability income, you might prefer to have the credit lines for backup.)

How you deal with your money is all at your discretion. I can tell you what I did, but I'm not in your situation and I probably don't deal with money the way you do. If you know a financial advisor, ask her/him for help. If you don't know anyone personally, some financial advisors give a 15-minute free consultation, so call around. Prepare for the meeting. Go in there with a list of all your debts, their corresponding interest rates, and payment due dates; your savings and its interest rate; and any retirement fund balances, their interest rates and penalties for early withdrawal.

Finally, a word of caution: It can feel overwhelming to look at your finances at the best of times, and more so when you are sick, but if you ignore them, they will grow into an unruly beast that can destroy your quality of life. Chip away at your financial puzzle each week. Make deadlines for decisions and applications and queries. Promise yourself to meet deadlines and follow through. If making doable goals and deadlines isn't your forte, ask a friend to help. Your financial conundrum *can* be managed. There is always a solution—you just need to invest some time and energy to find it.

Workers Compensation and Disability Insurance

Workers compensation and disability insurance companies have a lot more experience, power, legal resources, and know-how than the average newly chronically ill person. That doesn't mean you can't get compensation. It just means that you may have to participate in a difficult and unfair fight for compensation. I knew very little about this realm when I got CSS. I had always assumed my disability insurance would be there if I needed it, and that workers compensation was an organization that protected, and ensured fair compensation of injured workers. I was wrong on both counts. Needless to say, I've been attending the school of hard knocks for the past few years. This segment shares my lessons learned and top tips.

I lost the fight with my short- and long-term disability insurer in less than 6 months, appeals included. Backed by one of the biggest banks in Canada, the (non)insurer had a legal department, misinformation from GAS, and myriad loopholes on their side. They shrugged off all responsibility and put it on workers compensation who, at the time, had automatically accepted everything GAS had said (lies and all) and denied my claim. Nice pickle, eh?

You may wonder why I didn't choose to avoid workers compensation altogether and simply sue GAS. Smart thinking, but in Canada the deal is this: if you are unlucky enough to be injured at work, you cannot seek compensation directly from your employer. You must file a claim with a proprietary provincial workers compensation insurance corporation—I'll call them the WC—that is supposed to compensate injured workers in accordance with the province's Workers Compensation Act. This is a statutory scheme of insurance, which basically means the injured worker cannot expect full indemnity. In my experience, the Act's guidelines, within which the WC maneuvers, do not adequately protect or compensate injured workers. There are no hard deadlines, so the WC can take months or years to make a decision on a claim, and the worker has no real recourse. And any stress, financial loss, or misery the WC's tactics cause the worker is not compensable. The imbalance of power inherent in this system creates an abusive dynamic for a worker who is injured and in need of prompt and fair compensation.

The Act's criteria stating what the WC can and can't compensate is also inadequate. If you get MCS or ILS from a workplace injury and need environmental trigger-free housing or transportation, you won't be compensated for that because the Act doesn't contain relevant provisions in its law and policy. In fact, the Act's criteria focus more on acute care and are very thin on covering the ongoing care needs of workers whose injuries are chronic. The Act doesn't contain law and policy for most of my CS- and CSS-related expenses—physiotherapy equipment and treatments, acupuncture treatments, housing accommodation costs and losses, transportation accommodation costs, most of my medications and supplements, other related accommodations, and more—that's over $80,000 out of my pocket and gone. And that doesn't include the tens of thousands of dollars I've had to spend on lawyers fees, faxes, copies, postage, or the hundreds of thousands of dollars of wages I've lost. Nor does it take into account the hundreds of hours of my time spent on my compensation claim.

The Act's inadequacies and the WC claim process are nothing short of unconstitutional, in my opinion. When I asked a lawyer how to get the Act's law and policy updated to ensure prompt, fair, and adequate compensation for workers whose injuries include CS and CSS, she said, "lobby the government." Fun times, eh?

This is all very discouraging, and unfortunately, it can get worse. My province's WC has a claim process that I find confusing (and I'm a smart cookie) and adversarial and, in my opinion, the WC operates with an extreme bias against the worker. For example, the WC automatically believed *every*thing GAS told them, yet I was made to disprove what GAS said, as well as prove what I said. The WC has twisted my words around and tried to use them against me (to the point that I will not talk with them on the phone and must get everything in writing), has attempted to discredit me and my doctors, has spied on me, has pretended as if I am in perfect health and still asserts, at time of writing, that I should be working full-time as an office manager (despite letters dating back three years from my specialist describing and attesting to my level of debilitation). One doctor hired by the WC even claimed that I wasn't sick and was merely "on a diagnostic pilgrimage." (You know, I keep telling myself that will be funny one day, but it's not funny yet! Maybe tomorrow....) In short, I have found the WC and its claim process to be adversarial, biased against the worker, intimidating, demoralizing, exhausting, and inhumane. If the WC had dealt with my claim in a timely and fair manner, I would have received compensation within the first year of illness, I would not have lost my home or my savings, I wouldn't have had to hire a lawyer for appeals, I would not have had to suffer through years of financial duress, my CSS might not have developed so severely, and the list goes on …

Yep, going the WC route is a bummer, and dealing with other disability insurers can be too, especially when it comes to relatively new, unknown, and/or invisible conditions such as CS and CSS. My top lessons learned:

- **Persistence is key.** In my experience, the WC's goal is to *not* compensate you. They want you to give up and go away without getting what you need.
- Set alarms or calendar alerts or tie a ribbon around your finger—whatever it takes—but **do not miss a deadline on your claim.**
- **Buckle down** for a years-long battle, or dance, or however you see it. In my experience, the WC has done (and is still doing) everything possible to delay my claim.
- Emotional stress will only exacerbate symptoms, so it's best to **detach emotionally** from the claim process as much as possible.
- **Believe in who you are and what you are experiencing**, no matter what insurers throw at you.
- If you think you may have a human rights case, look into it right away. In my province, there is a short time window between the date the human rights infraction occurs and the complaint submittal date. (Remember, **don't miss a deadline**.)
- **Get everything in writing.** If the insurer is twisting your words around, do not answer the phone when they call. Respond to their voicemail in writing and request that they respond in writing, too. If you absolutely must talk to them on

the phone, take detailed notes and include the person's name and title, date, and time of call.

- **Be prepared** to take a financial hit. You won't know until the dust settles, but it's in your best interest to prepare for a loss.
- Use every ounce of **free legal help** you can. In many cases, this will amount to brief in-person meetings or phone calls with a legal advocate. This type of limited representation can be helpful, although I found that I needed full representation sometimes due to severity of my cognitive impairment.
- **Think hard before you hire a lawyer** to represent you. Lots of the admin on your claim can be done by you or a friend and save you thousands of dollars in legal fees, yet if the stress and energy toll of the claim is making you sicker, you may need to hire help.

Insurers will probably get under your skin, along with all the uncertainty surrounding your finances and medical condition. This can strip you down to a bare wire, but you have every right to seek compensation. You also have the power to change this awful process. Call and write letters to your elected officials demanding legislation that *cares* for and fairly compensates injured workers, and people with CS and CSS. If all injured workers and patients contacted their government leaders, we could get that ball a-rolling. Remember, you aren't alone, though it sure may feel like it, and I'm right here, talking to you.

Self-Care and Finances

Living with no job income can be pretty darn uncomfortable. Same with becoming able to provide for oneself financially. When GAS laid me off, I got another job right away and worked another eight months, my CSS worsening all the while, until I finally had to quit. From age 16, I had always worked, and I suppose I'd always imagined myself working until the day I dropped dead. I simply couldn't conceive of living with a chronic illness, or living long-term without working. My world-view has changed since then, of course. I've been unable to work now for three years. Yet I still try to "work," as you can see. Writing is work, and I am writing this book. But I can only do so in five to fifteen-minute intervals, a little bit on a good day, nowhere near enough to make a living.

Pre-CS, I believed that working, paying the bills, and being financially independent made me a good person. I found purpose and meaning in doing those things for myself, and taking responsibility for them formed a great part of my self-worth and sense of well-being. Maybe you're like that too, and it's as hard for you as it was for me to watch your fiscal status inexorably sinking into the red because of your illness. I found it very hard to feel good about myself and my finances at first. I felt like a failure, like I had failed myself. I had fear too. I feared dependency on others as much as I feared having no one to depend on. I feared being forced to live in someone else's space. I feared never having my own space again.

At some point while working on self-care, I realized that I hadn't failed myself. I had been as financially responsible as I could possibly be. I had lasted for years with no income, and with the added expense of high rent and a car! Pre-CS, I hadn't been able to even imagine doing that. Working didn't necessarily equate with self-care, I learned.

Taking care of me, and managing my responsibilities, that was self-care. I managed my money responsibly, and now I manage my debt responsibly. I fight for compensation and disability income no matter how soul-weary, scared, or intimidated I am. I do all I can to improve my financial outlook and sense of well-being. *That* is self-care.

Even in debt, we can practice self-care. Even in debt, we can have a positive sense of well-being.

Rethinking Money

I've had to give money a lot of thought since getting sick: first, to create a spending plan with no unnecessary expenditures; and later (after accepting the possibility that I might never be able to work for a living again), to make a long-term plan. I wanted to maintain my autonomy, I wanted to achieve and experience things that cost more than my basic life overhead, yet I had always believed that working was the only way to get "enough money." When I had to stop working, I had to confront that core belief. If work truly was the only way to get enough money, then I should not have enough money right now, yet I'm still here, with a roof over my head, with enough to get by. So where does "enough money" come from, and how much *is* enough?

Pre-CSS, I thought I had enough money in savings to support me through any job loss, but I didn't. I thought I had a good foundation for retirement, but CSS gnawed away at that too. I realized I knew very little about how to make enough money. I investigated, and that led to more questions: I had chosen to stay in the city for the short term, at least, because of the proximity to medical specialists, and because I love this city—my home— but did I want to stay here long-term now that I had CSS? Or did I want to live someplace with a lower cost of living? Or a slower pace?

This is another of those great transformational crossroads we inevitably come to when travelling the path of chronic illness. It's the perfect opportunity for a financial overhaul and examination of your longer-term quality of life. How do you know if you need an overhaul? Good question. Ask yourself these:

- Do you feel in control of your money?
- Do you feel you always have enough?
- Do you know how much your skills and energy are worth?
- Do you earn what you're worth?
- Do you have a sufficient retirement plan?
- Do you feel perfectly calm and confident when bills come due?
- Are your disability payments enough?

Talking about money can be uncomfortable, I know, but if you answered *no* to any of those questions, or if you simply want to learn more about money and managing it, I encourage you to explore this aspect of your life. Money is "just a tool. Creating and using money consciously and effectively is a skill some of us were taught and some were not—but if you weren't taught the skill, you still have time to learn."[104] Rethinking your beliefs about, and redefining your relationship with money can provide financial security and improve your quality of life. It can also erase a significant amount of mental stressors (intrinsic triggers), and thus reduce symptoms. Not sure where to start? Check Appendix F: Recommended Reading and Viewing for my go-to financial experts.

Review of Self-Care and Autonomy

- With CSS (or CS alone), self-care takes on an added dynamic that encompasses daily decisions about managing the illness. Bubble time, planning and pacing, meditation, mindfulness, medications, special diet, sleep hygiene, therapy, CBT, and any other treatments or strategies you use—anything you do to manage and improve your conditions—now belong in your self-care portfolio.
- If you didn't learn self-care skills when young, that's ok. It's not too late now.
- Getting back to basics means focusing on self-care skills. These are a portal to happier, healthier, and more mindful living.
- Self-compassion skills are necessary for connecting with yourself and with others, and for changing unhelpful thoughts and behaviors.
- Negative self-criticism is not helpful; nor are affirmations you don't believe. It's ok to take baby steps as you learn self-compassion. Demonstrating a willingness to show compassion to yourself is the first step.
- Chronic illness can cause a crisis of faith and provide an opportunity to examine one's spirituality and recover faith and a whole lot more.
- We can reestablish our sense of well-being by nurturing self-worth and self-compassion, working on mental health, focusing on the basics, recovering what we need and mastering self-care.
- Maintaining autonomy may seem like an enormous monster, but it can be managed with careful planning and research. Ask for help if you need it.
- Rethinking your relationship with money may provide you with financial and lifestyle options you'd never considered before.

> It helps,
> putting my hands on a pot, on a broom,
> in a wash
> pail.
> I
> tried painting
> but it was easier to fly slicing
> potatoes.
> —Rabia[105]

Where CS and CSS Science Is Headed

Because CS and CSS are so complex, research can/must take countless directions. For example, FM research over the past three decades has examined "characterization and management of symptoms, psychophysiology, [and] neuroendocrine-immune pathophysiology, including central sensitization mechanisms."[106] That's early research, on only *one* syndrome out of many, so can you imagine how sizeable the amount, and how divergent the subject matter of research must be in order for us to learn all we need to know about CS and CSS? Future research will focus on topics such as identifying biomarkers[107] for CS and CSS, the role epigenetics[108] may play, neuroplastic theory, neuroplasticity-based treatments, mindfulness and meditation, immunology and neuroendocrinology, neurosensory, chemical exposure and toxicity; neuroimaging; neurotransmitter, neuron and glial cell health and function, laryngeal processes, gut health, prescription medication treatments, the role infections may play, models of assessment and patient care, and more. I encourage you to keep up to date on current research and discuss findings with your medical provider. This can seem overwhelming, but above you'll find a bunch of keywords for internet searching. If you aren't sure how to conduct research, your local librarian may be able to offer you a crash course. What follow here are some highlights of recent CS- and CSS-related research and its future directions.

Unfortunately, the prevalence of CS and CSS is increasing. A 2016 report found that 8 of the global "top 12 disabling conditions are related either to chronic pain or to the psychological conditions strongly associated with persistent pain."[109] It is not yet known what percentage of those may be attributed to CSS, but after finding a prevalence of chronic pain with unknown etiology in low- and middle-income countries, the researchers recommended that "strategies for assessment and treatment of chronic pain worldwide should consider the possibility of prevalent CSS."[110] While CSS becoming a worldwide phenomenon is not great news, it isn't all bad. Increased prevalence can lead to a higher profile, more medical providers and researchers becoming aware of CS and CSS and the need for improving diagnosis and care, and further research.

Some research will focus exclusively on improving patient care methods. Models for uniform classification of symptom severity and quality of life need to be developed and refined to aid accurate and prompt diagnosis and treatment, and to optimize care practices with a focus on cost-efficiencies and meeting patient and medical provider needs, both in the short- and long-term.[111] A 2013 study evaluated the efficacy of a new screening tool called the *Central Sensitization Inventory* (CSI)—designed to help medical providers identify patients with one or more CSS—and found the CSI to "have high reliability and validity."[112] A later study worked on establishing and validating severity levels for the CSI to help medical providers assess patient response to treatment.[113] Meanwhile a 2016 study focused on creating and assessing efficacy of a *Sensory Hypersensitivity Scale* (SHS) and concluded that the SHS would require further research in order to determine if it could help diagnose CS.[114] A 2015 study found that "neuroplasticity mediators" (certain proteins and signal molecules) could help medical providers screen/identify CSS in patients and validate symptoms,[115] while a 2016 study concentrated on developing a method for classifying different types of pain (one of which was CS-based) to facilitate treatment of pain in cancer survivors.[116] A 2015 review developed and proposed an "integrated theoretical framework for ELBD [episodic laryngeal breathing disorders, one of which is ILS, to provide] "a preliminary systemic platform" for further research.[117] The standardized results these types of studies will eventually produce are important. They will not only assist in diagnosis and effective treatment and patient care, they will legitimize CS and CSS in the eyes of disability insurers and help patients get the financial support they need more quickly and easily.

Other important research areas include peripheral neuropathies (dysfunctions or diseases of peripheral nerves) and the spinal cord's dorsal (rear) horn (which contains the first pain synapse, or neuron junction/circuit. Many CSS patients experience "peripheral pathology," including nerve-related pain in the muscles and inflammation.[118] Recent studies have shown that damage to the peripheral nervous system can cause plastic change and alter the activity of glial and certain immune response cells, "which all contribute to central sensitization."[119] Remember when I mentioned cytokines in relation to inflammation?

Researchers have found that imbalance "between pro- and anti-inflammatory cytokines in the dorsal horn microenvironment appears to be causal in the chronicity of [neuropathic] pain states."[120] A recent report also focuses on activity in the dorsal horn, this time with regards to *trigger points*, or "hyperirritable" areas in muscle tissue "which usually have referred pain,"[121] which involves the sensitization of dorsal horn neurons. While a handful of studies support the theory that trigger points "induce" CS and that treatment of trigger points decreases CS, initial evidence indicates that CS "can also promote trigger point activity."[122] One report calls for further research in order to prove the authors' hypothesis that "proper [trigger point] management may prevent and reverse the development of pain propagation in chronic pain conditions, because inactivation of [trigger points] attenuates [CS]."[123] This looks to me like we will see more dorsal horn research in the quest for potential prevention of, and treatments for CS and CSS.

Another research thread appeared when CS was discovered in patients with osteoarthritis (OA) and rheumatoid arthritis (RA). This finding helped researchers understand why some patients don't respond to "nonsteroidal anti-inflammatory drugs or joint replacement surgery, and require therapy directed at CS."[124] Related evidence has shown that cannabinoids (chemical compounds found in marijuana) and synthesized cannabinoid medications "[inhibit] central sensitization and its contribution to the manifestation of chronic OA pain" by stimulating CB_2 (cannabinoid 2) receptors (cell membrane receptors in several body systems and predominantly in the immune system).[125] There are still many questions about CB_2 receptors, so we can expect related research to continue.

The father of CSS, Dr. Yunus, has additional suggestions for avenues of research related to CS and CSS, such as creating "an international society of central sensitization (ISCS) with its own journal related to CS" that could facilitate the development of "a uniform classification criteria for CS," for use by both medical providers and researchers.[126] Yunus also believes that increased funding and research should be directed towards "both basic science (including genetics, epigenetics, neuroendocrine, neurosensory, neurophysiology and immunology areas) and clinical (including psychobiological and epidemiologic) research" surrounding chronic pain.[127] Biomarker research and patient-centered treatment were also among his recommendations.[128]

What does all this mean for those with CS and CSS? Help is a-coming, from countless avenues, but not right away. What can folks with these conditions do in the meantime? We can continue to address our symptoms and CS- and CSS-related issues with the strategies and treatments at our disposal. We can keep our eyes on ongoing research, take part in studies as appropriate, and petition our elected leaders to increase CS and CSS research funding, public education, accessibility, and disability support for those with these conditions. We can keep improving our quality of life, our relationships, and our sense of well-being. And that's just a start. Nutshell, there's a lot we can do.

BOONS OF CHRONIC ILLNESS

I've spent a lot of time talking about the rigors and pitfalls inherent in adjusting to and living with CS and CSS, but I want to emphasize that amidst all the chaos, tumultuous emotions and disorienting change involved with these conditions, there be diamonds. I've sprinkled them throughout this book—bits of magic and revelations that only those who experience CS and CSS are able to glean. Maybe that's another of our super powers: we can see things from both inside and outside of the bubble.

I loved many things about my pre–CSS life. I loved being physically fit, strong and active. I loved dancing and singing and spending time in the mountains. I loved being social and the feeling of satisfaction I got when I did my job well. I loved the ease at which I could get my daily living activities done. I loved reading for hours and browsing in bookstores, travelling, gardening, and going to movies or the symphony. Yep, there was lots to love, but in some ways, my life was unbalanced and dysfunctional, and I never would have known if I hadn't gotten sick.

- Like my friendships. I gave and gave to those I considered friends, but when I couldn't give like that anymore, most of those people vanished. I had been playing the fool, for years. Now I have authentic, balanced, reciprocal relationships and am all the happier for it.
- And my relationships with myself and with money. I worked for my living but didn't really have clarity about my financial plan or future goals, beyond this vague idea of "retirement savings." CFS, especially, has forced me to get clear on my financial plan and on who I am, regardless of *what I do*. I have learned better self-care and, paradoxically, even though I'm chronically ill and in debt, my sense of well-being has flourished.
- And behavioral issues that held me back. Chronic illness has revealed and forced me to face fears, fears that were preventing me from reaching a level of personal freedom, strength and joy that I had never known.

Chronic illness has made me very aware of what being alive is, how long a day is, an hour, a minute. It has taught me how to enjoy *living,* or *being,* not just finding enjoyment and satisfaction in what I *do.* I've learned to slow down, to rest, to have some downtime every day. I've learned that I am strong, stronger than I ever imagined. (I am Titan Amy, after all. And if you've got CS, you are Titan Amy too.) Endless planning and prioritizing has illuminated what's most important to me, and I put those values first now. Instead of focusing on the bad stuff I pay attention to the good. I spend less time and energy being angry or sad, and I maximize the joy and wonder in my experience. I've learned which of my relationships are authentic and worthwhile. I cherish my independence even more than before, the good fortune of having a safe place to live and food to eat, the miraculous beauty of a halcyon, sunshiny day, easy laughter, an ocean breeze, the taste of a fresh-picked wild cherry, a friend's companionship, a catchy melody, the divinely mysterious way good things happen to me and to people I love, the vastness of the stars—I savor it all. CS and CSS have made all the things I love about life that much dearer and enabled me to consciously appreciate them. Sights and sounds, languages, tastes, smells and textures—I breathe them in and try them on for a moment. (Truth be told, I often take longer than that.)

I hope that this book has helped you to understand CS and CSS and the challenges inherent in life with these conditions, to move from crisis to stability phase as quickly and painlessly as possible, and to establish and work towards goals for healing and for improving all aspects of your life. I wish you luck as you work to increase health, abolish suffering, heighten pleasure, and come to enjoy the hard-won boons of this illness. This book is designed to serve you as an ongoing resource in several ways: the detailed

Index enables you to examine or review a particular factoid, treatment, or strategy; *Coping* offers compassion, support, and solutions; the *Appendices* provide travel tips, information for your medical providers and loved ones, a crash plan for singles, and reputable foundations for further research and support. And you can always flip to any page on a bad day just to hear my voice. You're not alone, and I'm right here, talking to you.

> Surrender what you want
> she said
> because you will lose it anyway.
> I was standing at the foot of the tree
> outside my apartment
> counting the leaves as they fell.
> It was that day in mid-autumn
> that comes every year
> when the winds surge up
> and strip the trees bare.
> Life is like this wind
> she said.
> I nodded and made another tally mark on my notepad.
>
> Consider what you need
> she said
> because you will have to fight.
> I was tying a bundle of twigs
> upright inside a vase
> stringing wee branches with lights.
> It was that day in late autumn
> that comes every year
> when the night eats day
> and I must prepare.
> Life is like these twigs
> she said.
> I nodded, inserted the plug and basked in the glow.
>
> Fight only when you must
> she said
> because you will be fighting all your life.
> I was stomping on crocus heads
> outside my apartment
> covering them with ice cubes
> whispering, *Too soon. Too soon.*
> It was that day in winter
> that comes every year
> when the frost feigns retreat
> then starves the keen bear.
> Life is like this frost
> she said.
> I nodded and went inside for more ice.
>
> Save something for later
> she says
> because time cannot be trusted.

I am sitting on the bow of a tree
across from my apartment
gleaning peaches to be canned.
It is a day like no other.
Summer leaves filter sunshine
mosaics on my skin.
Honeybees nuzzle
my ear as if I am a prize blossom.
I nod,
peaches in my mouth.
Sweet sticky juice runs down my chin.

Appendix A:
For Friends and Loved Ones—
Helping, Connecting and Coping

What can I do for my friend or loved one who has CS? Great question. If you are asking that question and reading this book because of someone you love, congratulations are in order! Most people shy away from illness or run screaming because they have no experience with, or don't know how to handle it. You've already taken the first big steps: acknowledging that your friend or loved one has an illness, and learning about it.

CS and CSS can throw the dynamic of even the most functional relationships askew. Spinning away from togetherness and towards to the horizon of separateness, how do you cope? And how do you keep your relationship intact? Because these conditions tend to present themselves differently in different people, and relationships all have different circumstances and needs, I can't offer you any exact advice. I can point you in general directions though. From there, it's up to you to communicate with the person with the illness to learn what exactly they need or want, and to express your needs and desires as well.

Here are my top tips for showing or providing support:

- Ask what you can do.
- Offer to pick things up for your loved one when you go shopping.
- Offer to drive your loved one to a medical appointment so s/he won't have to take transit, or offer to give her/his kids rides wherever they need to go.
- Bring food or meals over.
- Offer to do the dishes or laundry or other chores around the house.
- Offer to take your loved one's kids once a week, or on any crash day.
- Ask or talk about something other than her/his illness.
- Call her/him just to chat. Say, "Hey, whatcha doing?"
- Offer to post or pickup library items for your loved one.
- Make your self environmentally trigger-free and come to your loved one's bubble for tea.
- Make your home environmentally trigger-free and invite your loved one over.
- Make your home environmentally trigger-free and offer to be "inn-keeper" in case of emergency. (One of my friends has done this and offered to be my "emergency inn-keeper" at any time. If one of my neighbors replaces carpets or repaints and the fumes are entering my apartment, I have a safe place to stay

while I make a longer-term plan. I have had to evacuate suddenly on more than one occasion and having a friend willing and able to put me up in their bubble has kept me off the streets. I highly recommend this for anyone with environmental triggers who lives in close proximity to folks without CS, especially when renting in an urban area.)

- If your loved one says something like "That environment is not manageable for me at this time. Why don't you come here for coffee instead?" it's important to respect, and not scoff or minimize her/his needs. Setting limits regarding light, noise, time away from home, your favorite perfume or laundry products, etc. is what your loved one needs to do to get better, and to be able to spend time with you.

- Educate yourself about your loved one's condition(s). It's an investment in your relationship with that person that will pay off thousand-fold.

- Don't decide to "help" your loved one by wearing a fragrance you know triggers her/him, just to "see if s/he notices." Don't assume that if s/he says nothing when you do this, s/he doesn't smell it or isn't triggered by it. Believe me, s/he will notice. S/he may be too overwhelmed or too tired to say anything, or s/he may feel betrayed or hurt by your behavior and unsure how to address it. Your loved one needs to know s/he can trust you and also needs to know what s/he's walking into when meeting with you. If s/he's already been exposed to or impacted by a lot of triggers before meeting you and you're wearing a surprise fragrance, that could send her/him into trigger overload and cause a crash or relapse.

  Putting your loved one in a position where s/he has to keep reminding you that your fragrance is a trigger, or must endure unplanned exposure in order to spend time with you, is not a helpful thing for you to do. If you suspect your fragrance will no longer trigger your loved one and want to know if you can try wearing it in her/his presence again, *ask*. Communication is key.

- Know your loved one may look much healthier than s/he is.

- Help your loved one research and acquire affordable, safe, and trigger-free housing.

- Help your loved one research and apply for finances and disability options, fight for fair compensation, and stay afloat financially in the meantime.

- Help your loved one research and acquire a reliable, trigger-free used car so s/he can avoid environmental triggers on transit and conserve energy.

- Remember that symptoms shift from day to day. Plans you made with your loved one may get cancelled at the last minute. This can happen often and can be frustrating and leave you at loose ends. Prepare yourself. Have a good book with you or make a backup plan ahead of time, like going to a movie by yourself, or a walk, or whatever you enjoy. Let your loved one know that you need this and discuss it openly.

- Offer to come over and just spend time with your loved one. S/he may love the company.

- Be patient with your loved one—even if s/he isn't always patient.

- Don't try to fix things.

- Show you care for the person with CS.

- Read this entire book. The facts and creative bits will all help you understand CS and CSS on an intellectual as well as emotional level.

Ideas for support for *you*:

- Educating yourself about your loved one's condition(s) isn't just to help you communicate with and support her/him. It's also so you can support yourself. Your life, too, is affected by the illness, so the more you know, the better.
- Therapy (one-on-one and/or group) can help you work through the effects of the illness on your life.
- A support group for people who don't have CS but whose lives are affected by it can offer you support and inspiration, a place to brainstorm, and a sense of normalcy. Groups like Codependents Anonymous or Al-Anon may also be helpful, as they offer support and help you develop boundaries and communication skills.
- Journaling about your experience and feelings can help enormously.
- Meditation, Qi Gong, Yoga, music, CBT, and other strategies in this book are not just for those with CS and CSS—they can help you too.

Appendix B:
For Medical Providers
and Patients—CS-Friendly
Office Protocols

For many folks with CS, seeing a medical provider can be very challenging. Having to sit in waiting rooms, close to people with synthetically fragranced skin, hair, and clothing is the tip of the iceberg. New carpet, paint, or furniture, industrial cleaners used to sanitize the office… The list of inescapable environmental triggers is endless, and there are significant intrinsic triggers too, such as the physical and mental exertion it takes to get to the medical office, and any mental or emotional stressors regarding the appointment itself and the outcome… You get the idea? So how can the patient with CS and CSS navigate these environments with the least damage, and how can the medical provider help make office visits manageable?

Checklist for medical providers: how to make your office as friendly as possible for patients with CS and CSS:

- Use only *free and clear* cleaning products in your office.
- Do not use air fresheners or scented soap in your office bathrooms.
- Do not use off-gassing office products such as Sharpies, dry-erase pens, plastic binders, or copy machines, or at least ensure these are not in use anywhere near the reception area or where patients might come into contact with their emissions.
- Have a separate waiting area for patients who have environmental triggers. This area should have dim lighting, be quiet, and have no new/off-gassing furnishings, paint, or carpet. If there is HVAC here, ensure it's not venting in fumes or smoke from outside or another room.
- Develop a protocol with your reception staff that enables them to know when a person with environmental triggers is coming in, such as a special sticker on their patient file, or a special mark in the appointment book/booking program, so they may escort that person to a separate waiting area immediately upon arrival.
- Train your staff about CSS and CS, and why it's important for people with these conditions to avoid triggers. (Better yet, buy each staff member a copy of this book.)
- Adopt a "scent-free" policy for all staff (that includes laundry products). Note that while this will help to reduce trigger exposure, it doesn't necessarily make

your office "easily accessible" for your patients with CS. "Scent-free" means far more than abstaining from wearing perfume or cologne. It also includes scented shampoos and hairsprays, deodorants, nail polish, shoe polish, hand lotion, face lotion, sunblock, bleach, scented detergent and fabric softeners, cigarette smoke in clothing… "Scent-free" doesn't cover half the potential environmental triggers in an office, but it is an element you can control, and if you control what you can, you're doing all you can.

- Ensure that only older, off-gassed toys, books, and magazines inhabit your waiting room, and no newspapers.
- Adopt a "scent-free" policy for all clients/patients and put up posters or place pamphlets in waiting room that educate people about what "scent-free" means, including laundry products, and how it helps people with environmental triggers. People want to help others, so this small amount of education can go a long way.
- If you renovate your office in any way—paint, carpet, furniture, etc.—notify your patients with CS and CSS ahead of time so they may plan accordingly.
- Offer online video appointments or phone appointments as an alternative for patients with CS who you don't need to examine in person and who would suffer too greatly by having to come into the office.

Checklist for patients: ways to survive a visit to your medical provider's office with minimal trigger exposure and impact:

- Before making an appointment, ask questions to assess how triggerful or trigger-free the medical office may be. An easy way to do this is to compare the above list to your trigger list, and discuss possible accommodations with your doctor's staff. Remember, no place is perfect, and even if you go through this list, you may run into unexpected triggers. The goal here is to minimize potential known triggers as much as possible. So, if the office environment, along with whatever accommodations the staff is willing to make, will be manageable for you, great—make that appointment! If you feel it won't be manageable, you may wish to ask the medical provider to consult with you outside the office or online, or look for another medical provider.
- Be sure to rest sufficiently in your bubble pre- and post-appointments. Have a friend drive you so you can rest on the way.
- Use your scarf and nosegay strategies to manage environmentally triggered symptoms.
- Use strategies from this book to manage stress and anxiety.
- Visualize the office visit prior to going inside. Imagine it will be a success and that you will get what you need from the appointment without increasing symptoms.
- Remember that few people understand CS and CSS, and most will need some education, (even medical providers) but once they understand, many are very willing to help.

Appendix C:
For Medical Providers—
A Patient-Centered Approach

This segment is for medical professionals who want more information on how to provide the best care for patients.

CS and CSS are *chronic* conditions. Presently, treatments are "empirical" and "palliative" and have limited efficacy.[1] Because these conditions are not well known and because patients tend to "look fine," patients commonly experience invalidation/dismissal by friends and family, bosses, and medical professionals.[2] Patients must make accommodations and learn to adapt and self-manage the illness and all other aspects of their lives while contending with upsetting symptoms and social/professional fallout.[3] This is no easy task, and the challenge is compounded by lack of knowledge in both the medical and public sectors. If the medical provider does not recognize that CS and CSS affect people on multiple levels, "including physiological, behavioral, cognitive, affective, and social features," s/he will not completely understand or be able to address the patient's needs.[4] Nutshell, the variable nature of CS and CSS and their often far-reaching and severe impact upon patients necessitate individual assessments and a patient-centered approach in treatment, rather than one based on ideas of "patient uniformity" or "homogeneity,"[5] or on "the more specific bioscientific pathways typical for a pathologically-defined disease."[6]

Dr. Yunus confirms this in his 2015 review, stating that many of those with CSS have both functional and organic pathology, so dichotomy "should be abandoned…. Psychobiology is also biology."[7] Although CSS share some features, patients "represent a heterogeneous group … both across CSS conditions and within them."[8] In order to best serve them, the medical provider must widen the lens, look beyond symptoms to the whole person, and consider patient history and environment, support/resources (or lack thereof), psychosocial factors, and other life circumstances, all of which play a role in the patient's symptoms and CSS presentation.[9] While symptoms need to be addressed, the medical provider also should focus on how social, physical, and emotional function can be improved.[10]

Several psychological and social factors may contribute to the intensity and longevity of CS and CSS symptoms, including anxiety or depression; alcohol or drug abuse; "common cognitive and affective features," such as anger, "symptom appraisals and symptom beliefs," "catastrophic thinking and fear-avoidance," "hypervigilance" for symptoms, "perceived control versus helplessness," "self-efficacy," and "psychological (in)flexibility"; and symptom-related "social learning," "social stigma and skepticism," or "social support."[11]

Note that while psychosocial factors may worsen symptoms, they "rarely are the sole cause of the symptoms,"[12] and their impact varies. It's crucial that medical providers inform the patient of the role psychosocial factors can play; however, because of the stigmatization patients often experience, the patient may feel s/he is being dismissed by yet another medical provider (and consequently, may resist considering psychosocial factors and ways to address them).[13]

A 2008 study states that the "explanatory gap" (the space between a patient's expectations and a medical provider's understanding of the patient's experience and needs) is greatest when dealing with CSS and can negatively impact proper care.[14] The researchers propose that medical providers use a "psychosomatic framework" based on somatic awareness to explore and validate the patient's experience and learn what biopsychosocial factors need to be addressed, and thus bridge the gap.[15] The study also suggests that patients use somatic awareness to aid them in self-managing their condition(s), and that when patient and medical provider both use the technique, they can more easily identify and decide which treatments and/or resources may optimize the patient's development of self-management skills and progress toward health goals.[16] Self-management plays a crucial role in treatment and should include "education of the patient in self-management skills, cognitive behavioral therapy (CBT), exercise, and drug therapy."[17]

While somatic awareness can be a useful tool, it carries a negative connotation in many medical circles and has been used all too often to discredit patients with CS and CSS. Dr. Yunus urges medical providers to employ "both pharmacological and non-pharmacological" treatments and "person/patient-centered care," but to avoid "patient-blaming terms like somatization, somatizer and catastrophizing."[18] For more information on patient-centered care for those with CS and CSS, please see the works cited in this segment.

Appendix D:
For Singles with CS Who
Live Alone—A Crash Plan

It's not helpful to focus on the discomfort symptoms cause; however, those of us with CS and CSS can become accustomed to functioning with a consistent level of pain or debilitation and may brush off warning symptoms until they've become so severe that we crash. An unplanned crash can also occur, seemingly "out of nowhere," or it can be provoked by a new treatment trial. The problem for many single people who live alone is, there's no one there to notice how poorly we're doing, or to help if we have a severe crash. If we experience significant cognitive impairment when we crash, we may not be able to assess the situation accurately and may make poor care decisions.

The best way I've found to ensure my safety in such a situation is to create a Crash Plan and have it posted on the fridge at all times. Mine looks something like this:

1. With onset of severe symptoms, call someone and ask her/him to check on me daily, at least via phone.
2. Consult your "triage checklist" daily to determine where you should be. If you aren't able to make this assessment, have a friend look at the checklist and determine if you are ok at home alone or should be in hospital.
3. Eat. Check the "crash menu" on fridge for no-prep snacks/meals. Check the "crash grocery list" on fridge and order groceries if needed, or ask someone to bring some.
4. If necessary, call someone and ask them to come water plants, do dishes, or tend to the cat's needs if you can't do such things.

Crash Plan Resources

- Crash Menu and Grocery List: I have trouble thinking clearly and making decisions when in a crash, so I keep a crash menu and grocery list on the fridge with my Crash Plan at all times. These contain foods that require little prep and cleanup and hence are "crash-friendly." I always keep crash-friendly foods stocked in the apartment. If I start to run out, I refer to the crash grocery list to place a delivery order, or ask a friend to pick up.
- Triage Checklist: This has my medical care card/insurance number on it, my doctor's number, and that of the BC health hotline (811). The checklist contains my

functional norms. Comparing my functionality during crash to the norms helps me to determine my level of debilitation when I'm in crash and not thinking too clearly. If I'm functioning at a level significantly lower than that baseline, I call my doctor or the health hotline to discuss whether or not I am ok at home alone.

- Phone List: This contains names and numbers of folks who've agreed to be part of my Crash Plan, whom I can call for a ride to hospital or for help with food or cat, etc. I also include a cab company number or two, in case I can't reach anyone and need to go to hospital.

- Protocol for trying a new treatment: Before attempting any new treatment, I ask/do everything on this list to minimize crashes and maximize recovery in the event of a treatment-caused crash:

  ◻ Ask, what is the goal of this treatment and can the results be achieved in any other way?

  ◻ Research treatment thoroughly.

  ◻ Ask about/research "Die-off' and other side effects: what are they, how long do they last and how severe can they get?

  ◻ Ask, does treatment cause people to crash or increase symptoms?

  ◻ Ask, do I need to follow a special diet pre-, post- or during treatment?

  ◻ Ask, do I need to follow a special diet if things go wrong with treatment?

  ◻ Make grocery list of special diet needs for this treatment in case of crash and post this list with Crash Plan.

  ◻ Ask/research how to safely stop treatment suddenly if things go horribly wrong.

Appendix E:
Travel and Vacations
with CS and CSS

I recommend that those with CSS or CS alone avoid all travel while in *crisis phase,* when the central nervous system is ultra-reactive. Travel is stressful and tiring at the best of times, and travelling with CS and CSS can place an even greater strain on your central nervous system and take a huge toll on your health, setting you back for weeks or months. This can be discouraging and undermine any confidence you'd built up in managing your symptoms and condition(s). However, sometimes travel is unavoidable. You may need to see a distant medical specialist, get to a wedding or a funeral, or attend a special environmental-trigger-free Muse concert in Iceland just for fans with CS (*Please, Muse? Please?*).

I have managed trips in both *crisis* and *stability phases.* Keyword: *managed,* meaning that the trips weren't good for me and set me back, but I survived. For local events, I can often minimize impact enough that I'm merely planning for a relapse. For distant or longer events, I have to plan to crash. I do so only for a rare and super important event—life-changing and worthy of the sacrifice—like camping in front of the coliseum for a week to get tickets to see Virtue and Moir's last performance ever. (Really, Virtue and Moir channel some kind of wonderful divine when they skate. They have no equal and there never will be one.) Either way, the trip is managed primarily by—you guessed it—planning and pacing, and limiting trigger exposure and impact.

Planning and Pacing for Traveling and Attending Events with CS and CSS

With planned relapses or crashes, I do the following to minimize severity and duration of symptoms (note, this is not an exact science. I have learned over time roughly how certain types and durations of over-exertion will affect me, but wild cards abound when we leave the bubble, so there is no way to make precise estimations or guarantee results.) Whether I'm in *crisis* or *stability phase,* the process is the same:

- Before RSVP-ing, I examine the event location and itinerary. I locate a place that can serve as my bubble during the event, and I plan the event day(s) carefully, with built-in rest times during which I will detach from the action and stimulus of the event and go rest in my temporary bubble. If I come across anything unmanageable in this initial planning stage and can't find a solution (this can happen, albeit rarely) I let the people know I won't be attending. However, if I may attend …

- A month or two before the event, I mark off the days immediately prior to the event in my calendar. These will be intensive bubble days, during which I remain in my bubble, doing pretty much nothing besides resting, meditating, or visualizing (me lying on a tropical beach, completely stress-free), with as little sensory stimulation as possible. The theory behind this is that I am giving the nervous system a rest, decreasing stress, and "storing up energy" before the big event, so that the over-exertion and whatever other triggers involved in the actual event will impact me as little as possible. (The number of days to mark off depends on the anticipated trigger load. It's something you'll have to figure out for yourself, but I can give you an example so you know what it looks like: If the event is an outdoor wedding held a 20-minute drive from my bubble, I'll mark off three days pre-event and a week to ten days post-event, depending on how much socializing I plan to do at the reception. If I have to fly 12 hours and spend three days in a hotel and socialize all day every day, I'll mark off two weeks prior and eight weeks post-event.)

- When I plan the post-event recovery time, I check my calendar and defer any appointments or obligations until after the estimated recovery period.

- A month or two before the event, I prepare and freeze food and/or plan post-event grocery delivery so I don't have to shop or cook post-event and can concentrate on recovering from the crash as quickly as possible.

- Post-event, I return home, commence intensive bubble time until symptoms disperse, and savour my wonderful memories of the event. *Ahhhhh …*

Limiting Trigger Exposure/Impact While Travelling and Attending Events

Unless you've become a meditating ninja and can keep your stress low and friendly even while travelling or dealing with your Uncle Gabby at your cousin's wedding, travel is likely to cause an increase in symptoms and triggers. That is, even if you don't normally have environmental triggers, you may experience them while travelling or attending events because the impact of your intrinsic triggers (especially sleep and certain foods) will most likely increase, making your central nervous system more reactive than usual. So be prepared. Check out Table 10, re-read Chapter 2, and bring a scarf, just in case.

TABLE 10. TRAVEL TIPS FOR LIMITING EXPOSURE TO ENVIRONMENTAL TRIGGERS

	When in Crisis Phase	*When in Stability Phase*
Road Trips (Driving)	The car needs to be your safe bubble. Ensure you can be in it for as long as you need to without being triggered. Ask a trigger-free friend to drive with you so you can rest at least part of the time. If you have the money, you may consider renting a van conversion for the trip, so you 'have bubble, will travel.' (Always go to van	The car needs to be your safe bubble. Ensure you can be in it for as long as you need to without being triggered. A van conversion is the way to go in style, but it can be pricey. Ask a trigger-free friend to drive with you so you can rest at least part of the time. Bring music that makes you feel happy as well as calm. This is

(When in Crisis Phase)	*(When in Stability Phase)*
rental place prior to your trip to test the van for triggers. There may be cleaning products or new van smell, etc.) Bring music that makes you feel happy as well as calm. Having a vehicle you can use as your bubble is the best way to travel when in *crisis phase*, I believe, because you have the most control over your environment and you know you have a safe bubble no matter where you are travelling to.	still the best way for folks with environmental sensitivities to travel, I believe, because of environment control. Bring your nosegay diffuser, scarf, and room diffusers.

Flights

The only way I could get through flights without coughing myself unconscious or enduring both extreme nausea and a migraine was to drink a couple glasses of wine before getting on the plane and a couple more when I got on, wrap my scarf triple thick around my face, and fall into a drunken sleep. (I hated this and later discovered that valium or sleeping pills worked too.)	Depending on flight length and how close I am to the nearest super-scented person (if I am seated in unmanageable proximity to someone wearing heavy fragrance on skin or clothing I ask to move), I use scarf and nosegay diffuser, along with relaxed breathing and mind-distraction techniques. If I need more help than that, I will go for the alcohol, valium or sleep pill options.

Staying with Friends or Family

If you're invited to stay with friends or family, ask ahead of time if anywhere in their home has been painted, renovated or refurnished lately. Ask if they can refrain from doing laundry or using chemical products (including scented personal products) while you're there. Be sure to mention any other triggers you may have that people commonly use in their homes. When you arrive, if the place is workable, great. Use it as your bubble and be sure to rest in between short spurts of social time. However, if the place is unworkable for you, don't try to stick it out to be polite. This ends in badness for all involved. Just say thanks anyways and evacuate as soon as possible.	I do the same now, in *stability phase*. My goal is still to find a place that feels safe and in which I can rest with as little sensory stimulation as possible.

Staying in Hotels

Some hotels will accommodate when I request that they use free and clear or unscented cleaning products in my room prior to arrival. I also request a room that has not been renovated, painted or furnished in the past year, nonsmoking, no carpet perfume powders or air fresheners of any kind in the room. I also require a radiant heat source (in cold seasons) because forced air HVAC triggers me. I always get a room with a window that opens and that is located far from the pool and laundry. When I get there, I do a sniff test of the room. If it's unmanageable, but close, I ask to sniff another. If nothing works, I go stay someplace else.	I do all the same stuff as in *crisis phase*, plus, I bring my room-sized scent diffusers and use them to make the room smell like what I'm used to. My goal is still to find a place that feels safe and in which I can rest with as little sensory stimulation as possible.

What to Bring

No matter where you stay, you'll need to bring your own free and clear stuff. So, depending on trip length and what your triggers are, you may need to bring any or all of the following: hand soap, laundry soap, dish soap, towel and washcloth, bed	I bring everything I said in the left column, plus my room-sized scent diffusers. Sometimes I bring a fold-up single futon bed thing with just a sleeping bag instead of all bed linens. I bring my own food in a cooler too, when possible, so I don't have to shop.

	(When in Crisis Phase)	*(When in Stability Phase)*
	linens, duvet or blanket, shampoo/conditioner, lotion, sunblock, pillow, etc.	
Backup Accommodation Plans	Sleep in the car or rented van conversion. Sleep in a used (pre-outgassed) tent (clean, no mildew or dust) in someone's backyard. If no workable solutions available you can always return home earlier than planned. Sometimes we try and it doesn't work out. We can only do what we can do.	Sleep in the car or van conversion, or in a used tent. Call on a few friends or family members willing to host you, and see which place is the least triggerful or has the easiest space to convert into a temporary bubble. Be prepared to go home early if you can't make anything work.

The same principle applies with symptoms that aren't triggered by your environment. That is, you may not normally experience significant pain or fatigue-related symptoms, but travelling and attending events may cause them to present themselves. Again, I say, travel is not the best thing to be doing, especially in *crisis phase*. Put it off if you can, even for six months, or a year. That said, some travel may be un-put-off-able. You may need to get to the spaceport in New Mexico for your first-ever space tour. (*Virgin Galactic, here I come!*) To make that happen with the least amount of setback, you need to minimize trigger exposure and impact. Check out Table 11, re-read Chapter 3, and pace yourself.

TABLE 11. TRAVEL TIPS FOR LIMITING PAIN OR FATIGUE-RELATED SYMPTOMS

	When in Crisis Phase	When in Stability Phase
Road Trips (Driving)	When I was in *crisis phase*, I couldn't drive more than three minutes without losing concentration. **Learn your limits and do not go beyond them.** This is for your safety as well as that of others on the road. Ask a CS-free friend to drive you. Rent a van conversion so you can sleep while your friend drives, and/or sleep in it instead of a hotel. In addition, the vehicle needs to be your safe bubble. Ensure you can be in it for as long as you need to without being triggered, by scents, lights, road noise, temperature, etc. If you can enjoy music, then bring music that makes you feel happy as well as calm. Keep it at a low volume to avoid irritating your sensitive nervous system. At first sign of your warning signals, turn off the music. A road vehicle is the best mode of travel when in *crisis phase*, I believe, because you have the most control over your environment and you know you have a safe bubble no matter where you are travelling to.	Even if you are in *stability phase*, I highly recommend that you ask a CS-free friend to drive you. You want to save up as much energy as possible for the event you will be attending, and driving is a huge exertion, cognitively as well as physically. If you must drive yourself, know your cognitive limits and take rests appropriately. I once had to drive 120 miles and did so by spreading it over two days and stopping and resting every 20 minutes. In addition, the car needs to be your safe bubble. Ensure you can be in it for as long as you need to without being triggered, by scents, lights, road noise, temperature, etc. Rent a van conversion so you can sleep while your friend drives, and/or sleep in it instead of a hotel. If you can enjoy music, then bring music that makes you feel happy as well as calm. Keep it at a low volume to avoid irritating your sensitive nervous system. At first sign of your warning signals, turn off the music.
Flights	My specialist gave me a note stating that I couldn't walk from check-in counter to gate and required transportation. I also checked my bags. That eliminated a massive over-exertion involved in walking all the way to the gate and carting and monitoring my luggage. During flights I got inflammation and pain, so I did chair stretches often, stood and stretched when I could, and I took ibuprofen if I needed it. I also brought a reusable ice pack, which was	I do much the same on flights now, even out of *crisis phase*. My priority is getting through the journey with as few symptoms and as little upset to my central nervous system as possible. Then I can enjoy the event I'm heading to as much as possible.

	(When in Crisis Phase)	*(When in Stability Phase)*
	helpful until it warmed. For long flights, I carried the disposable single-use ice packs. When one warmed, I'd crack open another. I used earplugs to protect my fragile nervous system against the noise of engines, HVAC and people. I spent most of the trip resting with eyes closed. If the pain became intolerable I took a sleeping pill and slept the journey away. Yep, it was boring at times, but I found it crucial to block out as much sensory stimulation as possible.	
Staying with Friends or Family	I ask ahead of time about access to the home. Are there a lot of stairs involved? A big hill? Is there parking nearby? I also ask if the space contains any scent or sound triggers (newly painted or carpeted, or a drunken neighbor upstairs prone to angry or violent fits at 3 a.m.?) When you arrive, if the place is workable, great. Use it as your bubble and be sure to rest in between short spurts of social time. However, if the place is unworkable for you, don't try to stick it out to be polite. This ends in badness for all involved. Just say thanks anyways and evacuate as soon as possible.	I do the same now, in *stability phase*. My goal is still to find a place that feels safe and in which I can rest with as little sensory stimulation as possible.
Staying in Hotels	I ask ahead of time about access to the rooms and restaurants. Are there a lot of stairs involved? A big hill? Is there parking nearby? I also ask if the room contains any scent or sound triggers (newly painted or carpeted, or is the room near enough to the pool that children's gleeful screams and running feet would startle me all day long? I ask for a room as close to a side entrance as possible so I don't have to navigate the lobby or walk too far. I always get a room with a window that opens and that is located far from the pool and laundry. When I get there, if anything about the room is unmanageable, but close, I ask to see another. If nothing works, I go stay someplace else.	I do the same now, in *stability phase*. My goal is still to find a place that feels safe and in which I can rest with as little sensory stimulation as possible.
What to Bring	In *crisis phase,* I brought as little as possible. The less I had to carry or take my attention, the better. I brought the clothing I needed for the event, and wore my only other clothes on travel days. Earplugs. Sunglasses. My iPod and earbuds with classical music, calming music, and meditations on it. Pain medication and sleep aids as needed.	I bring my own food when possible, so I don't have to shop. I bring my yoga mat on longer trips, and some resistance bands, so I can stretch like I do at home. I bring a Qi Gong DVD too. Earplugs. Sunglasses. My iPod and earbuds with classical music, calming music, and meditations on it. Pain medication and sleep aids as needed.
Backup Accommodation Plans	Sleep in the car or van conversion. If no workable solutions are available you can always return home earlier than planned. Sometimes we try and it doesn't work out. We can only do what we can do.	Sleep in the car. Call on a few friends or family members willing to host you, and see which place is the least triggerful or has the easiest space to convert into a temporary bubble. Be prepared to go home early if you can't make anything work.

Appendix F: Recommended Reading and Viewing

The resources listed here are a starting point for those who would like more information about some of the topics covered in this book.

Diet

D'Agostino, Dominic, with Ari Meisel. "Podcast #44 with Dr. Dominic D'Agostino from University of South Florida College of Medicine." keto nutrition podcast. LessDoing.com (November 4, 2013).

FODMAP information: www.med.monash.edu/cecs/gastro/fodmap/.

The Institute for Functional Medicine Web site: www.functionalmedicine.org.

KetoCalculator: www.keto-calculator.ankerl.com/

Maintz, Laura, and Natalija Novak. "Histamine and Histamine Intolerance." *The American Journal of Clinical Nutrition* 85 (2007): 1185–96.

Mancinelli, Kristen. *The Ketogenic Diet: The Scientifically Proven Approach to Fast, Healthy Weight Loss.* Berkeley: Ulysses Press, 2015.

SIBO information: www.siboinfo.com/diet.html.

USDA Food Database Web site: www.ndb.nal.usda.gov/.

Wahls, Terry, with Eve Adamson. *The Wahls Protocol: A Radical New Way to Treat All Chronic Autoimmune Conditions Using Paleo Principles.* New York: Penguin Group, 2014.

Environmental Triggers, MCS and Tilt

American Lung Association's Web site. "Formaldehyde." Lung.org.

Environmental Health Association of Nova Scotia's Web site. "Get Rid of Chemical Fabric Softeners: Protect Your Health and the Environment." EnvironmentalHealth.ca (2007).

Integrated Chronic Care Service Web site. "Fragrance Free and Unscented Products That Contain Chemicals." www.cdha.nshealth.ca/system/files/sites/86/documents/fragrance-free-or-unscented-products-contain-chemicals.pdf.

_____. "Fragrance Free and Unscented Products Without Chemicals." www.cdha.nshealth.ca/system/files/sites/86/documents/fragrance-free-and-unscented-products-without-chemicals.pdf.

Martini, A., S. Iavicoli, and L. Corso. "Multiple Chemical Sensitivity and the Workplace: Current Position and Need for an Occupational Health Surveillance Protocol." *Oxidative Medicine and Cellular Longevity.* June 2013.

Miller, Claudia. "Chemical Intolerance: Words Are Everything." *The Human Ecologist* (Winter 2008): 13–7.

Sutton, Rebecca. "Don't Get Slimed: Skip the Fabric Softener." *Environmental Working Group* blog post (September 1, 2011). www.ewg.org/enviroblog/2011/11/dont-get-slimed-skip-fabric-softener.

Ziem, Grace. "Hazardous Substances," list of environmental triggers. www.chemicalinjury.net/hazardoussubstances.htm.

Financial Health

Debtors Anonymous Web site: www.DebtorsAnonymous.org.

Lorenz, Suzanne, and Sam Beasley. *Wealth and Well-Being Workbook: Overcoming Barriers to Financial Independence.* Chico: Any Wind Publishing, 2010.

Mundis, Jerrold. *Earn What You Deserve: How to Stop Underearning & Start Thriving.* New York: Bantam, 1996.

Housing

Earthship Biotecture Web site: www.Earthship.com.

Grozdanic, Lidija. "Europe's First Chemical-Free Housing." Inhabitat.com Weblog post (April 17, 2014).

MCS Housing information: www.mcs-america.org/index_files/MCShousing.htm.

Tiny House Movement information: www.en.wikipedia.org/wiki/Tiny_house_movement.

Medication and Supplement Research

Mayo Clinic: www.mayoclinic.org/drugs-supplements.
U.S. National Library of Medicine: www.nlm.nih. gov/medlineplus/druginformation.html.

Meditation, Mindfulness, Boundaries, Self-Compassion

Ashley-Farrand, Thomas. *Mantra Meditation for Physical Health.* Boulder: Sounds True, 2003.
Codependents Anonymous Web site: www.coda.org.
Hanson, Rick. *Buddha's Brain: The Practical Neuroscience of Happiness, Love and Wisdom.* Oakland: New Harbinger Publications, 2009.
Katherine, Anne. *Boundaries in an Overconnected World: Setting Limits to Preserve Your Focus, Privacy, Relationships, and Sanity.* Novato: New World Library, 2013.
_____. *Where to Draw the Line: How to Set Healthy Boundaries Every Day.* New York: Fireside, 2000.
Ladinsky, Daniel, trans. *Love Poems from God: Twelve Sacred Voices from the East and West.* New York: Penguin Compass, 2002.
McGonigal, Kelly. "How to Make Stress Your Friend." *TEDtalk* presentation (2013).
_____. *The Neuroscience of Change: A Compassion-Based Program for Personal Transformation.* Boulder: Sounds True, 2012.
_____, with Tami Simon. "Kelly McGonigal: The Neuroscience of Change." *Insights at the Edge* podcast interview. SoundsTrue.com (April 19, 2012).
Neff, Kristin. *Self-Compassion: The Proven Power of Being Kind to Yourself.* New York: HarperCollins, 2011.
Rousseau. Natalie. "The 30-Day Illumination Challenge," introduction to meditation online course.
Salzberg, Sharon. *Lovingkindness: The Revolutionary Art of Happiness.* Boston: Shambhala, 2002.

Neuroplasticity and CBT

Brain training exercises from Posit Science: www. brainhq.com.
Brain training geography puzzles: www.yourchild learns.com/online-interactive-maps.htm.
Doidge, Norman. *The Brain That Changes Itself: Stories of Personal Triumph from the Frontiers of Brain Science.* New York: Penguin Books, 2007.
_____. *The Brain's Way of Healing: Remarkable Discoveries and Recoveries from the Frontiers of Neuroplasticity.* New York: Penguin Books, 2016.
EEG Education & Research. Web site discusses neurofeedback and lists therapeutic applications of it, such as anxiety, CFS, chronic pain, depression, PTSD, migraine, and more: www.eegspectrum. com/therapeutic-uses/.
Genetic Testing information: www.23andme.com.
International Society for Neurofeedback & Research Web site: www.isnr.org.

Low Level Laser Therapy information: www.bioflex laser.com.
Moskowitz, Michael, and Marla Golden. Web site dedicated to treating chronic pain via neuroplastic change: www.neuroplastix.com.
Patel, Aniruddh D. *Music and the Brain.* Chantilly: The Great Courses, 2015.
Satterfield, Jason M. *Cognitive Behavioral Therapy: Techniques for Retraining Your Brain.* Chantilly: The Great Courses, 2015.

Organizations for CS Research, Treatment and/or Support*

Bateman Horne Center. Salt Lake City, UT, USA.
Centre for Complex Chronic Diseases. Vancouver, BC, Canada.
Chronic Fatigue Syndrome Advisory Committee. www.hhs.gov/ash/advisory-committees/cfsac/ about-cfsac.
Pacific Voice Clinic, and *Provincial Voice Care Resource Program.* Vancouver, BC, Canada.

*I listed only the organizations I have had contact with. There are many more. I suggest you search online for the one(s) most suitable and accessible for you.

Pain

Butler, David, and G. Lorimer Moseley. *Explain Pain.* Australia: NOI Group, 2013.
Moseley, Lorimer G. "Body in Mind: The Role of the Brain in Chronic Pain," presentation at *Mind and Its Potential* conference (2011).
_____. "Why Things Hurt." *TEDx Adelaide* presentation (2011).

Planning and Pacing

BMR Calculator: www.calculator.net/bmr-calculator. html.
CFIDS & Fibromyalgia self-help Web site. Various articles on planning and pacing strategies. www. cfidsselfhelp.org/library/topic/Energy+Envelope+ and+Pacing.
Heart Rate Calculator: www.ottawarun.com/heart rate.htm.

Qi Gong and Yoga

Holden, Lee. *Qi Gong for Health and Healing: A Complete Training Course to Unleash the Power of Your Life-Force.* Boulder: Sounds True, 2010.
Yee, Rodney. *Moving Toward Balance: 8 Weeks of Yoga with Rodney Yee.* Emmaus, Rodale Books, 2004.

Vocal Health

Rammage, Linda. *Vocalizing with Ease: A Self-Improvement Guide.* Vancouver, BC: self-published, 1996.

Chapter Notes

Chapter 1

1. Muhammad B. Yunus, "Editorial Review: An Update on Central Sensitivity Syndromes and the Issues of Nosology and Psychobiology," *Current Rheumatology Reviews* 11 (2015): 70.

2. Norman Doidge, *The Brain's Way of Healing: Remarkable Discoveries and Recoveries from the Frontiers of Neuroplasticity* (New York: Penguin Books, 2016), 39.

3. Muhammad B. Yunus, "Editorial Review: An Update on Central Sensitivity Syndromes and the Issues of Nosology and Psychobiology," *Current Rheumatology Reviews* 11 (2015): 78.

4. J. Nijs et al., "Brain-derived Neurotrophic Factor As a Driving Force Behind Neuroplasticity in Neuropathic and Central Sensitization Pain: A New Therapeutic Target?" *Expert Opinion on Therapeutic Targets* 19, no. 4 (April 2015): 565.

5. Muhammad B. Yunus, "Editorial Review: An Update on Central Sensitivity Syndromes and the Issues of Nosology and Psychobiology," *Current Rheumatology Reviews* 11 (2015): 70.

6. Muhammad B. Yunus, "Fibromyalgia and Overlapping Disorders: The Unifying Concept of Central Sensitivity Syndromes," *Seminars in Arthritis and Rheumatism* 36 (2007): 339.

7. *Ibid.*

8. L.L. Kinder, R.M. Bennett, and K.D. Jones, "Central Sensitivity Syndromes: Mounting Pathophysiologic Evidence to Link Fibromyalgia with other Common Chronic Pain Disorders," *Pain Management Nursing* 12, no. 1 (March 2011): 15.

9. Leah M. Adams and Dennis C. Turk, "Psychosocial Factors and Central Sensitivity Syndromes," *Current Rheumatology Reviews* 11, no. 2 (2015): 96.

10. *Ibid.*

11. *Ibid.*, 97.

12. Muhammad B. Yunus, "Fibromyalgia and Overlapping Disorders: The Unifying Concept of Central Sensitivity Syndromes," *Seminars in Arthritis and Rheumatism* 36 (2007): 349.

13. Ric Arseneau, "Hope for Patients with Fatigue, Pain, and Unexplained Symptoms," University of British Columbia Faculty of Medicine's thischangedmypractice.com (October 13, 2015): 1–3.

14. Leah M. Adams and Dennis C. Turk, "Psychosocial Factors and Central Sensitivity Syndromes," *Current Rheumatology Reviews* 11, no. 2 (2015): 99–100.

15. Mayo Clinic, "Chronic Fatigue Syndrome: Definition," http://www.mayoclinic.org/diseases-conditions/chronic-fatigue-syndrome/basics/definition/con-20022009, accessed July 12, 2016.

16. Mayo Clinic, "Myofascial Pain Syndrome: Definition," http://www.mayoclinic.org/diseases-conditions/myofascial-pain-syndrome/basics/definition/con-20033195, accessed July 12, 2016.

17. M. de Tommaso, and C. Fernández-de-Las-Peñas, "Tensions Type Headache," *Current Rheumatology Review* 12, no. 2 (2016): 127.

18. Mayo Clinic, "Migraine: Overview," http://www.mayoclinic.org/diseases-conditions/migraine-headache/basics/definition/con-20026358, accessed July 12, 2016.

19. National Heart, Lung, and Blood Institute, "What Is Restless Legs Syndrome?" http://www.nhlbi.nih.gov/health/health-topics/topics/rls/, accessed July 12, 2006.

20. National Sleep Foundation, "Periodic Limb Movements in Sleep," https://sleepfoundation.org/sleep-disorders-problems/sleep-related-movement-disorders/periodic-limb-movement-disorder, accessed July 12, 2006.

21. Integrated Chronic Care Service, "Multiple Chemical Sensitivity (MCS)," http://www.cdha.nshealth.ca/integrated-chronic-care-service-iccs/patients/multiple-chemical-sensitivity-mcs, accessed July 12, 2006.

22. Mayo Clinic, "Irritable Bowel Syndrome: Definition," http://www.mayoclinic.org/diseases-conditions/irritable-bowel-syndrome/basics/definition/con-20024578, accessed July 12, 2006.

23. Mayo Clinic, "Irritable Bowel Syndrome: Definition," http://www.mayoclinic.org/diseases-conditions/irritable-bowel-syndrome/basics/definition/con-20024578, accessed July 12, 2006.

24. BC Women's Hospital, "What Is Fibromyalgia," http://www.bcwomens.ca/health-info/living-with-illness/fibromyalgia, accessed July 12, 2016.

25. Mayo Clinic, "Post-Traumatic Stress Disorder: Definition," http://www.mayoclinic.org/diseases-conditions/post-traumatic-stress-disorder/basics/definition/con-20022540, accessed July 12, 2016.

26. L. Keefer et al., "Centrally Mediated Disorders of Gastrointestinal Pain," *Gastroenterology* 150, no. 6 (2016): 1408.

27. I. Sanzarello et al., "Central Sensitization in Chronic Low Back Pain: A Narrative Review," *Journal*

of Back and Musculoskeletal Rehabilitation, epub ahead of print (March 2016): [Abstract].

28. A. Akinci et al., "Predictive Factors and Clinical Biomarkers for Treatment in Patients with Chronic Pain Caused by Osteoarthritis with a Central Sensitisation Component," *International Journal of Clinical Practice* 70, no. 1 (January 2016): 31.

29. G. Di Stefano et al., "Central Sensitization as the Mechanism Underlying Pain in Joint Hypermobility Syndrome/Ehlers-Danlos Syndrome, Hypermobility Type," *European Journal of Pain*, epub ahead of print (February 2016): [Abstract].

30. C.M. Campbell et al., "An Evaluation of Central Sensitization in Patients with Sickle Cell Disease," *The Journal of Pain* 17, no. 5 (May 2016): 617.

31. K. Nishioka et al., "Fibromyalgia Syndrome and Cognitive Dysfunction in Elderly: A Case Series," *International Journal of Rheumatic Diseases* 19, no. 1 (January 2016): 21.

32. W.S. Reynolds et al., "Does Central Sensitization Help Explain Idiopathic Overactive Bladder?" *Nature Reviews Urology*, epub ahead of print (June 2016): [Abstract].

33. Leah M. Adams, and Dennis C. Turk, "Psychosocial Factors and Central Sensitivity Syndromes," *Current Rheumatology Reviews* 11, no. 2 (2015): 98.

34. Adam Hadhazy, "Think Twice: How the Gut's 'Second Brain' Influences Mood and Well-Being," *Scientific American* (February 12, 2010): 3.

35. *Ibid.*, 5.

36. *Ibid.*, 4–5.

37. *Ibid.*, 2.

38. *Ibid.*, 3.

39. John Richard Thompson, "Is Irritable Bowel Syndrome an Infectious Disease?" *World Journal of Gastroenterology* 22, no. 4 (January 2016): 1333–1334.

40. *Ibid.*, 1331.

41. Jan Bures et al., "Small Intestinal Bowel Overgrowth," *World Journal of Gastroenterology* 16, no. 24 (June 2010): 2983.

42. For more information on SIBO, visit http://www.SiboInfo.com.

43. For more information on Celiac Disease, visit http://www.Celiac.ca.

44. Centers for Disease Control and Prevention, "Chronic Fatigue Syndrome (CFS): General Information," http://www.cdc.gov/cfs/general/index.html, accessed May 2016.

45. *Ibid.*

46. *Ibid.*

47. *Ibid.*

48. *Ibid.*

49. *Ibid.*

50. Institute of Medicine, "Myalgic Encephalomyelitis/Chronic Fatigue Syndrome (ME/CFS) Key Facts," https://www.nationalacademies.org/hmd/~/media/Files/Report%20Files/2015/MECFS/MECFS_KeyFacts.pdf (February 2015): 1.

51. *Ibid.*

52. *Ibid.*

53. The Institute of Medicine, "Beyond Myalgic Encephalomyelitis/Chronic Fatigue Syndrome: Redefining an Illness" report brief, http://www.national academies.org/hmd/~/media/Files/Report%20Files/2015/MECFS/MECFS_ReportBrief.pdf (February 2015): 4.

54. Institute of Medicine, "Myalgic Encephalomyelitis/Chronic Fatigue Syndrome (ME/CFS) Key Facts," https://www.nationalacademies.org/hmd/~/media/Files/Report%20Files/2015/MECFS/MECFS_KeyFacts.pdf (February 2015): 2.

55. The Institute of Medicine, "Beyond Myalgic Encephalomyelitis/Chronic Fatigue Syndrome: Redefining an Illness" report brief, http://www.national academies.org/hmd/~/media/Files/Report%20Files/2015/MECFS/MECFS_ReportBrief.pdf (February 2015): 4.

56. Nicholas A. Ashford, and Claudia S. Miller, "Case Definitions for Multiple Chemical Sensitivity," in *Multiple Chemical Sensitivities: Addendum to Biologic Markers in Immunotoxicology* (Washington, D.C.: National Academy Press, 1992), 46.

57. "Multiple Chemical Sensitivity: A 1999 Consensus," *Archives of Environmental Health* 54, no. 3 (May/June 1999): 147.

58. *Ibid.*

59. *Ibid.*

60. *Ibid.*

61. *Ibid.*

62. G.E. McKeown-Eyssen et al., "Multiple Chemical Sensitivity: Discriminant Validity of Case Definitions," *Archives of Environmental & Occupational Health* 56, no. 5 (September–October 2001): 406.

63. Claudia S. Miller, "Toxicant-Induced Loss of Tolerance—An Emerging Theory of Disease?" *Environmental Health Perspectives* 105, supplement 2 (March 1997): 445.

64. M.D. Morrison, L.A. Rammage, and A.J. Emami, "The Irritable Larynx Syndrome," *Journal of Voice* 13, no. 3 (1999): 447.

65. Murray Morrison, and Linda Rammage, "The Irritable Larynx Syndrome as a Central Sensitivity Syndrome," *Revue canadienne d'orthophonie et d'audiologie* 34, no. 4 (Hiver 2010): 283.

66. *Ibid.*

67. *Ibid.*

68. *Ibid.*

69. *Ibid.*, 282–89.

70. R.F. Hoy, M. Ribeiro, J. Anderson, and S.M. Tarlo, "Work-Associated Irritable Larynx Syndrome," *Occupational Medicine* 60 (2010): 546–51.

71. L.A. Forrest, T. Husein, and O. Husein, "Paradoxical Vocal Cord Motion: Classification and Treatment," *Laryngoscope* 122, no. 4 (April 2012): 844.

72. Norman Doidge, *The Brain's Way of Healing: Remarkable Discoveries and Recoveries from the Frontiers of Neuroplasticity* (New York: Penguin Books, 2016), 267.

73. *Ibid.*

74. John Steinbeck, *East of Eden* (New York: Penguin Books, 2002), 22.

Chapter 2

1. Saul McLeod, "What is the Stress Response?" SimplyPsychology.org (2010) http://www.simply

psychology.org/stress-biology.html, accessed July 14, 2016.

2. P.C. Konturek, T. Brzozowski, and S.J. Konturek, "Stress and the Gut: Pathophysiology, Clinical Consequences, Diagnostic Approach and Treatment Options," *Journal of Physiology and Pharmacology* 62, no. 6 (December 2011): 591.

3. L.A. Jason et al., "Kindling and Oxidative Stress as Contributors to Myalgic Encephalomyelitis/ Chronic Fatigue Syndrome," *Journal of Behavioral Neuroscience Research* 7, no. 2 (January 2009): 3.

4. *Ibid.*

5. *Ibid.*

6. Kelly McGonigal, "How To Make Stress Your Friend," *TEDtalk* transcript (June 2013): 2–3.

7. Merriam-Webster, http://www.merriam-webster.com/dictionary/intrinsic, accessed June 2016.

8. Greg Charles Fischer, *Chronic Fatigue Syndrome: A Comprehensive Guide to Symptoms, Treatments, and Solving the Practical Problems of CFS,* 100–103.

9. Wikipedia, "Autonomic Nervous System," https://en.wikipedia.org/wiki/Autonomic_nervous_system, accessed July 14, 2016.

10. Aniruddh D. Patel, *Music and the Brain* (Chantilly: The Great Courses, 2015), 117.

11. Mayo Clinic, "Chronic Stress Puts Your Health at Risk," http://www.mayoclinic.org/healthy-lifestyle/stress-management/in-depth/stress/art-20046037, accessed July 14, 2016.

12. John Berger, *Pig Earth* (New York: Vintage Books, 1992), 2.

13. Kelly McGonigal, and Tami Simon, "Kelly McGonigal: The Neuroscience of Change" interview transcript, SoundsTrue.com *Insights at the Edge* (April 19, 2012): 12.

14. From the Penguin bestselling anthology: *Love Poems from God...* copyright 2002 by Daniel Ladinsky and used with his permission.

Chapter 3

1. This essay first published in *The Healing Muse,* Fall 2015 issue.

2. Orthostatic Intolerance is a condition in which symptoms worsen when a person stands or sits upright and improve when the person lies back down. One of the major symptoms of this condition is an abnormally rapid heart rate, known as tachycardia. This is one of those cases in which we have some symptom overlap, and the newness of these conditions and terminology can create some confusion as well. The Institute of Medicine lists Orthostatic Intolerance as a symptom of CFS, but Melissa Cortez, Director and Founder of the Autonomic Physiology Lab in Utah, sees Orthostatic Intolerance as not so much a symptom of CFS, but rather a condition that probably about 30 percent of those with CFS have. (She states this in her April 2016 Bateman Horne Center presentation "Remaining Upright: Approach to Orthostatic Intolerance.")

To make the matter more confusing, Orthostatic Intolerance is closely related to Postural Orthostatic Tachycardia Syndrome (POTS), which some consider to be a CSS in its own right, having some symptom overlap with CFS. (For more information about POTS please see *Appendix F: Recommended Reading and Viewing* at the end of the book.) Is POTS the same as Orthostatic Intolerance, and should we lump them both in as symptoms of CFS? Good questions, and luckily, not ones we need to answer right here. We can allow the research scientists time to find clarity. For now, let's just say that the three conditions all share the symptom of tachycardia, and if you experience an abnormally rapid heart rate with minimal exertion and/or postural change, you should notify your doctor.

3. Institute of Medicine, "Myalgic Encephalomyelitis/Chronic Fatigue Syndrome (ME/CFS) Key Facts," https://www.nationalacademies.org/hmd/~/media/Files/Report%20Files/2015/MECFS/MECFS_KeyFacts.pdf (February 2015): 1.

4. Centers for Disease Control and Prevention, "Fibromyalgia: Background," http://www.cdc.gov/arthritis/basics/fibromyalgia.htm, accessed July 15, 2016.

5. Centers for Disease Control and Prevention, "Chronic Fatigue Syndrome: Managing Activities and Exercise," www.cdc.gov/cfs/management/managing-activities.html, accessed July 15, 2016.

6. J.E. Sumpton, and D.E. Moulin, "Fibromyalgia," *Handbook of Clinical Neurology* 119 (2014): 513.

7. Christa Wolf, *In the Flesh,* trans. John S. Barrett (Jaffrey, NH: David R. Godine, Publisher, 2002), 96.

Chapter 4

1. Centers for Disease Control and Prevention, "Chronic Fatigue Syndrome: Managing Activities and Exercise," www.cdc.gov/cfs/management/managing-activities.html, accessed July 15, 2016.

2. The 2011 PACE trials (P.D. White et al., "Comparison of Adaptive Pacing Therapy, Cognitive Behaviour Therapy, Graded Exercise Therapy, and Specialist Medical Care for Chronic Fatigue Syndrome [PACE]: A Randomised Trial," *Lancet* 377 [2011]: 823–36) claimed that GET was an effective treatment for CFS, but these trials have been discredited. (If you'd like to learn more about the PACE trials and the ensuing controversy, David Tuller's blog list at http://www.virology.ws/mecfs is a good place to start.) As a consequence, many folks came to believe that *all* exercise, including GET, will harm folks with CFS. Do not make this mistake. The takeaway from the PACE trials is that GET cannot cure CFS, and that if GET is done incorrectly, or if one exercises/ exerts beyond one's functional capacity, this can worsen symptoms. But what if someone with CFS or other CSS uses GET appropriately? Read on and find out!

3. Many randomized trials have shown the benefits of exercise for those with CFS; for example, the Cochrane Collaboration's 2015 review (L. Larun, K.G. Brurberg, J. Odgaard-Jensen, and J.R. Price,

"Exercise Therapy for Chronic Fatigue Syndrome [Review]," *The Cochrane Library*, Issue 2 [2015], published by John Wiley & Sons, Ltd.) shows that exercise within the limits of one's functional capacity can improve symptoms and can even expand one's functional capacity somewhat. GET has helped me in this way and more: to recover some functionality following the deconditioning inherent in a crash or relapse, to maintain some muscle tone and strength, to increase my functional capacity to the degree that my brain and body allow, and to nurture and sustain a healthy mental outlook. Perhaps GET can help you with such things too. (As with any strategy, there are no guarantees, but when implemented properly, it may produce helpful results. Employ GET only within the limits of your functional capacity and under the supervision of a medical provider experienced with CSS.)

4. Centers for Disease Control and Prevention, "Chronic Fatigue Syndrome: Managing Activities and Exercise," www.cdc.gov/cfs/management/managing-activities.html, accessed July 15, 2016.

5. Mayo Clinic, "Fitness Training: Elements of a Well-Rounded Routine," www.mayoclinic.org/healthy-lifestyle/fitness/in-depth/fitness-training/art-20044792, accessed July 15, 2016.

6. Centers for Disease Control and Prevention, "Target Heart Rate and Estimated Maximum Heart Rate," http://www.cdc.gov/physicalactivity/basics/measuring/heartrate.htm, accessed July 15, 2016.

7. Mayo Clinic, "Target Heart Rate Tips," www.mayoclinic.org/healthy-lifestyle/fitness/in-depth/exercise-intensity/art-20046887?pg=2, accessed July 15, 2016.

8. Mayo Clinic, "Target Heart Rate Tips," www.mayoclinic.org/healthy-lifestyle/fitness/in-depth/exercise-intensity/art-20046887?pg=2, accessed July 15, 2016.

9. Melissa Cortez, "Remaining Upright: Approach to Orthostatic Intolerance," *Bateman Horne Center* presentation (April 2016) https://www.youtube.com/watch?v=_eydfpVtb0c, accessed July 14, 2016.

10. From the Penguin bestselling anthology: *Love Poems from God...* copyright 2002 by Daniel Ladinsky and used with his permission.

11. Wei Taotao, Chen Chang, Hou Jingwu, Xin Wenjuan, and Mori Akitane, "Nitric Oxide Induces Oxidative Stress and Apoptosis in Neuronal Cells" *Biochimica et Biophysica Acta (BBA)-Molecular Cell Research* 1498, no. 1 (October 2000): 72–79.

12. L.A. Jason et al., "Kindling and Oxidative Stress as Contributors to Myalgic Encephalomyelitis/Chronic Fatigue Syndrome," *Journal of Behavioral Neuroscience Research* 7, no. 2 (January 2009): 4.

13. Jie Xiao, Sheng Xi, Zhang Xinyu, Guo Mengqi, and Ji Xiaoping, "Curcumin Protects Against Myocardial Infarction-Induced Cardiac Fibrosis Via SIRT1 Activation in Vivo and in Vitro," *Drug Design, Development and Therapy* 10 (March 2016): 1267.

14. While there is no definitive treatment or solution yet for CS or CSS, some recent research supports the use of certain antioxidant supplements for decreasing symptoms. For example, results from a 2013 study, "demonstrated that [alpha lipoic acid] presents an antioxidant capacity and the ability to regenerate other antioxidants, which is essential to treat the central sensitization diseases." Translation: alpha lipoic acid has been shown to help the body increase its production of natural antioxidants and dispose of oxidants.

M. Durand, and N. Mach, "Alpha Lipoic Acid and Its Antioxidant Against Cancer and Diseases of Central Sensitization," [in Spanish,] *Nutrición Hospitalaria* 28, no. 4 (July–August 2013): 1031.

15. Christa Wolf, *City of Angels or, The Overcoat of Dr. Freud*, trans. Damion Searls (New York: Farrar, Straus and Giroux, 2010), 226.

Chapter 5

1. This essay was first published in *Folia Literary Magazine*, Winter 2016 issue.

2. Leah M. Adams, and Dennis C. Turk, "Psychosocial Factors and Central Sensitivity Syndromes," *Current Rheumatology Reviews* 11, no. 2 (2015): 96.

3. Merriam-Webster, http://www.merriam-webster.com/dictionary/emotion, accessed July 16, 2016.

4. Rachael E. Jack, Oliver G.B. Garrod, and Philippe G. Schyns, "Dynamic Facial Expressions of Emotion Transmit an Evolving Hierarchy of Signals over Time," *Current Biology* 24, no. 2 (January 2014): 191.

5. Anne Katherine, *Boundaries: Where You End and I Begin* (New York: Fireside, 2000), 67.

6. *Ibid.*

7. From the Penguin bestselling anthology: *Love Poems from God...* copyright 2002 by Daniel Ladinsky and used with his permission.

8. A version of this essay was published in TRANSITION Magazine, Summer 2016 issue.

9. Canadian Mental Health Association, "What Are Mental Illnesses?" http://www.cmha.ca/mental_health/mental-illness/#.Vz3D5yMrK00, accessed July 16, 2016.

10. BC Women's Hospital, "Symptoms of Fibromyalgia," http://www.bcwomens.ca/health-info/living-with-illness/fibromyalgia, accessed July 16, 2016.

11. National Association of Cognitive-Behavioral Therapists, "What is Cognitive-Behavioral Therapy (CBT)?" http://www.nacbt.org/whatiscbt-htm/, accessed July 16, 2016.

12. Jason M. Satterfield, *Cognitive Behavioral Therapy* (Chantilly: The Great Courses, 2015), 4.

13. Amy Wenzel, "Modification of Core Beliefs in Cognitive Therapy," in *Standard and Innovative Strategies in Cognitive Behavior Therapy*, ed. Irismar Reis De Oliveira (Rijeka, Croatia: InTech, 2012), 17.

14. Jason M. Satterfield, *Cognitive Behavioral Therapy* (Chantilly: The Great Courses, 2015), 4.

15. Amy Wenzel, "Modification of Core Beliefs in Cognitive Therapy," in *Standard and Innovative Strategies in Cognitive Behavior Therapy*, ed. Irismar Reis De Oliveira (Rijeka, Croatia: InTech, 2012), 17.

16. *Ibid.*

17. *Ibid.*

18. The 2011 PACE trials (P.D. White et al., "Comparison of Adaptive Pacing Therapy, Cognitive Behaviour Therapy, Graded Exercise Therapy, and Specialist Medical Care for Chronic Fatigue Syndrome [PACE]: A Randomised Trial," *Lancet* 377 [2011]: 823–36) claimed that a specific type of CBT was an effective treatment for CFS, but these trials have since been discredited. (If you'd like to learn more about the PACE trials and the ensuing controversy, David Tuller's blog list at http://www.virology.ws/mecfs is a good place to start.) To be clear, I am *not* claiming that CBT can cure CFS or other CSS. My intent is to introduce CBT as a strategy that may help you cope with the changes CFS or other CSS may cause in your life, and help you maintain and/or regain mental health. CBT has helped me greatly in coping with the huge losses and changes my CSS have caused, and has helped me to live a happier, more satisfied life. It has served me well as a coping technique and I hope it may serve you in that way too.

19. Sarah Baldwin-Beneich, "Full Mind," *Brown Medicine* (Winter 2015): 1.

20. Kristin Neff, *Self Compassion: Stop Beating Yourself Up and Leave Insecurity Behind* (New York: HarperCollins, 2011), 41.

21. *Ibid.*, 90–91.

22. Kelly McGonigal, and Tami Simon, "Kelly McGonigal: The Neuroscience of Change" interview transcript, SoundsTrue.com *Insights at the Edge* (April 19, 2012): 16.

23. *Ibid.*

24. Kristin Neff, *Self Compassion: Stop Beating Yourself Up and Leave Insecurity Behind* (New York: HarperCollins, 2011), 111.

25. Kelly McGonigal and Tami Simon, "Kelly McGonigal: The Neuroscience of Change" interview transcript, SoundsTrue.com *Insights at the Edge* (April 19, 2012): 13.

26. *Ibid.*

27. Eudora Welty, *One Writer's Beginnings* (Cambridge: Harvard University Press, 1995), 76.

28. From the Penguin bestselling anthology: *Love Poems from God...* copyright 2002 by Daniel Ladinsky and used with his permission.

Chapter 6

1. Norman Doidge, *The Brain's Way of Healing: Remarkable Discoveries and Recoveries from the Frontiers of Neuroplasticity* (New York: Penguin Books, 2016), 112.

2. *Ibid.*

3. Daniel K. Hall-Flavin, "Depression (Major Depressive Disorder)," from Mayo Clinic's Expert Answers, http://www.mayoclinic.org/natural-remedies-for-depression/expert-answers/faq-20058026, accessed July 17, 2016.

4. *Ibid.*

5. Mayo Clinic, "Melatonin," http://www.mayo clinic.org/drugs-supplements/melatonin/background/hrb-20059770, accessed July 17, 2016.

6. Mayo Clinic, "Weight Loss," http://www.mayo clinic.org/healthy-lifestyle/weight-loss/in-depth/metabolism/art-20046508, accessed July 17, 2016.

7. M.D. Mifflin et al., "A New Predictive Equation for Resting Energy Expenditure in Healthy Individuals," *The American Journal of Clinical Nutrition* 51, no. 2 (February 1990): 241.

8. Wikipedia, "Harris-Benedict Equation," https://en.wikipedia.org/wiki/Harris%E2%80%93Benedict_equation, accessed July 17, 2016.

9. Norman Doidge, *The Brain's Way of Healing: Remarkable Discoveries and Recoveries from the Frontiers of Neuroplasticity* (New York: Penguin Books, 2016), 109.

10. *Ibid.*, 111.

11. Norman Doidge, *The Brain That Changes Itself: Stories of Personal Triumph from the Frontiers of Brain Science* (New York: Viking Penguin, 2007), xiv–xv.

12. *Ibid.*, xv.

13. *Ibid.*

14. J. Nijs et al., "Brain-derived Neurotrophic Factor As a Driving Force Behind Neuroplasticity in Neuropathic and Central Sensitization Pain: A New Therapeutic Target?" *Expert Opinion on Therapeutic Targets* 19, no. 4 (April 2015): 565.

15. Norman Doidge, *The Brain's Way of Healing: Remarkable Discoveries and Recoveries from the Frontiers of Neuroplasticity* (New York: Penguin Books, 2016), 7.

16. *Ibid.*, 7–8.

17. *Ibid.*

18. *Ibid.*

19. Norman Doidge, *The Brain That Changes Itself: Stories of Personal Triumph from the Frontiers of Brain Science* (New York: Viking Penguin, 2007), 59.

20. Norman Doidge, *The Brain's Way of Healing: Remarkable Discoveries and Recoveries from the Frontiers of Neuroplasticity* (New York: Penguin Books, 2016), 8.

21. Norman Doidge, *The Brain That Changes Itself: Stories of Personal Triumph from the Frontiers of Brain Science* (New York: Viking Penguin, 2007), 68.

22. *Ibid.*, 71.

23. *Ibid.*

24. *Ibid.*

25. Norman Doidge, *The Brain's Way of Healing: Remarkable Discoveries and Recoveries from the Frontiers of Neuroplasticity* (New York: Penguin Books, 2016), 90.

26. Norman Doidge, *The Brain That Changes Itself: Stories of Personal Triumph from the Frontiers of Brain Science* (New York: Viking Penguin, 2007), 209.

27. *Ibid.*

28. *Ibid.*, 209–10.

29. *Ibid.*, xvi.

30. *Ibid.*, 243.

31. *Ibid.*, 242.

32. *Ibid.*

33. L.A. Jason et al., "Kindling and Oxidative Stress as Contributors to Myalgic Encephalomyelitis/

Chronic Fatigue Syndrome," *Journal of Behavioral Neuroscience Research* 7, no. 2 (January 2009): 4.

34. Bell et al., "Testing the Neural Sensitization and Kindling Hypothesis for Illness from Low Levels of Environmental Chemicals," *Environmental Health Perspectives* 105, supplement 2 (March 1997): 539–47.

35. L.A. Jason et al., "Kindling and Oxidative Stress as Contributors to Myalgic Encephalomyelitis/Chronic Fatigue Syndrome," *Journal of Behavioral Neuroscience Research* 7, no. 2 (January 2009): 2.

36. *Ibid.*

37. Norman Doidge, *The Brain's Way of Healing: Remarkable Discoveries and Recoveries from the Frontiers of Neuroplasticity* (New York: Penguin Books, 2016), 108–09.

38. D'Agostino, Dominic, with Ari Meisel, "Podcast #44 with Dr. Dominic D'Agostino from The University of South Florida College of Medicine" keto nutrition podcast, LessDoing.com (November 4, 2013), accessed July 18, 2016.

39. G. Morris, and M. Maes, "Mitochondrial Dysfunctions in Myalgic Encephalomyelitis/Chronic Fatigue Syndrome Explained by Activated Immune-Inflammatory, Oxidative and Nitrosative Stress Pathways," *Metabolic Brain Disease* 29, no. 1 (March 2014): 19–36.

40. M. Meeus et al., "The Role of Mitochondrial Dysfunctions Due to Oxidative and Nitrosative Stress in the Chronic Pain or Chronic Fatigue Syndromes and Fibromyalgia Patients: Peripheral and Central Mechanisms as Therapeutic Targets?" *Expert Opinion on Therapeutic Targets* 17, no. 9 (September 2013): 1081–89.

41. Norman Doidge, *The Brain's Way of Healing: Remarkable Discoveries and Recoveries from the Frontiers of Neuroplasticity* (New York: Penguin Books, 2016), 119.

42. *Ibid.*, 140.

43. L.A. Jason et al., "Kindling and Oxidative Stress as Contributors to Myalgic Encephalomyelitis/Chronic Fatigue Syndrome," *Journal of Behavioral Neuroscience Research* 7, no. 2 (January 2009): 4.

44. *Ibid.*

45. *Ibid.*

46. *Ibid.*

47. *Ibid.*

48. *Ibid.*

49. *Ibid.*

50. P. Forte et al., "Evidence for a Difference in Nitric Oxide Biosynthesis Between Healthy Women and Men," *Hypertension* 32 (1998): 730–34.

51. L.A. Jason et al., "Kindling and Oxidative Stress as Contributors to Myalgic Encephalomyelitis/Chronic Fatigue Syndrome," *Journal of Behavioral Neuroscience Research* 7, no. 2 (January 2009): 4.

52. *Ibid.*

53. R.A. Van Konynenburg, "Glutathione Depletion-Methylation Cycle Block, a Hypothesis for the Pathogenesis of Chronic Fatigue Syndrome" poster presented at the *8th International Conference on in International Association of CFS* in Fort Lauderdale, Florida (January 2007).

54. Minori Koga, Anthony V. Serritella, Marcus

M. Messmer, Akiko Hayashi-Takagi, Lynda D. Hester, Solomon H. Snyder, Akira Sawa, and Thomas W. Sedlak. "Glutathione is a Physiologic Reservoir of Neuronal Glutamate," *Biochemical and Biophysical Research Communications* 409, no. 4 (June 2011): 596.

55. *Ibid.*, 600.

56. Jaswinder S. Bains, and Christopher A. Shaw, "Neurodegenerative Disorders in Humans: The Role of Glutathione in Oxidative Stress-Mediated Neuronal Death," *Brain Research Reviews* 25, no. 3 (December 1997): 335.

57. Muhammad B. Yunus, "Editorial Review: An Update on Central Sensitivity Syndromes and the Issues of Nosology and Psychobiology," *Current Rheumatology* Reviews 11 (2015): 78.

58. L.A. Jason et al., "Kindling and Oxidative Stress as Contributors to Myalgic Encephalomyelitis/Chronic Fatigue Syndrome," *Journal of Behavioral Neuroscience Research* 7, no. 2 (January 2009): 12.

59. Terry Wahls, with Eve Adamson, *The Wahls Protocol: A Radical New Way to Treat All Chronic Autoimmune Conditions Using Paleo Principles* (New York: Penguin Group; 2014).

60. D'Agostino, Dominic, with Ari Meisel, "Podcast #44 with Dr. Dominic D'Agostino from The University of South Florida College of Medicine" keto nutrition podcast, LessDoing.com (November 4, 2013), accessed July 18, 2016.

61. *Ibid.*

62. Kristen Mancinelli, *The Ketogenic Diet: The Scientifically Proven Approach to Fast, Healthy Weight Loss* (Berkeley: Ulysses Press, 2015).

63. Norman Doidge, *The Brain's Way of Healing: Remarkable Discoveries and Recoveries from the Frontiers of Neuroplasticity* (New York: Penguin Books, 2016), 109.

64. *Ibid.*, 140, 143.

65. *Ibid.*, 141.

66. *Ibid.*, 142.

67. L. Assis et al., "Low-Level Laser Therapy (808 nm) Reduces Inflammatory Response and Oxidative Stress in Rat Tibialis Anterior Muscle After Cryolesion," *Lasers in Surgery and Medicine* 44, no. 9 (November 2012): 726–35.

68. T. De Marchi et al., "Low-Level Laser Therapy (LLLT) in Human Progressive-Intensity Running: Effects on Exercise Performance, Skeletalmuscle Status, and Oxidative Stress," *Lasers Medical Science* 27, no. 1 (2012): 231–36.

69. Y. Ide, "Phototherapy for Chronic Pain Treatment," *Masui* 58, no. 11 (November 2009): 1401.

70. Norman Doidge, *The Brain's Way of Healing: Remarkable Discoveries and Recoveries from the Frontiers of Neuroplasticity* (New York: Penguin Books, 2016), 110.

71. *Ibid.*

72. S. Enriquez-Geppert, R.J. Huster, and C.S. Herrmann, "Boosting Brain Functions: Improving Executive Functions with Behavioral Training, Neurostimulation, and Neurofeedback," *International Journal of Psychophysiology* 88, no. 1 (April 2013): 1–16.

73. Norman Doidge, *The Brain's Way of Healing: Remarkable Discoveries and Recoveries from the*

Frontiers of Neuroplasticity (New York: Penguin Books, 2016), 6–7.

74. *Ibid.*, 7–8.

75. *Ibid.*, 7.

76. *Ibid.*, 14.

77. *Ibid.*

78. *Ibid.*

79. *Ibid.*, 9.

80. *Ibid.*

81. *Ibid.*, 11.

82. *Ibid.*, 11–12.

83. *Ibid.*, 11.

84. *Ibid.*, 13.

85. *Ibid.*, 15.

86. *Ibid.*

87. Magdalena Sarah Volz, Vanessa Suarez-Contreras, Andrea L Santos Portilla, and Felipe Fregni, "Mental Imagery-Induced Attention Modulates Pain Perception and Cortical Excitability," *BMC Neuroscience* 16 (2015): 1.

88. *Ibid.*

89. Norman Doidge, *The Brain's Way of Healing: Remarkable Discoveries and Recoveries from the Frontiers of Neuroplasticity* (New York: Penguin Books, 2016), 14.

90. Norman Doidge, *The Brain That Changes Itself: Stories of Personal Triumph from the Frontiers of Brain Science* (New York: Viking Penguin, 2007), 202.

91. *Ibid.*, 202–04.

92. *Ibid.*, 203.

93. Norman Doidge, *The Brain's Way of Healing: Remarkable Discoveries and Recoveries from the Frontiers of Neuroplasticity* (New York: Penguin Books, 2016), 215.

94. *Ibid.*

95. *Ibid.*

96. *Ibid.*

97. From the Penguin bestselling anthology: *Love Poems from God...* copyright 2002 by Daniel Ladinsky and used with his permission.

98. Kelly McGonigal, and Tami Simon, "Kelly McGonigal: The Neuroscience of Change" interview transcript, SoundsTrue.com *Insights at the Edge* (April 19, 2012): 15.

99. *Ibid.*

100. Kristin Neff, *Self Compassion: Stop Beating Yourself Up and Leave Insecurity Behind* (New York: HarperCollins Publishers Ltd., 2011).

101. Kelly McGonigal, and Tami Simon, "Kelly McGonigal: The Neuroscience of Change" interview transcript, SoundsTrue.com *Insights at the Edge* (April 19, 2012): 14.

102. From the Penguin bestselling anthology: *Love Poems from God...* copyright 2002 by Daniel Ladinsky and used with his permission.

103. Suzanne Lorenz, and Sam Beasley, *Wealth and Well-Being Workbook: Overcoming Barriers to Financial Independence* (Chico: Any Wind Publishing, 2010), 4.

104. *Ibid.*, 5.

105. From the Penguin bestselling anthology: *Love Poems from God...* copyright 2002 by Daniel Ladinsky and used with his permission.

106. A.T. Masi, and A. Vincent, "A Historical and Clinical Perspective Endorsing Person-Centered Management of Fibromyalgia Syndrome," *Current Rheumatology Reviews* 11, no. 2 (2015): 86.

107. Studies have found several genes to be involved in oxidative stress and ion transport/activity in CFS patients. "Genes from the sympathetic nervous system ... [and] the immune system have also been implicated in CFS." [L.A. Jason et al., "Kindling and Oxidative Stress as Contributors to Myalgic Encephalomyelitis/Chronic Fatigue Syndrome," *Journal of Behavioral Neuroscience Research* 7, no. 2 (January 2009): 6.]

108. Epigenetics is the idea that "gene expression can be altered by specific experiences, and this in turn can lead to organizational changes in the nervous system." [Bryan Kolb, and Robbin Gibb, "Brain Plasticity and Behaviour in the Developing Brain," *Journal of the Canadian Academy of Child and Adolescent Psychiatry* 20, no. 4 (November 2011): 266.] Epigenetics in the context of CS and CSS basically means that if a gene is activated by an experience to contribute to CS and CSS, then deactivation of that gene by another experience would help correct CS and CSS.

109. T. Jackson et al., "Chronic Pain Without Clear Etiology in Low- and Middle-Income Countries: A Narrative Review," *Anesthesia & Analgesia* 122, no. 6 (June 2016): 2028.

110. *Ibid.*

111. A.T. Masi, and A. Vincent, "A Historical and Clinical Perspective Endorsing Person-Centered Management of Fibromyalgia Syndrome," *Current Rheumatology Reviews* 11, no. 2 (2015): 86.

112. Randy Neblett, Howard Cohen, Yunhee Choi, Meredith Hartzell, Mark Williams, Tom G. Mayer, and Robert J. Gatchel, "The Central Sensitization Inventory (CSI): Establishing Clinically-Significant Values for Identifying Central Sensitivity Syndromes in an Outpatient Chronic Pain Sample," *Journal of Pain* 14, no. 5 (May 2013): 438.

113. Randy Neblett, Meredith Hartzell, Tom G. Mayer, Howard Cohen, and Robert J. Gatchel, "Establishing Clinically Relevant Severity Levels for the Central Sensitization Inventory," *Pain Practice* (March 2016).

114. E.A. Dixon et al., "Development of the Sensory Hypersensitivity Scale (SHS): A Self-Report Tool for Assessing Sensitivity to Sensory Stimuli," *Journal of Behavioral Medicine* 39, no. 3 (June 2016): 537.

115. A. Deitos et al., "Clinical Value of Serum Neuroplasticity Mediators in Identifying the Central Sensitivity Syndrome in Patients With Chronic Pain With and Without Structural Pathology," *The Clinical Journal of Pain,* 31, no. 11 (November 2015): 959.

116. J. Nijs et al., "Pain Following Cancer Treatment: Guidelines for the Clinical Classification of Predominant Neuropathic, Nociceptive and Central Sensitization Pain," *Acta Oncologica* 55, no. 6 (June 2016): 659–63.

117. A.C. Shembel, M.J. Sandage, and Abbott K. Verdolini, "Episodic Laryngeal Breathing Disorders: Literature Review and Proposal of Preliminary

Theoretical Framework." *Journal of Voice* 30 (February 2016): 321.

118. Muhammad B. Yunus, "Editorial Review: An Update on Central Sensitivity Syndromes and the Issues of Nosology and Psychobiology," *Current Rheumatology* Reviews 11 (2015): 70.

119. Anna K. Clark, Elizabeth A. Old, and Marzia Malcangio, "Neuropathic Pain and Cytokines: Current Perspectives," *Journal of Pain Research* 6 (November 2013): 803.

120. *Ibid.*, 809.

121. C. Fernández-de-las-Peñas, and J. Dommerholt, "Myofascial Trigger Points: Peripheral or Central Phenomenon?" *Current Rheumatology Reports* 16, no. 1 (January 2014): 395.

122. *Ibid.*

123. *Ibid.*

124. Muhammad B. Yunus, "Editorial Review: An Update on Central Sensitivity Syndromes and the Issues of Nosology and Psychobiology," *Current Rheumatology* Reviews 11 (2015): 70.

125. J.J. Burston et al., "Cannabinoid CB2 Receptors Regulate Central Sensitization and Pain Responses Associated with Osteoarthritis of the Knee Joint," PLoS ONE 8, no. 11 (November 2013): 1, http://journals.plos.org/plosone/article/asset?id=10.1371%2Fjournal.pone.0080440.PDF.

126. Muhammad B. Yunus, "Editorial Review: An Update on Central Sensitivity Syndromes and the Issues of Nosology and Psychobiology," *Current Rheumatology* Reviews 11 (2015): 80.

127. *Ibid.*

128. *Ibid.*

Appendix C

1. Leah M. Adams, and Dennis C. Turk, "Psychosocial Factors and Central Sensitivity Syndromes," *Current Rheumatology Reviews* 11, no. 2 (2015): 96.

2. *Ibid.*

3. *Ibid.*

4. *Ibid.*, 103.

5. *Ibid.*, 97.

6. A.T. Masi, and A. Vincent, "A Historical and Clinical Perspective Endorsing Person-Centered Management of Fibromyalgia Syndrome," *Current Rheumatology Reviews* 11, no. 2 (2015): 86.

7. Muhammad B. Yunus, "Editorial Review: An Update on Central Sensitivity Syndromes and the Issues of Nosology and Psychobiology," *Current Rheumatology* Reviews 11 (2015): 70.

8. Leah M. Adams, and Dennis C. Turk, "Psychosocial Factors and Central Sensitivity Syndromes," *Current Rheumatology Reviews* 11, no. 2 (2015): 97.

9. *Ibid.*

10. D. Hoffman, "Central and Peripheral Pain Generators in Women with Chronic Pelvic Pain Patient Centered Assessment and Treatment," *Current Rheumatology Reviews* 11, no. 2 (2015): 146.

11. Leah M. Adams, and Dennis C. Turk, "Psychosocial Factors and Central Sensitivity Syndromes," *Current Rheumatology Reviews* 11, no. 2 (2015): 99–103.

12. *Ibid.*, 103.

13. *Ibid.*, 97.

14. Donald Bakal, Patrick Coll, and Jeffrey Schaefer, "Somatic Awareness in the Clinical Care of Patients with Body Distress Symptoms," *BioPsychoSocial Medicine* 2 (February 2008): 2.

15. *Ibid.*, 6.

16. *Ibid.*

17. J.E. Sumpton, and D.E. Moulin, "Fibromyalgia," *Handbook of Clinical Neurology* 119 (2014): 513.

18. Muhammad B. Yunus, "Editorial Review: An Update on Central Sensitivity Syndromes and the Issues of Nosology and Psychobiology," *Current Rheumatology* Reviews 11 (2015): 70.

Bibliography

Adams, Leah M., and Dennis C. Turk. "Psychosocial Factors and Central Sensitivity Syndromes." *Current Rheumatology Reviews* 11, no. 2 (2015): 96–108.

Akinci, A., M. Shaker, M.H. Chang, C.W. Cheung, A. Danilov, H. José Dueñas, Y.C. Kim, et al. "Predictive Factors and Clinical Biomarkers for Treatment in Patients with Chronic Pain Caused by Osteoarthritis with a Central Sensitisation Component." *International Journal of Clinical Practice* 70, no. 1 (January 2016): 31–44.

Arseneau, Ric. "Hope for Patients with Fatigue, Pain, and Unexplained Symptoms." University of British Columbia Faculty of Medicine Web site (October 13, 2015): 1–3. http://thischangedmypractice.com/hope-for-patients-with-fatigue-pain-and-unexplained-symptoms/ (accessed July 19, 2016).

Ashford, Nicholas A., and Claudia S. Miller. "Case Definitions for Multiple Chemical Sensitivity." In *Multiple Chemical Sensitivities: Addendum to Biologic Markers in Immunotoxicology*, compiled by National Research Council. Washington, D.C.: The National Academies Press, 1992.

Assis, L., A.I. Moretti, T.B. Abrahão, V. Cury, H.P. Souza, M.R. Hamblin, and N.A. Parizotto. "Low-Level Laser Therapy (808 nm) Reduces Inflammatory Response and Oxidative Stress in Rat Tibialis Anterior Muscle After Cryolesion." *Lasers in Surgery and Medicine* 44, no. 9 (November 2012): 726–35.

"Autonomic Nervous System." *Wikipedia*. https://en.wikipedia.org/wiki/Autonomic_nervous_system (accessed July 14, 2016).

BC Women's Hospital. "Symptoms of Fibromyalgia." http://www.bcwomens.ca/health-info/living-with-illness/fibromyalgia (accessed July 16, 2016).

_____. "What Is Fibromyalgia." http://www.bcwomens.ca/health-info/living-with-illness/fibromyalgia (accessed July 12, 2016).

Bains, Jaswinder S., and Christopher A. Shaw. "Neurodegenerative Disorders in Humans: The Role of Glutathione in Oxidative Stress-Mediated Neuronal Death." *Brain Research Reviews* 25, no. 3 (December 1997): 335–58.

Bakal, Donald, Patrick Coll, and Jeffrey Schaefer. "Somatic Awareness in the Clinical Care of Patients with Body Distress Symptoms." *BioPsychoSocial Medicine* 2 (February 2008): 1–6.

Baldwin-Beneich, Sarah. "Full Mind." *Brown Medicine* (Winter 2015): 1–4.

Bell, I.R., J. Rossi 3rd, M.E. Gilbert, G. Kobal, L.A. Morrow, D.B. Newlin, B.A. Sorg, and R.W. Wood. "Testing the Neural Sensitization and Kindling Hypothesis for Illness from Low Levels of Environmental Chemicals." *Environmental Health Perspectives* 105. Suppl. no. 2 (March 1997): 539–47.

Berger, John. *Pig Earth*. New York: Vintage Books, 1992.

Bures, Jan, Jiri Cyrany, Darina Kohoutova, Miroslav Förstl, Stanislav Rejchrt, Jaroslav Kvetina, Viktor Vorisek, and Marcela Kopacova. "Small Intestinal Bowel Overgrowth." *World Journal of Gastroenterology* 16, no. 24 (June 2010): 2978–90.

Burston, J.J., D.R. Sagar, P. Shao, M. Bai, E. King, L. Brailsford, J.M. Turner, et al. "Cannabinoid CB2 Receptors Regulate Central Sensitization and Pain Responses Associated with Osteoarthritis of the Knee Joint." *PLoS ONE* 8, no. 11 (November 2013): 1–9. http://journals.plos.org/plosone/article/asset?id=10.1371%2Fjournal.pone.0080440.PDF.

Campbell, C.M., G. Moscou-Jackson, C.P. Carroll, K. Kiley, C. Haywood, Jr., S. Lanzkron, M. Hand, R.R. Edwards, and J.A. Haythornthwaite. "An Evaluation of Central Sensitization in Patients with Sickle Cell Disease." *The Journal of Pain* 17, no. 5 (May 2016): 617–27.

Canadian Mental Health Association. "What Are Mental Illnesses?" http://www.cmha.ca/mental_health/mental-illness/#.Vz3D5yMrK00 (accessed July 16, 2016).

Centers for Disease Control and Prevention. "Chronic Fatigue Syndrome (CFS): General Information." http://www.cdc.gov/cfs/general/index.html (accessed July 15, 2016).

_____. "Chronic Fatigue Syndrome: Managing Activities and Exercise." http://www.cdc.gov/cfs/management/managing-activities.html (accessed July 15, 2016).

_____. "Fibromyalgia: Background." http://www.cdc.gov/arthritis/basics/fibromyalgia.htm (accessed July 15, 2016).

_____. "Target Heart Rate and Estimated Maximum Heart Rate." http://www.cdc.gov/physicalactivity/basics/measuring/heartrate.htm (accessed July 15, 2016).

Clark, Anna K., Elizabeth A. Old, and Marzia Malcangio. "Neuropathic Pain and Cytokines: Current Perspectives." *Journal of Pain Research* 6 (November 2013): 803–14.

Cortez, Melissa. "Remaining Upright: Approach to Orthostatic Intolerance," *Bateman Horne Center* presentation (April 2016). https://www.youtube.com/watch?v=_eydfpVtb0c (accessed July 14, 2016).

D'Agostino, Dominic, with Ari Meisel. "Podcast #44 with Dr. Dominic D'Agostino from The University of South Florida College of Medicine," keto nutrition podcast. LessDoing.com (November 4, 2013). http://www.lessdoing.com/podcasts/2013/11/04/podcast-44-with-dr-dominic-dagostino-from-the-university-of-south-florida-college-of-medicine (accessed July 18, 2016).

De Marchi, T., E.C. Leal Junior, C. Bortoli, S.S. Tomazoni, R.A. Lopes-Martins, and M. Salvador. "Low-Level Laser Therapy (LLLT) in Human Progressive-Intensity Running: Effects on Exercise Performance, Skeletalmuscle Status, and Oxidative Stress." *Lasers Medical Science* 27, no. 1 (2012): 231–36.

de Tommaso, M., and C. Fernández-de-Las-Peñas. "Tensions Type Headache." *Current Rheumatology Review* 12, no. 2 (2016): 127–39.

Deitos, A., J.A. Dussán-Sarria, Ad Souza, L. Medeiros, Mda G. Tarragô, F. Sehn, M. Chassot, et al. "Clinical Value of Serum Neuroplasticity Mediators in Identifying the Central Sensitivity Syndrome in Patients With Chronic Pain With and Without Structural Pathology." *The Clinical Journal of Pain,* 31, no. 11 (November 2015): 959–67.

Di Stefano, G., C. Celletti, R. Baron, M. Castori, M. Di Franco, S. La Cesa, C. Leone, et al. "Central Sensitization as the Mechanism Underlying Pain in Joint Hypermobility Syndrome/Ehlers-Danlos Syndrome, Hypermobility Type." *European Journal of Pain*, epub ahead of print (February 2016): [Abstract].

Dixon, E.A., G. Benham, J.A. Sturgeon, S. Mackey, K.A. Johnson, and J. Younger. "Development of the Sensory Hypersensitivity Scale (SHS): A Self-Report Tool for Assessing Sensitivity to Sensory Stimuli." *Journal of Behavioral Medicine* 39, no. 3 (June 2016): 537–50.

Doidge, Norman. *The Brain That Changes Itself: Stories of Personal Triumph from the Frontiers of Brain Science*. New York: Viking Penguin, 2007.

_____. *The Brain's Way of Healing: Remarkable Discoveries and Recoveries from the Frontiers of Neuroplasticity*. New York: Penguin Books, 2016.

Durand, M., and N. Mach. "Alpha Lipoic Acid and Its Antioxidant Against Cancer and Diseases of Central Sensitization." [In Spanish.] *Nutrición Hospitalaria* 28, no. 4 (July–August 2013): 1031–38.

Enriquez-Geppert, S., R.J. Huster, and C.S. Herrmann. "Boosting Brain Functions: Improving Executive Functions with Behavioral Training, Neurostimulation, and Neurofeedback." *International Journal of Psychophysiology* 88, no. 1 (April 2013): 1–16.

Fernández-de-las-Peñas, C., and J. Dommerholt. "Myofascial Trigger Points: Peripheral or Central Phenomenon?" *Current Rheumatology Reports* 16, no. 1 (January 2014): 395.

Fischer, Greg Charles. *Chronic Fatigue Syndrome: A Comprehensive Guide to Symptoms, Treatments, and Solving the Practical Problems of CFS*. New York: Warner Books, Inc., 1997.

Forrest, L.A., T. Husein, and O. Husein. "Paradoxical Vocal Cord Motion: Classification and Treatment." *Laryngoscope* 122, no. 4 (April 2012): 844–53.

Forte, P., B.J. Kneale, E. Milne, P.J. Chowienczyk, A. Johnston, N. Benjamin, and J.M. Ritter. "Evidence for a Difference in Nitric Oxide Biosynthesis Between Healthy Women and Men." *Hypertension* 32 (1998): 730–34.

Hadhazy, Adam. "Think Twice: How the Gut's 'Second Brain' Influences Mood and Well-Being." *Scientific American* (February 12, 2010): 1–8.

Hall-Flavin, Daniel K. "Depression (Major Depressive Disorder)." *Expert Answers*. http://www.mayoclinic.org/natural-remedies-for-depression/expert-answers/faq-20058026 (accessed July 17, 2016).

"Harris-Benedict Equation." *Wikipedia*. https://en.wikipedia.org/wiki/Harris%E2%80%93Benedict_equation (accessed July 17, 2016).

Hoffman, D. "Central and Peripheral Pain Generators in Women with Chronic Pelvic Pain Patient Centered Assessment and Treatment." *Current Rheumatology Reviews* 11, no. 2 (2015): 146–66.

Hoy, R.F., M. Ribeiro, J. Anderson, and S.M. Tarlo. "Work-Associated Irritable Larynx Syndrome." *Occupational Medicine* 60 (2010): 546–51.

Ide, Y. "Phototherapy for Chronic Pain Treatment." *Masui* 58, no. 11 (November 2009): 1401–06.

Integrated Chronic Care Service. "Multiple Chemical Sensitivity (MCS)." http://www.cdha.nshealth.ca/integrated-chronic-care-service-iccs/patients/multiple-chemical-sensitivity-mcs (accessed July 12, 2006).

Jack, Rachael E., Oliver G.B. Garrod, and Philippe G. Schyns. "Dynamic Facial Expressions of Emotion Transmit an Evolving Hierarchy of Signals over Time." *Current Biology* 24, no. 2 (January 2014): 187–92.

Jackson, T., S. Thomas, V. Stabile, X. Han, M. Shotwell, and K.A. McQueen, "Chronic Pain Without Clear Etiology in Low- and Middle-Income Countries: A Narrative Review." *Anesthesia & Analgesia* 122, no. 6 (June 2016): 2028–39.

Jason, L.A., N. Porter, J. Herrington, M. Sorenson, and S. Kubow. "Kindling and Oxidative Stress as Contributors to Myalgic Encephalomyelitis/Chronic Fatigue Syndrome." *Journal of Behavioral Neuroscience Research* 7, no. 2 (January 2009): 1–17.

Katherine, Anne. *Boundaries: Where You End and I Begin*. New York: Fireside, 2000.

Keefer, L., D.A. Drossman, E. Guthrie, M. Simrén, K. Tillisch, K. Olden, and P.J. Whorwell. "Centrally Mediated Disorders of Gastrointestinal Pain." *Gastroenterology* 150, no. 6 (2016): 1408–19.

Kinder, L.L., R.M. Bennett, and K.D. Jones. "Central Sensitivity Syndromes: Mounting Pathophysiologic Evidence to Link Fibromyalgia with other Common Chronic Pain Disorders." *Pain Management Nursing* 12, no. 1 (March 2011): 15–24.

Kolb, Bryan, and Robbin Gibb. "Brain Plasticity and

Behaviour in the Developing Brain." *Journal of the Canadian Academy of Child and Adolescent Psychiatry* 20, no. 4 (November 2011): 265–76.

Koga, Minori, Anthony V. Serritella, Marcus M. Messmer, Akiko Hayashi-Takagi, Lynda D. Hester, Solomon H. Snyder, Akira Sawa, and Thomas W. Sedlak. "Glutathione is a Physiologic Reservoir of Neuronal Glutamate." *Biochemical and Biophysical Research Communications* 409, no. 4 (June 2011): 596–602.

Konturek, P.C., T. Brzozowski, and S.J. Konturek. "Stress and the Gut: Pathophysiology, Clinical Consequences, Diagnostic Approach and Treatment Options." *Journal of Physiology and Pharmacology* 62, no. 6 (December 2011): 591–99.

Ladinsky, Daniel, trans. *Love Poems from God: Twelve Sacred Voices from the East and West.* New York: Penguin Compass, 2002.

Lorenz, Suzanne, and Sam Beasley. *Wealth and Well-Being Workbook: Overcoming Barriers to Financial Independence.* Chico: Any Wind Publishing, 2010.

Mancinelli, Kristen. *The Ketogenic Diet: The Scientifically Proven Approach to Fast, Healthy Weight Loss.* Berkeley: Ulysses Press, 2015.

Masi, A.T., and A. Vincent. "A Historical and Clinical Perspective Endorsing Person-Centered Management of Fibromyalgia Syndrome." *Current Rheumatology Reviews* 11, no. 2 (2015): 86–95.

Mayo Clinic. "Chronic Fatigue Syndrome: Definition." http://www.mayoclinic.org/diseases-conditions/chronic-fatigue-syndrome/basics/definition/con-20022009 (accessed July 12, 2016).

_____. "Chronic Stress Puts Your Health at Risk." http://www.mayoclinic.org/healthy-lifestyle/stress-management/in-depth/stress/art-20046037 (accessed July 14, 2016).

_____. "Fitness Training: Elements of a Well-Rounded Routine." www.mayoclinic.org/healthy-lifestyle/fitness/in-depth/fitness-training/art-20044792 (accessed July 15, 2016).

_____. "Irritable Bowel Syndrome: Definition." http://www.mayoclinic.org/diseases-conditions/irritable-bowel-syndrome/basics/definition/con-20024578 (accessed July 12, 2016).

_____. "Melatonin." http://www.mayoclinic.org/drugs-supplements/melatonin/background/hrb-20059770 (accessed July 17, 2016).

_____. "Migraine: Overview." http://www.mayoclinic.org/diseases-conditions/migraine-headache/basics/definition/con-20026358 (accessed July 12, 2016).

_____. "Myofascial Pain Syndrome: Definition." http://www.mayoclinic.org/diseases-conditions/myofascial-pain-syndrome/basics/definition/con-20033195 (accessed July 12, 2016).

_____. "Post-Traumatic Stress Disorder: Definition." http://www.mayoclinic.org/diseases-conditions/post-traumatic-stress-disorder/basics/definition/con-20022540 (accessed July 12, 2016).

_____. "Target Heart Rate Tips." www.mayoclinic.org/healthy-lifestyle/fitness/in-depth/exercise-intensity/art-20046887?pg=2 (accessed July 15, 2016).

_____. "Weight Loss." http://www.mayoclinic.org/healthy-lifestyle/weight-loss/in-depth/metabolism/art-20046508 (accessed July 17, 2016).

McGonigal, Kelly. "How To Make Stress Your Friend." *TEDtalk* transcript (June 2013): 1–8. http://www.ted.com/talks/kelly_mcgonigal_how_to_make_stress_your_friend/transcript?language=en.

_____, and Tami Simon. "Kelly McGonigal: The Neuroscience of Change," interview transcript. SoundsTrue.com *Insights at the Edge* (April 19, 2012): 1–20.

McKeown-Eyssen, G.E., C.J. Baines, L.M. Marshall, V. Jazmaji, and E.R. Sokoloff, "Multiple Chemical Sensitivity: Discriminant Validity of Case Definitions." *Archives of Environmental & Occupational Health* 56, no. 5 (September–October 2001): 406–12.

McLeod, Saul. "What is the Stress Response?" Simply Psychology.org (2010). http://www.simplypsychology.org/stress-biology.html (accessed July 14, 2016).

Meeus, M., J. Nijs, L. Hermans, D. Goubert, and P. Calders. "The Role of Mitochondrial Dysfunctions Due to Oxidative and Nitrosative Stress in the Chronic Pain or Chronic Fatigue Syndromes and Fibromyalgia Patients: Peripheral and Central Mechanisms as Therapeutic Targets?" *Expert Opinion on Therapeutic Targets* 17, no. 9 (September 2013): 1081–89.

Mifflin, M.D., S.T. St. Jeor, L.A. Hill, B.J. Scott, S.A. Daugherty, and Y.O. Koh. "A New Predictive Equation for Resting Energy Expenditure in Healthy Individuals." *The American Journal of Clinical Nutrition* 51, no. 2 (February 1990): 241–47.

Miller, Claudia S. "Toxicant-Induced Loss of Tolerance—An Emerging Theory of Disease?" *Environmental Health Perspectives* 105. Suppl. no. 2 (March 1997): 445–53.

Morris, G., and M. Maes. "Mitochondrial Dysfunctions in Myalgic Encephalomyelitis/Chronic Fatigue Syndrome Explained by Activated Immune-Inflammatory, Oxidative and Nitrosative Stress Pathways." *Metabolic Brain Disease* 29, no. 1 (March 2014): 19–36.

Morrison, Murray, Linda Rammage, and A.J. Emami. "The Irritable Larynx Syndrome." *Journal of Voice* 13, no. 3 (1999): 447–55.

_____, and Linda Rammage. "The Irritable Larynx Syndrome as a Central Sensitivity Syndrome." *Revue canadienne d'orthophonie et d'audiologie* 34, no. 4 (Hiver 2010): 282–89.

"Multiple Chemical Sensitivity: A 1999 Consensus." *Archives of Environmental Health* 54, no. 3 (May/June 1999): 147–49.

National Association of Cognitive-Behavioral Therapists. "What is Cognitive-Behavioral Therapy (CBT)?" http://www.nacbt.org/whatiscbt-htm/ (accessed July 16, 2016).

National Heart, Lung, and Blood Institute. "What Is Restless Legs Syndrome?" http://www.nhlbi.nih.gov/health/health-topics/topics/rls/ (accessed July 12, 2006).

National Sleep Foundation. "Periodic Limb Movements in Sleep." https://sleepfoundation.org/sleep-disorders-problems/sleep-related-movement-dis orders/periodic-limb-movement-disorder (accessed July 12, 2006).

Neblett, Randy, Meredith Hartzell, Tom G. Mayer, Howard Cohen, and Robert J. Gatchel. "Establishing Clinically Relevant Severity Levels for the Central Sensitization Inventory." *Pain Practice* (March 2016).

_____, Howard Cohen, Yunhee Choi, Meredith Hartzell, Mark Williams, Tom G. Mayer, and Robert J. Gatchel. "The Central Sensitization Inventory (CSI): Establishing Clinically-Significant Values for Identifying Central Sensitivity Syndromes in an Outpatient Chronic Pain Sample." *Journal of Pain* 14, no. 5 (May 2013): 438–45.

Neff, Kristin. *Self Compassion: The Proven Power of Being Kind to* Yourself. New York: HarperCollins, 2011.

Nijs, J., M. Meeus, J. Versijpt, M. Moens, I. Bos, K. Knaepen, and R. Meeusen. "Brain-derived Neurotrophic Factor As a Driving Force Behind Neuroplasticity in Neuropathic and Central Sensitization Pain: A New Therapeutic Target?" *Expert Opinion on Therapeutic Targets* 19, no. 4 (April 2015): 565–76.

_____, L. Leysen, N. Adriaenssens, M.E. Aguilar Ferrándiz, N. Devoogdt, A. Tassenoy, K. Ickmans, et al. "Pain Following Cancer Treatment: Guidelines for the Clinical Classification of Predominant Neuropathic, Nociceptive and Central Sensitization Pain." *Acta Oncologica* 55, no. 6 (June 2016): 659–63.

Nishioka, K., T. Hayashi, M. Suzuki, Y. Li, S. Nakayama, T. Matsushima, C. Usui, et al. "Fibromyalgia Syndrome and Cognitive Dysfunction in Elderly: A Case Series." *International Journal of Rheumatic Diseases* 19, no. 1 (January 2016): 21–29.

Patel, Aniruddh D. *Music and the Brain.* Chantilly: The Great Courses, 2015.

Reynolds, W.S., R. Dmochowski, A. Wein, and S. Bruehl, "Does Central Sensitization Help Explain Idiopathic Overactive Bladder?" *Nature Reviews Urology*, epub ahead of print (June 2016): [Abstract].

Sanzarello, I., L. Merlini, M.A. Rosa, M. Perrone, J. Frugiuele, R. Borghi, and C. Faldini. "Central Sensitization in Chronic Low Back Pain: A Narrative Review." *Journal of Back and Musculoskeletal Rehabilitation,* epub ahead of print (March 2016): [Abstract].

Satterfield, Jason M. *Cognitive Behavioral* Therapy. Chantilly: The Great Courses, 2015.

Shembel, A.C., M.J. Sandage, and Abbott K. Verdolini. "Episodic Laryngeal Breathing Disorders: Literature Review and Proposal of Preliminary Theoretical Framework." *Journal of Voice* 30 (February 2016): 321–25.

Steinbeck, John. *East of Eden.* New York: Penguin Books, 2002.

Sumpton, J.E., and D.E. Moulin. "Fibromyalgia." *Handbook of Clinical Neurology* 119 (2014): 513–27.

Taotao, Wei, Chen Chang, Hou Jingwu, Xin Wenjuan, and Mori Akitane, "Nitric Oxide Induces Oxidative Stress and Apoptosis in Neuronal Cells."

Biochimica et Biophysica Acta (BBA)—Molecular Cell Research 1498, no. 1 (October 2000): 72–79.

The Institute of Medicine. "Beyond Myalgic Encephalomyelitis/Chronic Fatigue Syndrome: Redefining an Illness." *The Institute of Medicine* report brief (February 2015): 1–4. http://www. nationalacademies.org/hmd/~/media/Files/ Report%20Files/2015/MECFS/MECF S_Report-Brief.pdf.

_____. "Myalgic Encephalomyelitis/Chronic Fatigue Syndrome (ME/CFS) Key Facts." *The Institute of Medicine* (February 2015): 1–2. https://www.national academies.org/hmd/~/media/Files/Report% 20Files/2015/MECFS/MEC FS_KeyFacts.pdf.

Thompson, John Richard. "Is Irritable Bowel Syndrome an Infectious Disease?" *World Journal of Gastroenterology* 22, no. 4 (January 2016): 1331–34.

Van Konynenburg, R.A. "Glutathione Depletion-Methylation Cycle Block, a Hypothesis for the Pathogenesis of Chronic Fatigue Syndrome," poster presented at the *8th International Conference of the International Association of CFS* in Fort Lauderdale, Florida (January 2007).

Volz, Magdalena Sarah, Vanessa Suarez-Contreras, Andrea L Santos Portilla, and Felipe Fregni. "Mental Imagery-Induced Attention Modulates Pain Perception and Cortical Excitability." *BMC Neuroscience* 16 (2015): 1–10.

Wahls, Terry, with Eve Adamson. *The Wahls Protocol: A Radical New Way to Treat All Chronic Autoimmune Conditions Using Paleo Principles.* New York: Penguin Group, 2014.

Welty, Eudora. *One Writer's Beginnings.* Cambridge: Harvard University Press, 1984.

Wenzel, Amy. "Modification of Core Beliefs in Cognitive Therapy." In *Standard and Innovative Strategies in Cognitive Behavior Therapy,* edited by Irismar Reis De Oliveira. Rijeka, Croatia: InTech, 2012.

Wolf, Christa. *City of Angels or, The Overcoat of Dr. Freud.* Translated by Damion Searls. New York: Farrar, Straus and Giroux, 2010.

_____. *In the Flesh.* Translated by John S. Barrett. Jaffrey, NH: David R. Godine, Publisher, 2002.

Xiao, Jie, Sheng Xi, Zhang Xinyu, Guo Mengqi, and Ji Xiaoping. "Curcumin Protects Against Myocardial Infarction-Induced Cardiac Fibrosis Via SIRT1 Activation in Vivo and in Vitro." *Drug Design, Development and Therapy* 10 (March 2016): 1267–77.

Yunus, Muhammad B. "Central Sensitivity Syndromes: A Unified Concept for Fibromyalgia and Other Similar Maladies." *Journal of Indian Rheumatism Association* 8 (2000): 27–33.

_____. "Editorial Review: An Update on Central Sensitivity Syndromes and the Issues of Nosology and Psychobiology." *Current Rheumatology Reviews* 11 (2015): 70–85.

_____. "Fibromyalgia and Overlapping Disorders: The Unifying Concept of Central Sensitivity Syndromes." *Seminars in Arthritis and Rheumatism* 36 (2007): 339–56.

Index

Numbers in **bold italics** indicate pages with charts, diagrams or tables.

IBS *see* irritable bowel syndrome
identity 2, 28, 63, 130–31, 135–36, 143; *see also* de-identification; loss
idiopathic 9
ILS *see* irritable larynx syndrome
immune function 14–15, 88, 183, 201–2, 229
immunology 200, 202
income assistance 194
infection 9, 16, 24, 88, 179, 201
inflammation 9, 12, 18, 24, 87–89, 110; author's 13, 26, 92–93, 154, 164, 219; decreasing 107, 115, 183, 201–2; diet and 25, 64; *see also* cytokines; dorsal horn
Institute of Medicine 1, 17, 88, 225*ch3n2*
insurance 7, 38, 90, 138, 142–43, 145, 152, 194, 196, 214; *see also* disability insurance; money; workers compensation
intensive bubble time *see* bubble time, intensive
interstitial cystitis 12, *34*
intrinsic trigger 34–38, *37*, 46, 61, 82, 93, 117, 120, 175, 178, 199, 210, 217; decreasing impact 38–39, 51, 68, 71, 90–91, 96–97, 103, 108; load 36, 122–23, 125, 141, 171; *see also* stressors; triggers
iodine 115–16
irritable bowel syndrome 10, 12–13, 16, 32, *33*, 88, 174, 186
irritable larynx syndrome 5, 13, 62, 83, 182, 186, 196, 201; complexity 24; definition 11, 21–24, 32; depression and 148; fear and 74; management 24–28, 68, 70, 73, 92, 114, 141, 155, 178; triggers 33, *33*, 36, *36–37*, 46–47, 122; voice loss 29; *see also* larynx; vocal therapist; voice; work-associated irritable larynx syndrome
isolation 55, 61, 101, 128, 149, 164, 167

joint hypermobility syndrome *see* Ehlers Danlos syndrome
joint pain *see* pain
journaling 129, 161–61, 164, 209; *see also* writing

Kabat-Zinn, Jon 153
Katherine, Anne 141, 222
ketosis 181–82, 221
kindling 178, 180
klonopin 180

Ladinsky, Daniel 222
larynx 11, 21–29, 32–33, 62–67, 73, 145–46, 201; *see also* irritable larynx syndrome; neck muscles; work-associated irritable larynx syndrome
laundry 81, 164, 207, 218, 220; facilities 45–50, 62, 79–80, 144; pacing and 56, *77*, 78–79, 104,

110, 112, 136, 152, 166; products 20, 36, 47, 117, 119, 161, 208, 210–11
legal assistance 194, 198
light therapy 183; *see also* low level laser therapy
limbic system 30, 32, 52, 63; *see also* amygdala; fear
LLLT *see* low level laser therapy
localized pain 11; *see also* pain
loneliness 5–7, 54–55, 87; *see also* depression; isolation; single life with CS
loss 6, 40, 76, 129, 135–38, 160, 164, 193; appetite 31; as change 140, 143; cognitive function 182; employment 20, 44, 88, 126, 194, 199; financial or material 49, 135–36, 148, 193, 195–96, 198; friends 131–35; identity 130–31; spiritual 41, 67, 76, 100, 136, 192; voice 22, 25, 29, 62–63, 142, 145; *see also* coping; de-identification; depression; identity; recovery
low back pain 13; *see also* chronic pain
low level laser therapy 183–84, 222; *see also* light therapy

mantra making 156–57; *see also* mantras
mantras 75, 86, 156–57, 160, 168, 222; *see also* mantra making
mask 39, 65–66, 74, 172; odors 114, 118, 125; *see also* nosegay; scarf
Maslow 67, 131, 145, 153
McGonigal, Kelly 35, 73, 156, 222
MCS *see* multiple chemical sensitivities
ME *see* myalgic encephalomyelitis
medical office policies 46, 160, 210–11
medical office survival 71, 73, 75, 121, 160, 210–11
medication *see* prescription medication
meditation 16, 44, 52, 122, 142, 150, 156, 161, 172, 179, 209, 217, 220; definition 58–59; mindfulness and 153–54; parasympathetic nervous system and 183; self-care and 186–87, 200; *see also* Rousseau, Natalie
melatonin 172–73
memory 11, 17, 87–88, 93, 104, 154, 164, 180, 185; senses and 32, 118, 170; *see also* cognitive impairment
mental health 12, 14, 54, 70, 77, 141, 162, 193, 200; maintaining 129, 147, 171, 227*ch5n18*; *see also* cognitive behavior therapy; mental illness
mental illness 145, 147–49, 160, 162, 171, 193; *see also* anxiety; cognitive behavior therapy; depression; mental health; stigma
mental practice *see* visualization

methylation 228
migraine 11, *34*, 74–75, 88, 92, 124, 164, 168, *218*, 222; *see also* headache; tension-type headache
Miller, Claudia S. 19, 221
mindfulness 3, 54, 186–87, 200, 222; practicing 153–55, 162, 172, 176; *see also* meditation; rumination
mitochondria 57, 179–81; *see also* brain health
mobility aids 158
money 80–82, 109; little 3, 40–41, 44, 72, 136–38, 145, 195; relationship with 199–200, 203; self-care and 23, 49, 113, 120, 160, 186, 217; sources 29, 175, 194; *see also* autonomy
Morrison, Murray 21–22
Moseley, Lorimer G. 222
Moskowitz, Michael 184, 222
multiple chemical sensitivities 1, 5, 13, 126, 137, 145, 166; definition 12, 18–20; symptoms 19–20, 32; *see also* bubble; environmental triggers; hyper-sensitivity to chemicals; symptoms; triggers
multitasking 12, 85, 93, 164; *see also* cognitive impairment
muscle pain *see* pain
muscle tension dysphonia 21
music 5, 54, 85, 100, 115, 168, *217–20*; for healing 55, 60–61, 154, 183, 209, 222
myalgic encephalomyelitis 1, 11, 17–18; *see also* chronic fatigue syndrome
myofascial pain syndrome 11, *34*

n-acetyl-l-carnitine 179
neck muscles 23, 26–27, 62–64, 66, 118; *see also* larynx
Neff, Kristin 153, 155, 188, 222
nerve cell 176; *see also* neuron
nervous system *see* autonomic nervous system; central nervous system; enteric nervous system; parasympathetic nervous system; peripheral nervous system; sensitized nervous system; sympathetic nervous system
neurobiofeedback 183–84, 222
neurocognitive disorders 13
neuroendocrine 200, 202
neurofeedback 183–84, 222
neuromodulation 184
neuron 13, 15, 202; cell health and 179–80, 201; neuroplasticity 176–79, 184–85; *see also* nerve cell
neurontin 180
neuropathic pain 10; *see also* chronic pain; neuroplasticity
neuroplasticity 32, 39, 92, 115, 201, 222; basics 176–77, 185–85; chronic pain and 184–85; for healing 60, 119, 177–78, 200;